Noble
Conspirator

---◆---

Noble Conspirator

FLORENCE S. MAHONEY

and the Rise of the National Institutes of Health

———◆———

Judith Robinson

THE *F*RANCIS PRESS

Washington, D.C.

Printed in the United States of America

FIRST EDITION

LIBRARY OF CONGRESS CATALOGING-IN-PUBLICATION DATA

Robinson, Judith
    Noble conspirator: Florence S. Mahoney and the rise of the National Institutes of Health / Judith Robinson.-- 1st. ed.
      p. cm.
    Includes bibliographical references and index.
    ISBN 0-9665051-4-X (hardcover)
      1. Mahoney, Florence S. (Florence Stephenson) 2. Medicine --United States--Biography. I. Title.

R133.M24 R63 2001
610'.7'2073--dc21
[B]

                                        2001040385

Jacket design by Ann Aspell
Interior design by Andrea Gray

Published by The Francis Press
Washington, D.C.
www.francispress.com

Contents

Preface

———◆———

*T*ELLING THE STORY OF FLORENCE MAHONEY and the history of the National Institutes of Health was a long-desired labor of love for the author. For many years, Mrs. Mahoney had talked of putting her memories on paper and organizing a lifetime of archives. When the project finally went forward, many people were pleased that the record at last would be completed.

Florence Mahoney's reputation was well known and respected in Washington and familiar to me, a former legislative aide to United States Senator Gaylord Nelson of Wisconsin, a far-sighted lawmaker who led early efforts to protect the environment, consumer rights, public health and those in need. I worked on a number of biomedical research and health initiatives with which Mrs. Mahoney was associated. I felt fortunate to have the opportunity to write her biography, a particular pleasure because it involved reliving many experiences in the national legislature.

Mrs. Mahoney agreed to an objective biography and cooperated fully in its preparation by allowing extensive access to her personally and to her private papers. She participated in many hours of taped conversations (in 1998), time that the author treasured. Quotes attributed to her that are not specifically cited are from those interviews. She wanted to record the history of the National Institutes of Health from her experiences, emphasizing that it be largely "about the issues" rather than her personal life, and factually correct. A vast amount of information therefore was researched and put together in what we hope is a readable story about an exciting and important aspect of American policymaking.

Numerous people pertinent to the story, from a president's daughter to White House aides and cabinet secretaries, generously consented to interviews for the biography, for which we are grateful. Virtually everyone who was contacted (more than twenty interviews were conducted) was delighted to talk about Florence Mahoney, happy to recollect both her personality and her accomplishments and to shed light on them from a variety of perspectives. Thanks to all who helped in that regard. They are identified as quoted.

Talton Ray, publisher of The Francis Press, contributed extensively by locating and assembling material related to legislation and federal funding of biomedical research in which Mrs. Mahoney played a significant part. He also gathered information about the events and people in the early years of her life that influenced her inclination and ability to play the advocacy role that she did.

Besides Mrs. Mahoney's private papers (cited as FM Personal Papers), other resources included papers that she had archived at the National Library of Medicine (cited as FM Papers, National Library of Medicine); selected materials from the Mary Woodward Lasker Papers, Columbia University; Mike Gorman Papers, National Library of Medicine; James M. Cox Papers, Wright State University; Margaret Sanger Papers, Smith College; and relevant materials from the libraries of Presidents Harry S. Truman, John F. Kennedy, and Lyndon Baines Johnson.

In addition to the many people who offered either personal interviews or written materials, certain contributors to Mrs. Mahoney's story deserve special thanks: Mrs. Margaret Truman Daniel; Bruce Babbitt, secretary of interior in the Clinton administration; former members of Congress; and congressional and National Institutes of Health (NIH) staff. Former NIH Deputy Director John Foord Sherman, Ph.D., and medical historian Stephen P. Strickland, Ph.D., author of *Politics, Science and Dread Disease* (1972), provided valuable assistance in reviewing facts and adding information to the manuscript.

Florence Mahoney's story perpetuates her legacy as an energetic, prescient, thoughtful, warm individual who combined personal attributes with determined advocacy to lead, persuade, and convince policymakers from science laboratories to the White House to promote biomedical research and discoveries. It has been an enlightening and exciting journey through one of this nation's most significant sagas. It also is a story that could happen only in America, with its open and responsive system of democratic government.

Judith Robinson
October 2000

Introduction

---◆---

FLUSH FROM VICTORY IN WORLD WAR II, Americans were turning their attention to long-neglected domestic problems. The war had revealed that Americans were far less healthy than thought. Nearly one in three draftees examined for military induction had been rejected as physically or mentally unfit to serve. The war effort had demonstrated great success with government-funded health and scientific research to benefit servicemen, but what was to be done in peacetime for the civilian population? Very little biomedical research was being funded by the government on such things as heart disease — the number one cause of death. A few far-sighted people, determined to change that situation, in 1947 succeeded in getting Congress to authorize funds earmarked to study heart disease. It was a modest beginning but a step with enormous implications.

"It was quite late in the session when we got the heart bill through, close to when Congress was to adjourn," explained one who backed the measure, Florence Mahoney. To be funded, however, the bill still needed to go through the appropriations process. "President Truman was in San

Francisco, campaigning. I was at Governor Cox's house in Dayton, and I called Clark Clifford, who was with the Truman campaign, and asked him, 'If we send the bill out there, can you get Mr. Truman to sign it so we can get it back in time to get appropriations?' He said to send it.

"So I got the bill sent out on a White House courier plane. There were three hours difference in time from the west coast to Ohio, and I kept Governor Cox and the valet awake all night with phone calls — they rang in different rooms all the time — trying to get through to San Francisco" to confirm that Clifford had been successful in his mission, Mahoney remembered with amusement. "The governor complained about being awakened all night. I told him, 'Never mind — that bill might save your life one day'."

Clifford succeeded, and the National Heart Institute was born. What previously had been simply a National Institute of Health was now plural.

Who was Florence Mahoney and why could she claim the attention of a president, a governor, and their closest advisors? This book tells the story of a remarkable, public-spirited woman who became a unique "people's lobbyist" and helped stimulate the explosion of medical research that fundamentally changed postwar America.

As an unpaid advocate, Florence Stephenson Mahoney would play a key role in reshaping how the federal government set priorities and allocated money for biomedical research, resulting in taxpayer support and generous funding to ease suffering and lengthen lives. The legacy of her efforts today is the greatest biomedical research aggregation in the world — the United States' National Institutes of Health (NIH).

Florence Mahoney was able to quietly exert a profound influence on national research policies by using her native intelligence and strong character to acquire knowledge, skills, and contacts, and by close friendships with people who made key policy decisions and respected her views. She educated, cajoled, and persuaded presidents, cabinet secretaries, congressional leaders, and aides to take up her causes. They listened, the public backed them, and the results are evident in the lives of people worldwide today.

The unusual story of Mahoney's lobbying on behalf of the public interest, laced with personal anecdotes about many of the players, offers a unique insider's view into the workings of the American system of government during more than three decades after World War II.

Various currents merged in Mahoney's early adult life to shape her personality as an effective advocate. She studied physiology and kinesthesiology (the study of muscles) and earned a college certificate in physical education. As an adventurous young woman in the 1920s and 1930s, she developed a life-long passion for exercise and healthy living, augmented by an insatiable thirst for new information. As the wife of a newspaper publisher, she observed firsthand how power was exercised and media could be used. As a mother she investigated health issues, discovering little-known but innovative research efforts throughout the world, which she began to discuss with people who might share her visions of expanded medical research.

In the early 1940s Mahoney fortuitously teamed up with another astute woman with similar goals and tenacity, Mary Woodward Lasker, who benefitted from the fortune of her husband, advertising mogul Albert Lasker. Although Mary Lasker was often more publicly visible and widely acknowledged by the media for her crusades to advance medical research, Florence Mahoney was the quiet but effective partner with extensive access to the ears and minds of people in positions of power. While both possessed uncommon determination and persistence, their differing styles complemented one another and made for a formidable team.

Washington, D.C., was deluged with lobbyists in the postwar years — spending a billion dollars a year by 1950 — but very few had altruistic motives, and even fewer were women. Those facts make Mahoney's and Lasker's work all the more extraordinary. Mahoney developed the intimate dinner party in the nation's capital to a fine art of political influence, not unlike eighteenth-century French women whose *salons* were centers of intellectual and political life in Paris. Mahoney's small gatherings, however, always had a specific purpose: She introduced policymakers, scientists, and doctors to one another and gently guided conversation to subjects that concerned her, usually the nation's health and the need for federal funding of research. With thought-provoking but non-judgmental observations, Mahoney had an "uncanny way of persuading you to do things, even if you didn't agree with her," as one of her protégés put it. While Washington has known many lobbyists and nonprofit advocates with virtuous agendas, rarely has there been one who had such regular access to the highest levels of the executive and legislative branches.

The work of these two intrepid women would have far-reaching effects. A modest federal endeavor to support medical research had begun with the establishment of the National Institute of Health in 1930, but that was all. Only with strong government funding, Mahoney and Lasker perceived, could research into the causes and cures of major diseases be greatly expanded. They set about in a deliberate way to build up the NIH and watched it grow, thanks in great part to their indomitable efforts, from one institute with a budget of less than $3 million to a giant complex encompassing twenty-five research facilities and an annual budget of $16 billion by the turn of the millennium.

Mahoney's crowning achievement was a single-handed campaign to establish an Institute on Aging within the NIH in the early 1970s. "This is not about living longer — it's about being healthy while you're here," she told skeptics who sniffed that "nobody wants to live *that* long." The president, government officials, and biomedical interest groups opposed her but Mahoney persisted. She finally prevailed with Congress, and despite presidential efforts to kill the bill twice, the institute came into being in 1974, inaugurating a new era of research in the field of gerontology and health issues related to aging.

People worldwide can thank Florence Mahoney for her lifelong dedication to promoting biomedical research, from which all humankind benefit.

Noble
Conspirator

◆

1

Early Awakenings

———————◆———————

FLORENCE AMELIA SHEETS WAS BORN "out in the country some-place" near Muncie, Indiana, on April 20, 1899, the eldest of three daughters born to Abraham L. and Julia T. Stephenson Sheets. The child was named for an aunt. Florence, who used her mother's maiden name as part of her own as an adult, was proud of her ancestors, and with justification. Her father had been born in Indiana, but her mother's birthplace was West Virginia, where her Scottish ancestors, the Clendenins, had lived since before the American Revolution. The Clendenins fought in the Seven Years War (1756–63) and built Fort Lee (also known as Fort Clendenin), the first structure on the site of what would become the city of Charleston, West Virginia. They became large landholders and prominent community leaders. The family's fortunes radically changed when Florence's Grandfather Stephenson, a plantation owner in the Ohio River Valley, signed a note for a local merchant who, alas, went bankrupt. There was a lawsuit, and as the person liable for the note, Stephenson had to sell his large property to pay the creditors.[1]

3

"That's why they went to Indiana," Florence remarked. "My Grand-father Stephenson really died of a broken heart."

Florence was a bright, perky girl with large eyes and a serious look on her face in a photo taken of her as a child with her parents and one of two sisters.

She described her father as a farmer, although the family also had a house in town about two miles away. Of her youth on the farm she re-membered riding horses "a little bit," and dairy cows that provided milk for the family, but no chickens, pigs, or beef cattle. It was "a 'city' farm, mostly. I suppose it was for grain. I think they had quite a lot of land."

Muncie, where Florence spent her first seventeen years, was a small, closely knit community of some 30,000 people where neighbors knew one another. They were predominantly White and American-born, the family the center of life in neat clapboard or stone houses on quiet, elm-shaded streets with tidy front yards. Florence's father, like most of the men, was the family breadwinner.[2]

It was a town in which residents looked after those in need largely through volunteer agencies like Ladies' Aid societies. There were no Social Security or government-run health insurance programs, no public welfare, no drug-abuse treatment centers or halfway houses for mentally disturbed or criminal elements because there was little drug abuse or violent crime. Public "general" hospitals and clinics to which physicians donated time provided health care for the poor, and private or church-sponsored hospitals served those with money or insurance coverage.

Florence's family were people of some means, but they lived unosten-tatiously and without trappings of wealth. "It was very social in my family," she remembered of their entertainments. Her mother had two brothers and four sisters, but because her father was the only one of his siblings to marry, her cousins were all on her mother's side. "Everybody used to have dances all the time. We used to go to a social club. We didn't drink at all. I never thought about it. Everybody who lived around us were all friends or relatives, and they had all the land around."

Politics was not part of Florence's early life. "As a child I never knew anything about politics, I didn't even know there were two parties. I don't think people were very interested in politics at that point." Her mother and aunts, of course, could not even vote in national elections until passage of the national women's suffrage amendment in 1920.

"My father more or less had what he wanted" and chose not to go to college. Her mother, too, did not have a formal college education. "They had their own schoolhouse" when growing up in Virginia, and in her mother's hometown "everybody was *snobbish*" about women who desired something different from the norm. "In Muncie, Indiana, they thought that women shouldn't go to university, and they didn't."

Early influences

The lives of women were closely proscribed in those days. They were expected to be married homemakers and mothers. If a woman were forced to work for a living, the most respectable option was to be a teacher.

Mrs. Sheets was typical in most respects — "quiet, peace-loving, and gentle," according to her daughter. "I don't think she was really strong enough. I thought my aunts were stronger than my mother. But, of her sisters, she was much more independent." All the women, though, had presence. "I had four aunts who never married, and I *loved* them — they were absolutely fantastic, very strong." The presence of so many independent-minded women in this close extended family was formative of Florence's character. "All my life, I never seemed to suffer being a woman. I just went ahead and did what I wanted anyway. I wasn't scared of anybody."

She remembered clearly the first time she ever had any social conscience. "My friend had a pony cart, and we used to go riding. You didn't go very far when a little child, of course. There was an orphans' home nearby, which we passed once. We didn't know what it was, so one time we thought we'd stop and find out. We went in and I'll never forget it; I can *still* see it. *Everything* was *gray*. Even the *children* were all gray. It was all so depressing. That was my first feeling of social conscience." She was about ten years old at the time — "obviously old enough to drive a pony cart," she laughed. "I would drive it myself."

The image of the children singing the spiritual "Old Black Joe" was particularly impressed on her memory — "I still can't hear it without crying." Her mother had evinced sadness about the orphanage. She also had taught Florence that human nature made people ostrich-like, hiding their heads in the sand when it came to accepting "anything new." The grayness of the orphanage overwhelmed the little girl, and in the back of her mind she must have fixed a determination to try something "new" to brighten people's lives and make them healthier, to devise different, better, and more humane ways of caring for people.

Florence began her education at a small private school, then with her sisters went to public schools in Muncie. Her first two years of high school, while a new one was being built, were held in a building "right across the street from where we lived in town, so everybody gathered on our porch before classes." When she graduated from Muncie High School in 1917, her yearbook recorded that she "loved pleasure."[3]

A new idea was being implemented in schools at the time, one which particularly appealed to Florence: the concept that bodies as well as minds need training. She took particular pleasure in gymnasium courses.

Religion, like politics, did not play a strong role in her formative years. Although raised in a Protestant faith, Florence was introduced to some radical ideas about organized religion by her uncle Hiram Stephenson. He read her the works of Robert Green Ingersoll (1833–99), an irreverent, witty American writer and orator known as "the great agnostic," who gained a popular following. "He said wonderful things," she recalled of the impact that Ingersoll had on her thinking. One view that stayed in her mind was that those who called themselves "'Christians' were not the ones who were dropping money in beggars' hats. He probably didn't say it exactly that way, but that was the idea. 'You just watch them — they go right by,' when there were a lot of beggars on the streets."

Ingersoll's views about the status of women may have had a strong impact on young Florence, as well. He was unusually outspoken for the post-Victorian period, stating openly that women were virtually slaves unless they could control childbearing. He championed equal opportunity with men at every level, including the right to vote, and was a close friend of suffrage advocates Susan B. Anthony, Carrie Chapman Catt,

Lucretia Mott, and Matilda Joslyn Gage. "In my judgement, the woman is the equal of the man," he wrote, and certainly not "the intellectual inferior.... If there is any man I detest, it is the man who thinks he is the head of a family — the man who thinks he is 'boss.'" Ingersoll blamed the Bible for sustaining oppressive attitudes toward women and Blacks, noting that it spoke of women "simply as property — as belonging absolutely to the man." He also believed that organized religion repressed new ideas such as scientific discoveries. Science, Ingersoll said, was "the only possible savior of mankind" and when applied to birth control could "put it in the power of woman to decide for herself whether she will or will not become a mother." He also favored the option of divorce.[4]

Those were strong sentiments at a time when people were expected to believe blindly in the awful power of the Bible's words. Ingersoll was fond of saying that if *he* were designing the world, he "would make *good health* catching instead of disease" [emphasis added].[5] Such ideas could not but have impressed the adolescent Florence deeply, as they did another young woman whose life was changed by Ingersoll: Margaret Sanger, who also would figure prominently in Florence's future.

Small-town life, if comfortable and unhurried, nevertheless imposed constraints that the independent-thinking Florence Sheets felt at an early age. Rules of social behavior were rigid, and class distinctions clear between rich and poor, White and other ethnic groups. Florence would leave Muncie "far behind," as she put it many years later; "it didn't have any bright stars."

Acutely aware that women had few options other than to be schoolteachers, Florence chose another avenue of study. Following high school she entered the Battle Creek Normal School of Physical Education for women, which was associated with a sanitarium operated by John Harvey Kellogg (1852–1943), older brother of cereal king W. K. Kellogg (1860–1951). "The word 'sanitarium' was never mentioned in the school name, but all the doctors who were teachers were from Kellogg's." There were related schools for nursing and nutrition — "they called it something else then." The sanitarium, Florence recalled, "had many soldiers" injured in World War I as well as other patients. "We had all our meals

and studies at the sanitarium. That's where I was going to be a vege-
tarian," she laughed of her brief experience with the "wonderful food,"
although she did not continue the practice.

"I went there because I did *not* want to be a schoolteacher, and it was
the only thing you could *do* if you were in school in those days. I had seen
Pavlova dance when I was thirteen, and I was *mad* about dancing, mad
about all kinds of exercise. I would have preferred going, at that point, to
a school like Harvard, which had the Sargent school that focused on
physical education similar to Battle Creek's, but this was at the end of the
war, and my father said, 'not for a while.'" [6]

Florence did not waste time on regrets. The school in Michigan "was
really wonderful. In fact, it worked out fine. The faculty were all doctors;
it was sort of a minor medical school." In her final year there, 1919, the
influenza epidemic peaked and Florence volunteered to help the sick.
Subsequent polio epidemics also called on her newly acquired training.
"I and others learned a great deal about the importance of muscles and
health. When the muscles atrophied, doctors used physical therapy to
combat it. It opened up a whole new field."

She spent two summers and two winters at the Normal School,
taking courses in kinesthesiology and anatomy leading toward a certificate in physical education, which she received in 1919. Armed with her
certificate, Florence embarked on her first job — teaching physical education in Moose Jaw, Saskatchewan, a booming railroad town in the
southern part of the Canadian province.

"I could hardly wait to get out of school," Florence said of why she
took the job teaching dance and other physical activities at a health
center operated by the Young Women's Christian Association (YWCA).
"My father was upset about it, but anyway I *did* go. I taught everything
— dance, sports." It was early evidence of the spirited young woman's
curiosity and fearlessness, characteristics that would serve her well
throughout her life.

"Demonstration of Physical Work is Great Success" a headline in a
Moose Jaw newspaper read. "What can be accomplished by children of
all ages was ably demonstrated by the gymnasium classes of the Young

Women's Christian Association last evening, under the capable direction of Miss Florence Sheets, physical director of the Association. The program opened with a march and kindergarten songs by the little tots. . . . Each succeeding number was equally well received, and demonstrated skill on the part of both director and class." [7]

When Florence Sheets, then in her early twenties, set foot in Moose Jaw, its 20,000 citizens included a large contingent of railroad men, prostitutes, and bootleggers serving the demands of American Prohibition, although respectable citizens predominated and, as in Muncie, one could go out of the house and leave the doors unlocked without fear of being robbed. The town also had a lively social life, with movies, dance halls, an aquatic club, and dances sponsored by local women's clubs. [8]

Florence relished the freedom of working for herself and for nine months endured simple dormitory conditions, antipathy toward Americans from Canadians still bitter about their neighbors' late entry into World War I, even the climate — "It was so bloody cold you couldn't believe it! And you had to stand up for America; they didn't like us because it was so soon after the war in which many Canadians had been killed. So you had to be very low key." People nevertheless warmed to the attractive American with the cheerful personality, "and I had a good time while I was there. The people were so nice, I loved it before I left." Besides, she could indulge her love for dancing. "They had dances all the time, everybody danced. You never thought about being cold then. It just seemed natural."

"When I was a reporter on the Moose Jaw *Times*, a very shapely young doll came to our Canadian prairie town to teach physical robustness," newspaper columnist George Dixon later wrote of seeing Florence in those days. "She was a wonderful ad for it. Today she is in Washington, but still concerned about health. She has become one of the nation's leading do-gooders." Dixon, who became a personal friend, went on to describe their social life in Moose Jaw:

I will not tell you how long ago it was that Florence Stephenson Mahoney mushed into Moose Jaw because I am no cad . . . All I care to recall is that we used to go to Temple Gardens every Saturday night and one-step madly to the newest popular song, "The International Rag," which had such up-to-the-minute lyrics as "German counts and Russian czars, men that own their motor cars . . . "

But she was a spirited creature then, and she is now . . .

Mrs. Mahoney's girlhood ambition was to study medicine, but she got side-tracked on ballet and physical health. She joined an organization which aimed to establish health centers across the continent. That's how she came to Moose Jaw.

When I met her she was teaching young women how to look and feel their best. She had our plains girls throwing themselves out in a most fancy manner. [9]

In 1924 Florence went to Europe with two girlfriends. She studied dancing in London with a woman who "learned to do it for her health. She was much older and taught this strange kind of dancing — you raised your arms," she demonstrated. It was a special technique that "I'd never seen before." The teacher "just moved up, she didn't push up, she just lifted her arms. She had learned that she could change her health if she did certain things" in dancing that benefitted the body. "From then on I realized the value of exercise and teaching that to people."

During her sojourn in England, the father of one friend told his daughter to "be sure and take the girls" for a ride in his airplane "so they asked me to go along" on a flight across the English Channel. "It was just the three of us" and the pilot — "I think there might have been a pilot," she laughed. They wore no goggles in the open cockpit, soaring low over the water and fields, landing at Paris' Le Bourget air field. "It isn't very far across, to tell you the truth," she commented wryly of the heady experience. "All I remember is how *exhilarated* I felt when we went to the Ritz Bar afterward!" It was another fearless adventure that she pooh-poohed. "None of the girls had any fear. We were looking for excitement. Didn't think anything about it at *all*."

In New York the following year, Florence began taking lessons at night with an Italian ballet master, Luigi Albertini, whose pupils included several well-known ballerinas and dancer Fred Astaire. "There were only professional students in the class, all serious. I was the only dumb one there. I remember he had a stick with which he would strike people on the backs of their legs if they made mistakes. But it was *wonderful* exercise," which she would practice all her life. "I liked all kinds of sports, tennis, anything athletic." She lived with several other girls on 49th Street (behind St. Bartholomew's church) and during the day volunteered at the Institute for Crippled and Disabled, where her conscience again was awakened by the horrors she saw. [10]

"One time I went over to a little girl sitting in a wheelchair and asked if I could get or do something for her. She said she'd like a glass of water. All I found was a dirty tin cup hanging in the sink. I took the water to her — and she didn't have any *arms*! That was the end of my volunteer work at the hospital. It was a very depressing place to work, but it started me on my interest in doing something *important* instead of just having a good time."

She "took all kinds of medical courses," auditing evening sessions designed for physicians, "and I kept on taking them, too," beginning a lifetime of continuous medical education. "I never wanted to be a doctor," she admitted, despite what Dixon had written. "I was interested in science — everything connected with science. I'd have been awful taking care of people. I didn't want that. I just liked learning about science" as it affected the human body. If she had briefly considered the possibility of being a doctor, she "knew it was hopeless" to expect it as a career for women at the time. In retrospect many years later, Florence found it "amazing" that such avenues were not readily open to women as they would be one day. She might have been a scientist, "so long as it didn't interfere with having *fun!*" she exclaimed, recalling with delight her experiences as a young woman in New York City in the 1920s.

"Everybody knew everybody, more or less, in the same group of people." One member of their set was a man ten years older than Florence who was to become her husband, Daniel J. Mahoney. He had been married to the daughter of James Middleton Cox (1870–1957), owner of the Cox newspaper chain, and worked for the company. Daniel Mahoney was a World War I veteran with a "wonderful war record," Florence knew. "He was very handsome and very nice — and he *loved* Florida," she said of the large, blond, outgoing Irishman who had been put in charge of the Miami *Metropolis* when the Cox company acquired it in 1923 and renamed it the *Daily News*.

Like Florence Sheets, Dan Mahoney was a product of the Middle West, born October 13, 1889, in Springfield, Illinois, one of seven children of Irish parents. He had only limited schooling before going to work, first as an apprentice engineer with the Southern Pacific Railroad in Mexico from 1903 to 1913, and then as sales manager for the Locomobile Corporation in Denver. He signed up as a scout with General John J. Pershing during the punitive expeditions against Mexican revolutionary "Pancho" Villa in 1916–17, then entered the army to serve in World War I. Just before leaving for Europe in 1918, he married Helen Cox. He served with the American Expeditionary Force infantry, beginning as a first lieutenant, saw action at the Argonne Forest and St. Mihiel, and rose to captain with the Army of Occupation after the war ended. He joined Cox's News League at Dayton in 1919 as national advertising manager and became the company's general manager in 1925 and its vice president in 1930, in which post he oversaw the development of the *Miami Daily News*. He became its vice president and general manager in 1935 and publisher in 1951.[11]

Marriage in Miami

Florence had begun to "winter" in Florida, where she conducted a "health studio" in her apartment, doing physical examinations and counseling friends on diet and nutrition. Miami in those years was a vibrant place. Miami Beach recently had been developed by flamboyant entrepreneur Carl Fisher, who, like Florence, had grown up in Indiana. Seeing rich possibilities for wealthy vacationers who were beginning to flock to the area, he drained a mile-long, swampy, mosquito-ridden spit of land across Biscayne Bay. Where palmetto scrub once had flourished, large homes and a grand hotel now rose on the beach front. The swampy sandbar became a tropical paradise. "Carl Fisher — the man who took Florida from the alligators and gave it to the Indianans," Will Rogers joked, "discovered that sand could hold a real-estate sign."[12]

Into this lively and speculative environment in 1923 had come James Cox and Daniel Mahoney, widowed by the death of his first wife in 1921. It was a place of polo matches and tea dances, fast boat trips across the bay, golf on newly built courses, swimming at bathing pavilions — in short, an American "Riviera."[13]

Dan Mahoney recalled on a radio program in 1953 how fledgling the small town had been at the time he arrived: "When I first glimpsed Miami, they were selling lots from upturned boxes on Flagler Street. My first trip to Miami Beach was over the old Collins wooden bridge. I purchased my first home on North Bay Road.... There was only one home between mine and St. Francis Hospital at that time on Miami Beach."[14]

He would have seen rows of tall masts and long bowsprits hanging over the waterfront in the newly dug Miami channel, the last sailing schooners bringing lumber from the north to build the boom town. The advent of Prohibition in 1919 had helped, not least because Miami was a convenient port for illegal rum running.[15]

By the autumn of 1926 Florence Sheets and Daniel Mahoney decided to marry and planned a New York wedding the following spring. Nature, though, dramatically altered their course. A horrendous hurricane blew through the Florida coast on September 17–18, requiring Mahoney's presence at the newspaper. The couple moved their wedding forward and at noon on Wednesday, October 13, Daniel's 37th birthday, the couple were married at Gesu Catholic Church in Miami. According to a newspaper announcement, Florence wore a brown lace dress that she had ordered especially from a dressmaker — "I was very particular about clothes" — and a large-brimmed hat.[16]

"I was a newspaper wife," Florence said of the small social world in which she found herself, made lively by frequent visits from friends and notables migrating south for the climate and sunshine. "It was charming. Everybody knew everybody then." She often took business guests of her husband's to the horse races at Hialeah, and occasionally yachting — "I hated boats, such a bore!" For a while she played golf, but that, too, was not active enough. "I quit after I got a 99, when I broke 100. I was good at the long game but I hated putting."

Relationship with Cox family

The Cox family, particularly James Cox, was an integral part of the Mahoneys' lives. Cox had been a congressman and three-term governor of Ohio. In 1920 he was the unsuccessful Democratic candidate for president of the United States (with former Assistant Secretary of the Navy Franklin Delano Roosevelt as his running mate) against fellow Ohioan Warren G. Harding. Dan Mahoney had been a constant companion on that campaign and now was a top executive in the newspaper company.[17]

After Cox's defeat for the presidency, he had devoted his energies to his newspaper company, the News League. On a vacation to Miami in the winter of 1923, he had been impressed with its physical beauty, climate, and booming growth. "It looks like another Los Angeles," he wrote journalist Arthur Krock. Cox decided to expand his chain into Miami and bought the *Metropolis* that year. "Any city growing as Miami is needs a vigilant press," he said, announcing that the paper would "uphold the principles of Jeffersonian Democracy and devote itself to the public interest." Mahoney, who negotiated the purchase, wrote Cox that their rival, the *Miami Herald*, remarked the day afterward that the *Metropolis* had passed "from a purely Southern man . . . to a purely Northern man," which would produce "a distinctive change in Southern journalism." That included unionized press men and catering to "the working people" who Cox knew bought and read his papers, which he wanted to be "champions of the rights of the weak."[18]

The Cox newspaper company had started with the Dayton *Daily News* (which Cox acquired in 1898) and at various times included, besides the Miami paper: the Springfield, Ohio, *Press-Republican*; Canton, Ohio, *Daily News*; and Dayton *Journal-Herald*. In 1939 Cox expanded his Southern holdings by buying the *Atlanta Journal,* which led reform campaigns against traditional Georgia political "machines" like that dominated by long-time Governor Eugene Talmadge (1933–37, 1941–43). The *Journal* was followed in 1950 by purchase of the *Atlanta Constitution,* which became associated with civil rights and other good-government reforms. Cox newspapers for many years dominated journalism in Dayton, Springfield, and Atlanta.[19]

Mahoney was Cox's right-hand man ("did everything for him for a long time," according to Florence) and Dan's growing power in the city afforded her entrée and introductions to influential people and political life.

"We all called him 'Mahoney,'" she explained of her popular husband. "He was very much a people's person," sociable and fond of golf with his many friends. At one point friends suggested that he run for the United States Senate, but his wife vigorously objected. "I was not going to be in politics," she stated. "He had plenty to do outside" the political arena. It was an ironic statement, considering her own future involvement in that world.[20]

When Daniel Mahoney had been put in charge of the Miami paper, which had been named the *Miami Daily News,* Cox had emphasized that it was to be "helpful to everything that advances the good of the community." Mahoney undertook the job with gusto, and the paper became the leading one in the city in the 1920s and a potent political influence. Cox himself wrote in his autobiography that Mahoney was "one of the best public relations and sales executives in the country."[21] During Mahoney's tenure, the *Miami Daily News* won two Pulitzer Prizes, one in 1938 for an exposé of corrupt city administration and again in 1960 for a series on exploitation of migrant workers.

Mahoney was especially proud of his role directing a newspaper campaign against organized crime that operated in the region beginning in the 1920s. Legalized gambling and horse racing attracted not only the wealthy but gangsters and racketeers exploiting Prohibition and the 1929 stock market crash who moved to the sunny southland bringing speakeasies and casinos with them, to the horror of residents like Mahoney and his neighbors.[22]

Among other things, the *Miami Daily News* campaigned against horse racing at Hialeah in 1927: "Do you want your children to see wide-open gambling? Do we want to send out the word that Dade County extends open arms to the gambling element of all the world, with their camp followers?" one editorial asked.[23]

The Hialeah track nevertheless was allowed to continue operating, despite legislative efforts to shut it down. Florence took special note of the fact that bribes, which were openly publicized, influenced the legislature to legalize pari-mutuel betting in 1931. She saw "how people operated; there were all kinds of politics around." The track's millionaire owner, Joseph E. Widener, reportedly spent $50,000 to insure the bill's passage. He celebrated his success with friends, who threw a $100,000 party in the midst of the Depression during which Widener's horses, draped in red and white racing stripes, were paraded around the New York Biltmore Hotel ballroom. It was a rude awakening about politics and money to the girl from Muncie.[24]

Mahoney, dubbed "Little Tammany" by another rival newspaper, the Miami Beach *Tribune*, gained a reputation as a fearless "mafia" buster for defying even Al Capone, who had moved to Miami about the same time as Mahoney and hung around the Jockey Club, reputedly fixing races. Mahoney got his newspaper to disparage the mobster's residency, and mysterious telephone callers began asking if Mahoney wanted to be measured for a coffin. To one he replied that he would "like to meet at any hour, at any place, the man who thinks he's big enough to put me in it." Soon afterward, at a Miami Beach party, the big Irishman found that Capone was present. He announced to the host in a loud voice, "Get that bum out of here or I'm leaving." Capone left. The newspaper kept up its pressure to clear the area of known gangsters, exposing a gambling syndicate that controlled Miami Beach politics. The group finally asked Mahoney for a truce meeting, which he set up in an auditorium used by the *Daily News*–owned radio station WIOD. The group loudly blamed the *Daily News* for bad publicity the Beach had gotten, discouraging tourists. Mahoney then let loose a tirade — "in his most colorful language, and it was plenty colorful," according to a *Daily News* reporter — saying the paper would not be intimidated nor cut back its campaign, which effectively brought the syndicate to terms. Mahoney subsequently was one of the founders of the Greater Miami Crime Commission.[25]

Mahoney was characterized by local media as a "man who was . . . big physically and in public deeds, and was never dull. Beloved by his colleagues on the *Miami Daily News*, venerated by the community he helped so much to build and held in awe by elements which didn't agree with him." He was known as "Irish Mahoney" and later "Uncle Dan." His life as a soldier, political power-broker, crime fighter, and "roaring newspaperman in the rugged old tradition," as he was described in the *New York Times*, was the stuff of legends in Miami. During hurricanes, Mahoney set up a coffee urn and bar in the *Daily News* building from which he personally served up stiff restoratives to soggy, tired reporters as they came in from covering the story.[26]

Dan Mahoney in the 1930s and 1940s wielded considerable power with his newspaper and was credited with delivering Democratic votes from low- and middle-class sections of Miami through World War II, after which the *Miami Herald* regained dominance. [27]

Florence, by association with her husband and the world in which they lived, also became astute at politics. She first had been awakened to the subject immediately after World War I. "It was not until the campaign to ratify the League of Nations came along that I got involved," she said. Before that, "I didn't know anything about politics, didn't pay attention to politics. But I was fascinated by the issue when I first heard about the League of Nations and President Wilson's horrible problem" getting the U. S. Senate to approve America's participation in it. "I couldn't understand how anyone could be against the League. I was in school then and had read all about it. I wondered how anybody could be so *stupid* not to let it happen, to let it die. When Wilson died, I was heartbroken."

When she later overheard a conversation between Idaho Republican Senator William E. Borah, a chief opponent of the League, and Cox, sitting on the porch at a guest ranch that they visited in Stanley, Idaho, Mahoney reflected that, although diametrically opposite in political views, both men had "been through a historical period. It was fascinating" to hear them talk; "they had been such enemies. I don't think they'd ever met before." She realized that she was witnessing history being made. At the same time; she noted that they all were privy to "the most *beautiful* view," characteristic of her ability to couple political events with personal observations and a sense of beauty and art, a trait that would become a feature of her personality.

Family and the West

In 1927 Florence gave birth to the first of two sons, Daniel J., Jr. The second, J. Michael Mahoney, was born a year and a half later, in 1929.

In those years she and the boys often went to Idaho for the summer. "From my Moose Jaw experience, which was my first in the West, I knew that I loved the West" with its expanses of land. A friend of her husband's owned a dude ranch along the Salmon River. She began taking the boys there. They rode horseback, fished, hiked, and helped neighbors during roundup time, benefitting from the fresh air, healthy food, and exercise that their mother championed.

Ever vigilant about the health of the children, Florence had taken note of the fact that undulant fever could be caught from diseased cows, so one summer she contacted the Idaho health and agriculture departments, asking that they test the cows on the ranch. "They found that a lot of them had tuberculosis. The neighbors had to destroy their cows, so I was not very popular. For a long, long time — we had so many children there and they drank so much of it — I boiled tubs and tubs of milk every day on the stove to try to pasteurize it." It was an early instance of activism that would presage changes in policy as the problem caught the attention of public health officials.

When the ranch owner decided to sell in 1937, the Mahoneys bought the property and subsequently acquired a neighboring ranch with a wide creek running through it. For many years they went to the ranch in early July and stayed "until after the round-up, in September."

W. Averell Harriman, who as chairman of the board of Union Pacific Railroad developed the Sun Valley recreation area in 1936, was one of the Mahoneys' Idaho friends. "He used to fly out to Idaho when nobody else was flying out there. He used to fly himself in his own plane," Florence remembered of the dashingly handsome future statesman. Harriman invited her and her sons to visit Sun Valley soon after it opened. To their delight, "he sent us on his private train car—they called it *his* train — and when we landed out there, you couldn't get up to the lodge because there was no transportation and no roads so they took us up by 'stage' [an old touring bus]." Her friendship with Harriman would come in handy.[28]

Young Daniel, though, suffered bouts of pneumonia and asthma. A physician in Florida prescribed a dry climate for the boys. Their mother found the Arizona Desert School in Tucson and sent them there. She spent the first year near them, and from there they went to a boys' preparatory school in New Hampshire, Phillips Exeter, which their mother let them choose over one that she preferred where the headmaster was a psychologist. "I'd always believed in psychiatry," she said, and even had sent one of her sons for a consultation before he first went away to school to help ease the trauma of leaving home.

An inveterate note-taker, Florence early began recording tidbits of information that interested her or sparked her curiosity. "I used to write down anything that I thought was intelligent that I didn't know about." One note to herself concerned childhood mental health and the influence of guilt and fear, which, she recorded, "create unsocial behavior and destroy the ability to use intelligence."[29]

On a visit with the headmaster at the school of her choice, she was impressed when he confided that he could readily spot troubled students and help them. She also observed that the headmaster's wife treated with kindness one boy who had fallen asleep in class — she signaled the other students to be quiet when they got up to leave so as not to waken the tired boy. "Isn't that wonderful?" Mahoney thought to herself, a manifestation of her empathy with people's feelings and needs, her preference for kindness over harsh, unfeeling behavior, and the thoughtful sensitivity for which she would become noted.

At Exeter, however, she had an early encounter with recalcitrance at changing ways. During a board of trustees meeting that she had been invited to attend, a discussion arose about a boy who had had problems and how the school should deal with such students. "I had been realizing how young they were when they were sent away to school," so Mahoney promptly suggested, "Why don't you get a good psychologist?" and named a man who had made a reputation during World War II.

"We don't want our boys going around saying they have to go to a *nut* doctor!" someone retorted. "'If that's what you think,'" Florence responded, "'I wouldn't want my boys here.' Isn't that fantastic?" she reflected many years later, "a *nut* doctor!" — and at one of the outstanding schools in the United States. The school nevertheless acted on her suggestion. "The next time I saw them, they told me that everybody was so upset at what I said that they got somebody immediately," which gratified her.

The Mahoney boys completed their high school education at Exeter. From there each went on to Ivy League universities, Daniel graduating from Yale in 1950 and Michael from Princeton in 1952. After receiving a law degree from the University of Virginia in 1953, Daniel joined the *Springfield News* as a police reporter and subsequently moved to the business side of the company. He became president of the Cox newspapers in Dayton in 1968. He later moved to Florida and served as publisher of the *Palm Beach Daily News* and the *Palm Beach Post*. Daniel died of cancer in Palm Beach on January 4, 1997, at age 69. Michael, after a career in the air force with the Strategic Air Command and as an intelligence officer in Korea, also worked for Cox, starting as a writer on the Springfield paper, then at the *Atlanta Journal* and *Constitution* as well as for Cox-owned television stations. In 1960–62 he went to Africa as a foreign correspondent based in Accra, Ghana. Among his dispatches was a seventeen-part series covering the continent. In retirement he pursued a study of schizophrenia, sparked by an interest developed while covering mental-health issues for the Atlanta papers. He also established generous scholarships at the University of California in memory of promising students who died in tragic circumstances, as his youngest daughter's best friend had in an automobile accident in 1980.[30]

Florence Mahoney had quietly pursued various interests while a mother of two young boys and wife of a busy newspaper publisher. Once the children were in school and she was confident they were secure, she began to become involved in more extracurricular activities. She believed in the "definition of a parent" that she once had seen and written down: "Like the old Roman gods, they should be present but out of sight and available upon demand." Heeding that advice, she became increasingly busy with causes that concerned her. Her husband supported and even helped her in several early activities.[31]

Florence and Daniel Mahoney had an understanding that "when the children grew up, we'd do what we wanted." In 1950 they were divorced. A few days after the proceeding in Florida, she wrote a close friend, "I feel very well and that sense of freedom is really something. I want to thank you for all your sympathetic interest these past few years." Florence moved quietly from Miami Beach to Washington, D. C., to begin a new life on her own. She found a house overlooking the Potomac River in Georgetown. "I was determined to be where I had a view." A few years later she purchased the neighboring house and there settled in for a lifetime. Its portals would welcome hundreds of people who themselves were making history.[32]

2

Of Saints and Santa Claus – New Perspectives

———————◆———————

*F*LORENCE MAHONEY PERCEIVED EARLY ON the advantages that stemmed from her connection to a distinguished political and newspaper family. She hit it off with Cox — "we always called him the Governor" — a supportive mentor who jokingly but affectionately dubbed her "Doc."

"I spent a lot of time with the Governor. He said that I knew more about politics than either Mahoney or Jim," Cox's son. "I was interested in all sorts of things," and the earnest young woman and savvy old politician spent many hours discussing topics of mutual interest. She in turn admired Cox, "an extremely intelligent man" who "was the first governor who ever did anything about health. He did something about tuberculosis in the 1930s. So he was always interested and he loved to talk about health things." At age 75, Cox wrote, "To me, health is a matter of maintaining a rhythmic way of living. Except for rhythm and the balance which rhythm keeps, the world would collapse." Mahoney herself might have expressed such sentiments. Because of her husband's close relationship with the Cox family, the Mahoneys often visited the Cox estate, "Trailsend," outside of Dayton.[1]

Mahoney also shared Cox's optimistic view of human nature. In his autobiography Cox said, "Human nature may not change, but intelligence can and does increase. It is clear now that with the new destructiveness of war, nations must conform to the demands of decency and humanity or perish at each others' throats.... Despite past and present discouragements, I still have faith in the ultimate good and progress of mankind."[2] Mahoney recognized that he was a dynamic politician who was genuinely "interested in improving everything. He also had this wonderful feeling about people — he was absolutely fascinated about what they were doing. He would ask millions of questions and identified with people extraordinarily well." His newspapers reflected his progressive views, ones that Mahoney shared. "The Governor was a very forthright Democrat."[3]

Cox also had a sense of humor, another thing that made him appealing to Mahoney, whose own humor was a delight, full of perky, ingenuous, but usually prescient remarks that produced a sparkling laugh from her and her listeners. "About Florence Mahoney," Cox wrote a mutual friend in 1946, "I can give you no guarantee as to what city or country her mental compass points to."[4]

He could be jokingly irreverent about the mass of information that she constantly foisted on him, grudgingly tolerant of her persistence. "Tell Doc I turned her hormones book over to Sharkey," he wrote Dan in one letter. "He thinks it is all baloney and I guess he's right. I don't know why she didn't keep it for Mahoney," Cox added, humorously suggesting that Dan himself might benefit from his wife's proselytizing. Cox gently chafed her a few weeks later about her lay medical advice in a letter addressed to "Mrs. Doc Mahoney" at their M-M Ranch in Idaho:

I have often wondered just what currents of life constituted a legitimate function for me. I have one this morning which is, that if it weren't for me, you wouldn't be able to clean up your

wastebasket. How many other people suffer from your imposi-
tions? I hope they are as cheerful about them as I am.

My suggestion would be that you apply your medical research
genius to Uncle Dan Mahoney. What status will you have among
those in the profession who really count if you continue your wide
studies to the neglect of Uncle Dan? This might not be attributed to
neglect. Some might be unkind enough to think that your preach-
ments spring from a lack of fundamental medical knowledge.
There is a hint for you.[5]

Deluged with mailings from her, Cox at one point asked in jest, "Will
you please give your son Daniel, who by reason of seniority may be a little
more responsible than his junior brother, a suggestion that he go into
Stanley and get a large waste basket and direct your attention to it every
time you start mailing a letter to me? He will get the point. Maybe he can
entrust you with the meaning of it all, and you may find that by trimming
the surplus contents that the postage charges can be reduced. We must
all begin habituating ourselves to economies."[6]

Of something that she told him had "brought about a precipitation of
tears," Cox gently remonstrated, "There was probably too much poetry
in it for a practical person like you." And he joked about her home town,
writing that "the Delta Airways line which has been granted service
rights from Chicago to Miami will go through Muncie. It would seem
that your old habitat is looking up."[7]

He nevertheless took Mahoney seriously, communicated with her
regularly in an affectionate tone, and passed on information that she
shared with him to his newspaper editors for possible follow-up stories.
"I have turned over your suggestion to [Dayton *Daily News* editor]
Walter Locke," Cox said in 1945 as Mahoney was embarking on efforts
to bring attention to cancer research. "It looks like the cancer thing is on
the boom in the country. I am glad it is." In another letter he enclosed
"some literature on the cancer subject. I suppose this is one way of
keeping you quiet." Polio was another incurable disease that greatly

frightened people. "Here's a chapter for your book of knowledge," Cox mused in the summer of 1946 after she had informed him that she was planning to raise Arabian horses. It concerned a letter from "a Dr. Wishnack of Miami Beach in which he said that he has for years tried to prove his theory that Polio is carried by the common 'horse' or 'stable' fly — that in every case he ever treated, he traced the source of infection to this pest. I don't know what you are going to do about this but get suits of mosquito bar and cover your chargers with DDT."[8]

Cox obviously enjoyed their relationship, urging Mahoney in one letter to "Fill up your mind with interesting anecdotes, news and whatnot, then call me." As the war wound down, he confided to her that it would leave a lot of people in military and government jobs with little to do. A friend had told Cox "that things were shifting so fast in New York that they were dizzy. They are all delighted with Truman. He is keeping things moving. He is doing exactly as I thought he would. You know, I said there would be train loads of bureaucrats leaving Washington." Mahoney herself would soon have close ties to the new president.[9]

Taking a dare

Mahoney for her part was frank with Cox, undaunted by his friendly if sometimes sardonic remarks. "I told him one time that I thought the women's pages were awful," referring to their trivial content devoted largely to frivolous society activities of the rich. "I complained that society reporters and gossip columnists wrote about ladies wearing pink hats when there were all kinds of serious things that were going on in the world."

In response to her complaints, Cox "said, in effect, 'If you think you're so smart, why don't you do it yourself?'" She took up the challenge and in 1946 began writing a weekly column, "About People," which she continued for some ten years, much of the time using the pseudonym "Mary Marley," which she made up in order not to be identified as the publisher's wife. The columns ran on Sundays in the *Miami Daily News*.

At one point, Cox sent her a thoughtful letter concerning a regular contributor to the Atlanta *Journal*, Violet Moore, who "interests me tremendously because of what she sees and how she tells about it . . . she says she tries 'to see more deeply into the familiar and give it recognition.' . . . I told her the difference between her and the average columnist is that the columnist sits in his easy chair and writes his own emotions . . . Violet Moore sees what is going on and then writes about it in unusual but very attractive words."[10]

Mahoney took note and tried to include subjects that she thought important. One column for example, had a section on birth-control advocate Margaret Sanger, another championed Eleanor Roosevelt's causes, and another mentioned former Senator William Benton, who, Mahoney wrote, "will be remembered as the Senator who was convinced . . . that Senator Joseph McCarthy should be expelled from the U. S. Senate. He was the first one who came out against McCarthy on the Senate floor."[11]

"I think things like that in *any* column are interesting," she said of her subjects. "I wrote about things that *I* would be interested in reading." She plugged the book *Anatomy of Peace* when its author Emery Reeves showed up in Florida in 1946, telling readers that it had "created such a stir that it is appearing currently in three installments in the *Reader's Digest* . . . . The book, as you know, was recommended by Einstein in his one press interview as a 'must' on everyone's reading agenda."[12]

She interspersed serious topics with accounts of famous people whom she knew, "but they weren't just about people in society." Of diplomat and politician Chester Bowles and Senator Benton, who had been advertising partners, she wrote: "Both men promised themselves that when they made a million, they would quit and go into government service," which they dutifully had done. Another column dealt with the Arizona mining town of Jerome, named for Eugene Jerome, a cousin of Sir Winston Churchill's mother Jenny Jerome. "Aren't they more interesting than most columns you read?" Mahoney wondered years later, proud of the fact that women's pages had evolved into more serious news. She credited a discussion between her husband, herself, and

Washington Times-Herald publisher Cissy Patterson with stimulating a trend to change the quality of women's pages.[13]

Politicians were favorite subjects. "Did you know," Mahoney asked readers as Congress was reconvening in January 1949, "that the new freshmen are largely ex-college athletes and ex-professors?" She mentioned, among others, Eugene McCarthy, Democrat of Minnesota, "a professor of sociology and a high school principal at 25 . . . Peter Rodino, Junior, Democrat of New Jersey, a law school professor and much-decorated veteran of WW II . . . Gerald Ford, Republican from Michigan, U. of Mich.'s star player in 1934 and later assistant football coach at Yale . . . . This must make our own ex-Marine and Florida U. athlete George Smathers feel pretty ancient as a senior representative in his middle 30s . . . . Also young Jack Kennedy who was a champion swimmer at Harvard." In 1953 she wrote "Barry Goldwater, the new Senator from Phoenix, Arizona, says that Jack Kennedy is the hardest working Senator. Jack has his office nearby and Barry has yet to find him not burning the night oil as he passes by en route to dinner. Jack flies down to weekend with his family at Palm Beach any time he can manage. Some have gone so far as to link Jack's name as a running mate with [Adlai] Stevenson in '56. Two bachelors on the ticket might be confusing, though."[14]

"Margaret Truman is doing a television show with Milton Berle next week with fun lines," Mahoney revealed in a 1953 column filed from New York City, and "James (Scottie) Reston, *New York Times* political correspondent, will probably get a Pulitzer for getting Stalin to answer his questions." Soon afterward she reported that Truman "was being congratulated on her shows by all and sundry at a large Safeway super market in Washington where she was shopping last Saturday afternoon with her hostess [Mahoney?]. One woman said, 'You mean you have to shop like the rest of us?' and Margaret answered, 'I certainly do.'"[15]

Mahoney also noted Truman's presence at a post-Eisenhower-election gathering of 600 Democrats, "who counted out $24 each for a bit of lunch . . . to hear the junior Senators philosophize re: the future of the now-dormant Democratic Party. Object of the luncheon was to put

pennies in the coffer to pay off late debts." At the same time, she remarked on the rising number of women in high places: "Now that President Eisenhower has women cabinet members [Oveta Culp Hobby,
Secretary of Health, Education and Welfare], a woman ambassador
[Clare Booth Luce] and a woman representing us at the coronation [of
Queen Elizabeth] and the U. N. [unclear whom she meant], the girls see
the handwriting on the wall and toiling in the fields will not be such a
chore."[16]

Mahoney's inside knowledge of the White House was apparent in
reports like a 1953 account of Mrs. Eisenhower's first press conference in
the room where President Roosevelt had broadcast his "fireside chats."
"When Mamie Eisenhower called on Mrs. Truman just before the inauguration, they spent most of the time trying to figure out where they
could put the Eisenhowers' big double bed in what was then President
Truman's bedroom." She reported a month later that, "from Mamie's
friends, one hears that she does as much work from her bed in the
morning as possible, answering letters by the score, that the First Lady
has 100 hats and 200 bed jackets and that she plays canasta in the
solarium almost every afternoon. The solarium is reached by a ramp
from the second floor and is also used for family breakfasts."[17] Mahoney
regularly attended such press conferences and heard speakers at the
National Press Club.

New perspectives

During the early 1940s Florence Mahoney met another man who would
influence her thinking, the author Philip Wylie, a novelist whose non-
fiction book *Generation of Vipers*, first published in 1943, created a
sensation for its brutal assessment of American society. At the time,
some of his predictions were thought to be "bordering on insanity," as
Wylie himself said in an introduction to a revised edition in 1955. The
book was "dashed off," he admitted, between May 12 and July 4 the year
after Pearl Harbor and the United States' entry into World War II, and
Wylie had "come home to Miami Beach" after a stint in "government
war information" work that had left him "ill, discouraged and frus-

trated." *Generation of Vipers* was a "private catharsis, a catalogue of what I felt to be wrong morally, spiritually and intellectually with my fellow citizens." He was surprised that "millions shared my vexations and anxieties." By his own admission, the book had "become a kind of 'standard work' for Americans who love liberty, detest smugness and are anxious about the prospects of our nation."[18]

Mahoney, who had the good fortune to meet Wylie in Miami and cultivated his acquaintance, was attracted to his iconoclastic style, courage, independence and broad knowledge of government and technology. "People were always coming to Miami Beach during the war" and asking to meet the author, including politicians and government officials for whom he sometimes wrote speeches. Mahoney considered him "an absolutely brilliant man, very quiet and sensitive. When Truman's people came down on their way to Key West, they always wanted to talk with Wylie, he knew so much about so many subjects involving the government. I knew him originally as a social friend."[19]

Mahoney shared Wylie's views about the danger of survival in the atomic age and his irreverence about many popular American attitudes, including the prevalent image of "Mom." Wylie criticized the "psychic umbilicus by which millions of moms hold millions of grown American men and women in diseased serfdom." But he admitted that "Criticism ... and the doubt out of which it arises are the prior conditions to progress of any sort." He confessed to looking for "what's wrong" rather than championing "what's right."[20]

In such concepts Mahoney found justification to pursue untried paths and to force changes in areas that she had come to believe needed changing, to challenge icons, whether individual or philosophical.

Saints, psychiatrists, and Santa Claus

One youthful experience that made a lasting impression on Mahoney had spurred her to act on the problem. "The first time that I got interested in birth control was when I volunteered to work in the Crippled and Disabled Hospital in New York." Because she was trained in kinesthesiology, she was asked to test the muscles of children who had had polio to determine which ones might need remedial therapy. "The mothers would come in with four or five children, all hanging on each other, and I'd take care of them." It particularly struck her that "they were *always* asking what rich people did in order *not* to have children. I must say, I didn't know anything about it either," she laughed, "and I didn't get into that, but at least I understood their problem. That's when I heard about Margaret Sanger and thought she was a *saint.*"

Mahoney found it hard to get anyone even to discuss the subject aloud, especially men. "Women never talked about birth control with men" in those days, and "most men wouldn't talk about it at *all,*" she noted, adding that "men are always so busy discussing the things they're interested in anyway."

It was through Cox's son that Mahoney met the woman who was unafraid to speak out on the touchy subject — Margaret Sanger. Her son Stuart had been a student with Jim Cox Jr. at Yale and had become a doctor. During the war, Stuart was stationed with the army in Miami, where one day young Cox "said to me, 'You're so interested in all these things, you should know my roommate's mother — she went to jail several times because of birth control.' I was absolutely *fascinated* that anybody would be put in jail for *anything! Horrible* thought! I wouldn't be *that* courageous. She went to jail every time she opened her mouth. So he introduced me to Margaret Sanger's son. That's how I got to know Margaret Sanger."

Coincidentally, both women had been greatly affected by the ideas of Robert Ingersoll, whom Sanger credited with stirring her philosophy about the importance of controlling birth rates and thus liberating women. Mahoney found her "very attractive, very refined, very sophisticated, small woman. And she never raised her voice but she got things done." Mahoney did not actively participate in Sanger's organization, Planned Parenthood, but became an avid fan. "The only thing I could do to help her was to be her friend at that time."

Mahoney, however, began her own work to enlighten people about the need for birth control, using her political contacts to spread the Planned Parenthood word. "I knew the governors of Florida and Georgia, and I wanted them to put birth-control programs" in their states. "But everybody was scared to mention it. You can't believe how people were frightened" to discuss the subject publicly. "When I asked the governor of Florida [Millad F. Caldwell, 1945–49] if he'd do something about putting birth control in the child health and welfare clinics, he said he would be glad to do it — if we could make it retroactive!" she laughed recalling his joke.

During the war Mahoney also met another innovator in medical practices — Dr. Howard A. Rusk — who she at first thought had been a medical student whom she had met while in college. "I read in the paper in Miami that there was a Doctor Rusk in Florida who was in charge of wounded veterans. He had a new idea — that people in 'sick bay' should gradually start exercising" to improve their rehabilitation (early ambulation after surgery, a new concept at the time). "Of course, I thought that was *wonderful*. So I called him one day and asked if he were the same person I'd met at the University of Michigan Sigma Chi house. He said 'No, but I'd like to talk to you anyway.' So I said, 'Come tomorrow morning for breakfast. Mahoney was there and we had a wonderful time — that's how I happened to meet Howard Rusk," who ultimately gained fame as a pioneer in rehabilitation methods.

"I went to see what he was doing and was fascinated because he had these soldiers who had been ill or had fractures working out of wheelchairs and gradually getting their strength back." Mahoney introduced Rusk to wealthy and influential people like John Oliver LaGorce, longtime head of the *National Geographic*, and Bernard Gimbel of department store fame — "we were all great friends" — who later would be helpful in raising money for Rusk's Rehabilitation Institute. "We *all* raised money for him," Mahoney said.[21]

Mental health reforms, too, occupied her attention. The Mahoneys in 1939 had gone to Atlanta with Cox for the December 15 gala premiere of the film *Gone with the Wind*, coincidentally a few days after Cox had acquired the *Atlanta Journal* and just after war erupted in Europe. They were introduced to the book's author, Margaret Mitchell, a former reporter on the paper (writing under the name Peggy Mitchell, 1922–26).

Florence Mahoney found a simpatico person in Mitchell, whom she described as down-to-earth and unassuming, and talked to her about raising money for a mental-health clinic. Mitchell, well-connected socially in her native Atlanta, referred Mahoney to a local banker, Tom Glenn, who "said that if we could find a psychiatrist, he would pay his salary." Mitchell added that she would "paint the place myself" if it opened. "I'll never forget her saying that," Mahoney mused of the encounter. Alas, psychiatrists were in growing demand and "I couldn't get anybody who'd go to Atlanta. They were all preoccupied."

From making suggestions she turned to more purposeful advocacy, concentrating particularly on mental-health and birth-control programs. Using a Cox press pass, she began in the 1940s to attend governors' conferences to "just try to *teach* them about having mental-health clinics." At the time there were virtually no non-institutional programs anywhere in the nation, and there was little interest in psychiatry as a public-health treatment. The mentally ill were warehoused in state insane asylums with minimal care.

As Miami began to fill with war casualties, Mahoney became acquainted with a growing number of psychiatrists stationed in the area. "All the hotels were taken over during the war," many for treatment of injured veterans. "I suggested to one psychiatrist, who knew the technique of hypnotism, that he go and talk to the soldiers" in an effort to help them recover from their trauma. "So he did. It was great fun" that he took her suggestion to heart, and she took him to an armed-services hospital in Coral Gables. "But then, sometime afterward, the Secret Service came to call on me and said that they had had a complaint about a psychiatrist who was doing hypnosis to help casualties. Somebody in the government complained about it — I think the psychiatrist had put it down as his background," causing an uproar in the ranks of commanders. Mahoney found it amusing that the results of her idea had caused such a stir.

"I was willing to suggest *anything* at *any* time that I thought was going to help anybody," she said.

At a meeting of psychoanalysts that she attended in New York in 1946, Mahoney heard a talk by a Canadian psychiatrist, Dr. Brock Chisholm, "who knew about getting soldiers back into combat long before Americans knew about it. It was the most wonderful speech I'd ever heard. I bought many copies afterward and gave them to people. I talked so much about it" that people either grew weary of hearing it or took notice.

Chisholm had gained infamy for soft-spoken but controversial pronouncements, sometimes chilling and enraging, on topics ranging from war and overpopulation to superstition. He was described as "a slight, friendly man" and "indefatigable speaker" who "rarely replied to his critics" but continued "to advance his basic ideas that the human race must achieve emotional health and learn to live in harmony — or perish." Such were the ideas that stunned Mahoney as she sat in the audience at the Waldorf Astoria.

Mahoney's "notes from the speech" reflected her deep interest in what Chisholm had said. "We are the wrong kind of people," she wrote. "Can we hope in a few years to change? . . . All patterns tried and none worked yet and no indications any will work in the future. Any war anytime . . . will be a world war. Will make atomic bomb look like child's play, will be mass murder worked on and planned by scientists, all populations of some countries or continents will be wiped out. This is biologically wrong, but people still unimpressed and actually making money for personal reasons (Goethe and Schiller). Living in the future means living AT ALL. We are the people who are wrong, must change our children, men are ostriches (hide head in sand when anything wrong). We must understand other peoples and their hopes and problems . . . their religions, points of view. Attitudes instilled in us before age of 6. Our own consciousness still undeveloped. Essential we must get on with everyone else . . . We are WORLD CITIZENS whether we like it or not . . . . How capable are we of re-educating ourselves? . . . Most dangerous person in the world is one who 'shoots off his mouth' and does not know what he is talking about . . . . We have blind spots. OUR ONLY SALVATION — world citizens who can think of cause and effect, people who are capable of . . . honest thinking. Guilts and fears impressed upon us in childhood creating unsocial behavior and destroys ability to use intelligence."[22]

A favorite theme of Chisholm's was the training and development of children, who would "make or destroy the world as they come to adulthood," but whose teachers and mentors, like psychiatrists and social workers, were paid far less than entertainers and sports figures. The only hope for world peace, he believed, was "a new concept [in] upbringing" that taught children "compassion, tolerance and understanding," allowing them freedom from taboos in order to develop imagination. Instead, they were exposed to "pathological sore spots" in their culture such as "the Santa Claus myth" and superstitions like the number 13 being bad luck. There was hardly a hotel in New York that had a 13th floor, he pointed out: "The implications of this are enormous and disturbing, and nobody is doing anything about it."[23]

Not long after such perspectives had been planted in her mind, Mahoney one afternoon noticed a hulking figure taking a walk near her house in Miami Beach. She recognized Winston Churchill, who was visiting a Canadian friend a block from the Mahoney home. "I used to see him quite often; he was right there, just down the street from where we lived at Miami Beach." Churchill had stopped in Florida en route to Fulton, Missouri, where he was to give what would become his famous "Iron Curtain" speech on the state of postwar Europe. "I was just walking," so she joined the former prime minister, an opportunity not to be missed to ask him about the psychiatrist from one of Britain's commonwealth countries who was attracting so much attention.[24]

"Mr. Churchill, did you ever hear of a Dr. Brock Chisholm?" she asked him.

"Ohh, yes, my deaahh — a *crackpot*, you know. Doesn't believe in Santa Claus!" Churchill snorted.

"His *exact* words," Mahoney remembered of the encounter. "And then he gave me a slap on the back, just for fun, that almost knocked me down! The next day he left for the speech that he made in Missouri."

Indeed, Chisholm, then Canada's deputy minster of health and welfare, had created a sensation in 1945 when he first remarked that any child who believed in Santa Claus would "refuse to think realistically when war threatens." Even if Churchill, as "almost everybody did," had placed him in the "crackpot" file, Mahoney was a fan of Chisholm's bold outspokenness, although she acknowledged that "it shocked people to say they shouldn't believe in Santa Claus. But it made *such* sense" to her. Chisholm also spoke of the "dangers of wars," she noted of his larger theme, but critics picked up only on the Santa Claus point. The outcry worldwide was so fierce as to provoke demands in the Canadian Parliament that Chisholm resign, which he refused to do.[25]

Advocacy to activism

Although *Reader's Digest* was not a publication that Mahoney read regularly — "I never went out any place where I didn't take something to read" — an article in a September 1948 issue caught her eye: "Oklahoma Attacks Its Snake Pits," a condensed account of deplorable conditions in state mental hospitals by a *Daily Oklahoman* newspaper reporter named Mike Gorman. The mentally ill, he had written, were treated "little better than in the times when they were chained in cages and kennels, whipped regularly at the full of the moon and hanged as witches." The story was not, as an editor's note warned, "easy or enjoyable reading." It graphically described a lack of state supervision and clinics to diagnose and treat children, and the squalor and "hopelessness" suffered by adult patients. Mahoney was so struck by the article — which she noted had appeared in a conservative newspaper, spearheading reforms — that she got in touch with Gorman and said she would like to talk to him.[26]

"I gave the story to Mahoney and asked if they could use it in our newspapers, and I offered to pay Gorman's salary for two weeks if he would come to Miami" and do a similar exposé in Florida. Dan Mahoney called Gorman's publisher and "after much heming and hawing," Gorman later said, "my publisher told me, 'You can go for thirty days.'" The Miami newspaper agreed to pay Gorman on a short-term basis, but "the things that he found were so *awful* that he stayed for six weeks," as

Mahoney remembered. She and Gorman quickly realized that they both were on a mission. It was to be a fateful alliance.[27]

Gorman was a feisty redhead of Irish descent from New York City, with a tough-talking irreverence to match his brash self-confidence (he wore his Phi Beta Kappa key to signal his election to the scholarly fraternity). If a bit "manic," Mahoney realized, "he was extremely intelligent" and had great energy. The two immediately felt a rapport. "Mike would take no nonsense," and his sometimes rough edges were enhanced by "this horrible humor that was so cutting." "Salty," one historian called him; "about forty percent bluster and sixty percent substance," a National Institutes of Health official thought.[28]

Gorman, after war service, in 1945 had joined the *Daily Oklahoman*. "He was a sort of romantic person," Mahoney thought, "and he wanted to change his lifestyle, I think, so he took this job in Oklahoma. He'd probably never been out of New York except for the service." Gorman himself told an interviewer, "I didn't want to go back to the *New York Herald Tribune*. After almost four years overseas, New York City didn't look pretty to me at all, and I wanted to see the country." During his five years on the Oklahoma paper he started a series of investigations of mental-health care, culminating in the book about Oklahoma's "snake pits." He subsequently undertook studies in other states. "My managing editor was getting itchy because I was spending a lot of time out of town." Florida would be the seventh state in which he covered the subject.[29]

"I sat down with a couple of reporters from the *Miami Daily News* who were indifferent to what I was doing. There was generally an indifference to mental illness in those days. It was just too easy to think of the state's taking care of the mentally ill in one big building, keeping them off the streets," as Gorman put it. "But this hospital in Florida, called Chattahoochee, turned out to be horrendous — it was just about the worst I'd ever seen. There were 6,000 patients in it. And I'd seen some real *beauts* already, naked patients lying in their own filth with attendants who were only paid $60 a month, people taken fresh off railroad trains and being put to work as attendants in a mental institution. Some of the *patients* there were filling in as attendants. I had seen enough not to be easily shocked, but what I found at Chattahoochee shocked me."[30]

Gorman's series in 1949 was "sensational," according to Mahoney, "headlines every day." It increased the *News'* circulation by 30,000, he recalled, "and they sure needed it" because the *News* ran behind the rival *Herald* at the time. That pleased Cox, "a real charmer" with whom Gorman shared an interest in politics.[31]

After that, "Florence and I got to be great pals," Gorman said. "I met everybody who was a mover and shaker, and I told her she should come with me to the legislature in Tallahassee, which was a typical small, old state capital," to seek funding for improvements in mental-health care. "So she went with me. That was really her forté," or would become one, cajoling people of influence.[32]

Mahoney had been observing how her husband got "money for various projects" by putting pressure on those in power, and she enlisted his help — "He was never against anything in the health field." Dan Mahoney, "because he knew all the politicians in Florida," smoothed the way for Gorman and her to talk to state legislators. The foray was successful beyond their expectations. Several million dollars were added to the budget, possibly "the first money ever appropriated in any state for mental-health alone," Florence noted with pride, crediting Gorman, and her husband's connections, with their success.

"The most tired I've ever been in my life — there were two times — once was coming back from trying to get money for the mental-health facility in Florida," Mahoney recalled of that first political effort. "The second time was staying up late dancing at a Culver Institute graduation, slinking around on my feet with all those boys," she laughed about the youthful experience. "Those are the two times I remember being so tired I just didn't think I could *walk*." Her efforts paid off, though, "more or less. We got the money" for a small facility in Miami. "Nobody started mental-health clinics willy-nilly" in those days, she pointed out, and the National Mental Health Association, with which she "tried to do business . . . had no money at all" and was of little help.

Friends and politicians

Because Miami since the 1920s had been a popular destination for people seeking sunshine, and many political and famous figures made it a holiday retreat, the Mahoney home became a place where interesting people met — particularly Democratic politicians.

One of those with whom they became acquainted was a dazzlingly attractive young navy officer from Massachusetts whose father, another Democratic Party backer, had personal motives tied to high ambitions for his sons — Joseph Patrick Kennedy, the prewar U. S. ambassador to Britain, who maintained a residence in Palm Beach. Twenty-seven-year-old John Fitzgerald "Jack" Kennedy was recovering from injuries suffered when the PT boat that he had commanded was cut in two and sunk in war action off the Solomon Islands in August 1943. He shared with Florence Mahoney a keen intellect and sense of humor as well as respect for her crusading tinged with gentle sardonicism, addressing her as "Madame Mahoney."

His father, Joe Kennedy, with department-store owner Bernard Gimbel, brought the young man to the Mahoney's house one day on a visit to see Dan. The older men went off to a room to talk, leaving Jack alone with Florence. "He completely, utterly impressed me," she recalled of that first meeting. "He could do *anything*, I thought at the time. He had just come back from the Pacific. He asked more interesting questions than I have ever heard from anyone — he had such a broad range of interests." The two became instant friends and Jack a frequent visitor, whom Michael Mahoney as a boy remembered seeing at the house.

"Due to the magnificent miscoordination of the mailing service of the United States Navy, I didn't receive your letter till just today, as it has been to Miami and back," Kennedy wrote Mahoney in a personally typed note, replete with errors, from his summer home at Hyannisport, Massachusetts, in 1944. "I hope I haven't missed you and that you haven't wended your way through Greater Bston [*sic*], distributing pamphlets as you go," a reference to her constant handing out of birth-control materials that she pressed on Kennedy. He gave her the family compound's private telephone number, saying "We always answer the phone when somebody calls," and conveying "My best wishes to mrs. [sic] Ripley who may or may not accept them, depending on what kind of a humor she's in. Affectionately, Jack."[33]

In September of that same year, three weeks after his older brother Joe had been killed on a bombing mission from England to a German target in France, Kennedy typed another letter to Mahoney, who had sent condolences from the ranch in Idaho. He again blamed "that superhuman ability of the Navy to screw up everything they touch — even the simple delivery of a letter frequently over-burdens this heaving puffing war-machine of ours. God save this country . . . from those patriots whose war cry is, 'what this country needs is to be run with military effenciancy [sic].' Anyways, thank you very much for your thought. Joe's loss has been a great shock to us all. He did everything well and with a great enthusiasm, and even in a family as large as ours, his place can't ever be filled, and he will always be missed. But thank you for your sympathy." He went on,

> In regard to the fascinating subject of my operation, I should naturally like to go on for several pages on a subject of general interest like this — but will confine myself to saying that I think that the doc shaould [sic] have read just one more book before picking up the saw. It may have to be done again. I got out of the hospital the other day and go back the nineteenth. If you are in Bosoton [sic] that day, I should love to see you. Otherwise you can get me on the phone [at Hyannis].[34]

Mahoney had mentioned to Kennedy several books she thought would be of interest to him, including an autobiography by British diplomat Baron Robert Gilbert Vansittart, an outspoken advocate of "hard peace" with Germany. She also suggested several works by Karl Menninger, the noted psychiatrist and co-founder of the well-known clinic in Topeka, Kansas. Kennedy, whose Harvard honors thesis, *Why England Slept*, on the British failure to anticipate the rising dangers of

Nazi Germany, had been a best-seller when published in 1940, told her,

> I have read Mr. Vansittart's book — I imagine that a great deal of his force comes from his remembrance of his son, and what the Germans did to him. In regard to Monsieur Menninger's Love against Hate and Man against himself [*sic*], I shall put them on my Fall reading list, and from the titles, I feel sure that they will enable me to dominate the annual meeting of the Boston psychiatric association.
>
> Thanks again for writing — please remember me to Dan and the boys.
>
> Affectionately,
> Jack[35]

Mahoney's friendship with Kennedy, which continued to be warm and close throughout their lives, was to have unforeseen ramifications.

Another political friendship that grew in the mid-1940s also was important to Mahoney. That was with incumbent Democratic Senator Claude Pepper, a Miami Beach neighbor. Pepper was an ardent advocate of social reforms who had served in the U. S. Senate since 1931. "We *all* liked him, and the [Cox] papers supported him," Mahoney said.[36]

An avowed liberal in his leanings, Pepper often was at odds with prevailing views. He spoke at a Congress of Industrial Organizations (CIO) rally in 1942 that called for aid to Russia to divert German forces to the eastern front, an appearance that later would be used against him in charges that he was sympathetic to Communism. FBI Director J. Edgar Hoover even placed the congressman under surveillance, telling him, when Pepper complained, that it was for his own protection because the agency had evidence of threats against his life. The agent assigned to watch him ironically became a House colleague, George Danielson (Democrat of California), who later confessed the fact to Pepper. Characteristic of his sense of honor, when the Senate in 1942 voted to exempt its members from wartime rationing, Pepper's was one of only two dissenting votes.[37]

Through such Democratic acquaintances Mahoney also developed contacts, beginning in 1945, with the nation's most powerful man, President Harry S. Truman, his wife Bess, and daughter Margaret. The Trumans began coming to south Florida in 1946, the year after he became president, when his doctor decreed a vacation to cure a persistent cold and cough.

"It was no small task to find a place that could accommodate 20 or 30 reporters, a staff of 16, and another 15 or 16 Secret Service men," Margaret Truman recalled in a biography of her father. "After some investigation, Dad made a choice which he never regretted—the submarine base at Key West, Florida. On November 18 [1946], he wrote his mother and sister from there, obviously delighted with the place." Truman stayed in the commandant's house, joking that he "did not 'rank' anyone out of his house." He also liked the privacy of the place, resolving on his first visit to avoid seeing "outsiders": "From now on I'm going to do as I please and let 'em all go to hell," he told his mother and sister. "At least for two years they can do nothing to me and after that, it doesn't matter." There he fished, swam, relaxed, and played jokes on reporters and aides, handing out cards that read, "DON'T GO AWAY MAD — JUST GO AWAY."[38]

Bess and Margaret sometimes joined him at Key West, notably in November after the 1948 presidential win over Thomas Dewey, when Truman told his sister Mary that he "must have signed 5,000" thank-you letters for congratulations sent to him. They went again that winter after finding the White House was falling apart and had be gutted and rebuilt.[39]

Mahoney noted the visits in her weekly column: "The presidential party will arrive here Feb. 11 and stay until Feb. 25, during which time President Truman will be cruising in nearby waters," she reported in 1946. "White House headquarters will be in the duPont building, press correspondents in the McAllister," she added.[40]

In addition to meeting the Trumans, she got to know Clark M. Clifford, then counsel to the president, Mathew J. "Matt" Connelly, and other aides during those years when they were on what Margaret Truman termed "hard-working vacations" in which "everybody had a good time, too." Clifford, Mahoney wrote in a 1949 column, "is always re-

ferred to by the press as the President's handsome special counsel —
true, but he must get weary of the same adjective always."[41] These were
the people involved in planning postwar programs, spurred by Truman's Senate committee report on conversion to a peacetime economy
(1943–44). Their interests would consume Mahoney, as well.

It was the introduction to an odd couple outside the world of politics,
however, that would forge a special relationship destined to change
Mahoney's, and the nation's, future.

3

Benevolent Plotters

───────────◆───────────

*M*ARY LASKER HAD NOT YET BEEN recognized as a health activist when Florence Mahoney first met her in the early 1940s. Indeed, the word "activist" had yet to be applied to the kind of advocates that she and Mary would become—unknown to them at the time. While Mary would be important to Mahoney's future activities, her husband Albert Lasker, too, was significant, not only because he shared Mary's interests but because his wealth provided her with opportunities for beneficial works and important contacts with people in power — an essential ingredient for success in the kinds of endeavors on which she and Mahoney were about to embark.

Pioneering advertising tycoon Albert Lasker had been a close friend of Governor Cox and the Mahoneys since the 1920s. Lasker built an ocean-front house on Collins Avenue and for many years spent much of each winter there. He shared with Mahoney and other neighbors outrage over the invasion of the area by known gangsters like Al Capone. Lasker sold his house about 1945 (Florence tried to get Dan to buy it), but the friend-ship with the Mahoneys would take on new dimensions.[1]

Born in 1880, Albert Davis Lasker showed an entrepreneurial bent from his youth. He owned his own business by age 16 and was briefly a reporter before entering the advertising business in 1898 with the Chicago agency Lord & Thomas, which he bought in 1908. He was a registered and active member of the Republican Party (although in 1944 he confided to friends that he was voting for Roosevelt and in 1948 he voted for Truman).[2]

Lasker was credited with devising "modern" techniques to sell products actively rather than passively, in contrast to nineteenth-century advertising. He favored catchy phrases that he utilized to advantage. His largest account, beginning in 1922, was the American Tobacco Company, maker of *Lucky Strike* cigarettes. Lasker's innovative merchandising for a variety of other consumer products made them household words.[3]

The politician and the businessman

The 1920 presidential fight between two Ohioans brought out another aspect of Albert Lasker's advertising skills for which he would be credited as a forerunner. He took charge of promoting Warren Harding — who was loath to leave his Marion front porch — against Governor Cox. Lasker began to "humanize" Harding as a trustworthy, down-home Middle Westerner who would not rock any boats.[4]

Cox had told people during the campaign that he "hated" Lasker, even thought he was a "sinister" influence on the Republican party. But astonishingly, the day after the election, he telephoned the advertising executive. "I'm Jim Cox — remember me?" were his opening words to an amazed Lasker. Conceding that he had expected to lose but not by such a large margin, Cox then went on to attribute the Republicans' success to the publicity that Lasker had orchestrated, personalizing his candidate. Cox wanted to meet the man who was in large part responsible for the Democrats' loss.[5]

"I'd like to salvage something out of this defeat, and perhaps we could be friends," he told Lasker, who readily accepted the invitation, even canceling a meeting with Harding to join Cox. The two men quickly overcame their political differences and became lifelong pals, a friendship that by association had ramifications for Florence Mahoney.[6]

After his first wife's death, Lasker was briefly married to actress Doris Kenyon (in 1938). The following year, on April 1, he walked into Twenty One restaurant in New York City for lunch with World War I hero William "Wild Bill" Donovan, a mutual friend of his and Dan Mahoney's. At a nearby table sat two women whom Donovan knew and introduced to Lasker. After lunch he exchanged a few words with one of them, an attractive woman with bright blue eyes and an engaging smile. He turned to Donovan and asked to learn more about her.[7]

Partner and helpmate

Mary Woodward Reinhardt also noticed the tall, 59-year-old Lasker, who promptly called friends and asked if they would arrange invitations so the two could meet properly. They almost instantly were attracted to each other.

Mary Woodward was born in Watertown, Wisconsin, in 1901, the daughter of a banker and civic-minded mother, Sara Johnson, who had led campaigns for the town's first public library and two public parks. Mary attended the University of Wisconsin, then Radcliffe College, where she majored in art; she graduated *cum laude* in 1923 and did postgraduate work at Oxford.

Having suffered several serious illnesses as a child, Mary had memories of being badly stricken by the 1917–18 influenza epidemic. She and Lasker both had become frustrated that doctors seemed unable to cure sick people. "I'm infuriated when I hear that anyone's ill, especially when it's from a disease that virtually nothing is known about," she often told people.[8]

Rebelling against her parsimonious father, Mary decided to make money in order to be independent. She took a job at a gallery in New York that dealt in "modern" painting and in 1926 married its owner, art dealer Paul Reinhardt, one of the first to introduce twentieth-century French painting to America. Her job was to arrange benefit loan exhibitions and sell French masters and other works to collectors and museums. During that period she acquired a number of paintings by Impressionists that would be greatly valued in time, and she continued to collect art throughout her life. But the Reinhardts divorced in 1934, and Mary had to make a living on her own in the midst of the Great Depression.[9]

She conceived an idea to promote inexpensive dress designs decorated with photos of movie stars and launched "Hollywood Patterns," which became a hit in poor economic times when women turned to making their own clothes. Mary had become a successful businesswoman in her own right, and her bright personality and forthright capabilities attracted the wealthy Lasker, who also shared an interest in collecting art.[10]

Though considerably different in age (Mary was twenty years younger than Lasker), the two quickly realized that they were well matched. She was beautiful and smart and could stand up to his strong personality. They also respected one another. Lasker, however, demurred for a time, his confidence in marriage shaken by the previous one, and his health suffering from a malfunction of adrenal glands just as war in Europe was breaking out. Mary, manifesting a determination that would become her trademark, located the physician best known for treating Lasker's problem. She also recommended that he see a psychoanalyst to address his mental sufferings. He finally was persuaded and later said that analysis "taught me to forgive myself." Of Mary he confessed to his friend and biographer John Gunther, "All she did was keep me from losing my mind." Fifteen months after they had first met, Albert and Mary were married, on June 21, 1940.[11]

In 1942 Lasker suddenly announced to Mary one day that he had decided to give up the advertising agency that he had built up over forty-four years. He had gone to work for $10 a week. By the time he retired at sixty-two, his fortune was estimated at $80 million. He did not want the company name to continue, however, so Lord & Thomas was liquidated and a new company, operated by Lasker's associates, was set up to carry on with old accounts.

"I simply wish to take an intellectual and mental vacation," Lasker explained publicly of the surprising decision. "I am going to devote my time to matters concerning public welfare." Privately he told an old friend, "The Lasker of the advertising business died in 1942. I never think of him, and I'm not sure I ever knew the man."[12]

A major influence on Lasker's future would be his new wife's interests. Her frustration with medical care drove her to question what was going on in the health-research field if people continued dying, *ad infinitem*, of the same diseases. She also worried about those who could not afford to get medical care or whose life savings were wiped out by the costs of prolonged illness. She once was asked by a close friend for a $500 loan to send her mother to a hospital for cancer treatment. The money, though, came too late and had to be used for the woman's funeral. That was a turning point, Mary told *Time* magazine in 1948. When Albert Lasker asked her, soon after they met, what she wanted most out of life, she said that she wanted to see what could be done about making health insurance more widely available so that even those who could not afford care could get it and secondly that she wanted to promote research on major diseases like cancer and tuberculosis.[13]

Lasker, who had served in several high-level federal posts over his career and managed millions in government budgets, countered that private-sector spending for biomedical research would not have a significant impact. What was needed was the largesse of government coffers — huge sums of money from the taxpayer-supported "kitty." And "I'll show you how to get it," he offered.

Learning something about politics would be essential, he added.

The Albert and Mary Lasker Foundation

Mary's desires may have been the reason behind the important step that Lasker took immediately after giving up his business. He set up a foundation, named for himself and his beloved wife, with a purpose unique at the time: to *stimulate* federal government support of biomedical research. The Lasker Foundation would provide "seed" money with the object of encouraging government follow-up on research projects that showed promise. The couple's initial focus was on birth control and mental health; they also gave grants for work on heart disease, particularly arteriosclerosis. When their cook and another servant to whom they were devoted died of cancer, however, they added cancer research to their priorities. Cancer would be a central focus of both their efforts henceforth: Albert's brother Harry had died of it in the 1930s, and Mary had lost close friends to it. She was obsessed with the disease and why it could not be cured, ironic considering that Albert had made much of his fortune popularizing cigarettes, which by the early 1960s were blamed for causing lung cancer.[14]

The foundation, beginning in 1944, also gave annual awards recognizing significant new contributions in various health fields. That was a reflection of Mary's desire to leave money at her death for pioneers in medicine. Why not do it while she was alive, a lawyer suggested? The award program was instituted, Mary said, to "give encouragement to people in medicine as the Pulitzer Prize has in journalism." Albert was reticent about the publicity that necessarily accompanied such awards, and at first refused to appear at ceremonies or to meet winners.[15]

Biomedical research awards were given for "a major contribution to the struggle against killing or crippling diseases." Others were made in the fields of public health and administration and for medical journalism and media coverage. Although not financially large — awards ranged from $500 to $2,500 as of 1952, rose to $15,000 and by 2001 to $50,000 — they were considered prestigious among recipients' peers because they were judged and selected by professional organizations separate from the foundation, such as the American Public Health Association, National Committee against Mental Illness, American Heart Association, Planned Parenthood Federation, and others. By 1998, 59 of the nearly 300 Lasker awardees also had won Nobel Prizes.

"Benevolent plotters"

One of Lasker's first tasks in retirement was to spearhead a revamping of the American Society for the Control of Cancer, as it was then called, beginning in 1943. He perceived that if advertising methods were applied to a massive fundraising campaign, capitalizing on the public's willingness to donate to disease-oriented organizations such as the March of

Dimes for polio, more money could be raised than the society had ever seen. It traditionally held annual fund drives, but to the Laskers' amazement none of the money raised each year — about $350,000 — was spent on research. Part of the problem admittedly was a lack of breakthroughs in cancer research. "If there are no leads, let us make them," Mary stated.[16]

Most of the society's money went to running the organization and a 30,000-member "Women's Field Army" that rang doorbells every year in a cancer "drive" to collect funds. The society had been instrumental in pushing for the establishment of the federal National Cancer Institute (NCI) that Congress first authorized in 1937, the only disease-related government research agency in existence in the early 1940s. Even NCI spent less than $600,000, mostly for patient care rather than research.

Lasker offered to contribute to a national drive on the condition that one quarter of new money raised would go for research, the balance for public education. The offer was accepted and the Laskers and others put up $80,000 to pay for the drive. "To raise money you have to have it," Albert was fond of saying. The campaign was scheduled to last a month, beginning April 1, 1945.[17]

Lasker recruited other corporate executives, most notably Elmer H. Bobst, head of a pharmaceutical company, who had managed a successful War Bond campaign in New Jersey. Like Lasker, he brought a commercial approach to the cancer effort. "I decided to . . . run it like a business with a well-planned 'sales' campaign," Bobst said in his autobiography, astonished to find that "the entire federal medical research program in all areas in the early '40s was only $2 million — far less than the research budget of even a medium-sized pharmaceutical company." Bobst and the others whom Lasker recruited were men who were not afraid to ruffle feathers in accomplishing their objective. They would soon override the society's entrenched, largely physician-dominated leadership.[18]

While "good men," the doctors "didn't understand fundraising or promotion, or even money," according to Bobst who, with Lasker, undertook to change that state of affairs. In a coup they replaced the society's leaders with lay people (the professionals would act as scientific advisors). The organization's objectives were redefined to focus on the causes and cures of cancer through research, educating the public to the life-saving advantages of early detection and diagnosis (then believed to save one third of victims' lives), and expanding a program to supply hospitals with equipment and services. Naturally, the group's actions created dissension, frustrating Lasker so much that he retired from the active fight and Bobst appointed Mary to his place on the executive committee. "With her help," Bobst recorded, "I took control of the society." The "Women's Army" was disbanded, and new fundraising approaches started that concentrated on wealthy donors, communities, advertising, contests, and civic organizations.

"The task of education was perhaps the most urgent then, because cancer still was and is ... the most frightening word in medicine, almost unmentionable in private conversation," Bobst noted. When Mary began a campaign to publicize on the radio the importance of getting regular medical examinations to detect cancer, she was told that the "c" word was taboo, even improper, on the air despite the fact that cancer was the second leading cause of death in the United States. That led to the Laskers' calling in media executives like the heads of NBC and CBS and popular radio stars like Bob Hope and Fibber McGee and Molly to talk about the drive. A three-part series about it in the *Reader's Digest* also brought in money.

Florence and Dan Mahoney chaired the cancer fundraising campaign in the Miami area, increasing donations from fewer than $1,000 the year before to $55,000. Florence also remembered watching Walter Winchell broadcast one night from the *Miami Daily News* tower where she, Dan, and Cox had gone to observe the famous commentator. Winchell had "gotten on the bandwagon" by then, she noted, "and made a thing of raising money for the Damon Runyon Fund," named for the New York writer who had died of the disease. Before that, Winchell had told her, "You never, *never* mention" cancer on the air.[19]

Back in New York, the result of the Lasker-Bobst cabal — who dubbed themselves "benevolent plotters" — was an incredible increase in donations to the cancer society. Four million dollars was raised in just one month, of which $1 million would go to research, a large sum at the time and comparable to half of what the entire federal government was spending on cancer research. Cancer no longer was unmentionable. It also was evident that people would rally behind such efforts when motivated and convinced of their potential success. But private funding would not do what the Laskers and their allies envisioned; the federal government had to become the fulcrum for massive research programs. They realized, though, that if people would donate large sums out of their private pockets, surely they would back the use of taxes for expanded government programs.[20]

Flush with their success, the Laskers now wanted a role in deciding how the society's money would be allocated. They wanted the organization to back federal appropriations for agencies like the National Cancer Institute, an idea that raised the ire of many in the medical community who associated government funding with "socialized medicine." The society ultimately lent its weight to the concept, testifying before Congress, which would have far-reaching effects. Its name was changed to the American Cancer Society, fundraising reached $10 million the next year (1946), and it adopted as a slogan Mary's exhortation, "If there are no leads, let us make them." Mary Lasker would sit on its board for the rest of her life.[21]

The Lasker-Bobst-led core group would go on to "revolutionize American medical education, research and health care," Bobst felt. They were "united in one purpose: to stimulate federal support of medical research and education . . . [which] required enormous voluntary expenditures of time and energy." The "benevolent plotters" also included people whose names would come to be well known: Doctor Alton Ochsner, the first physician to establish a link between cancer and smoking, in 1954; Doctor Michael E. DeBakey, a pioneer in heart-transplant surgery; and Anna Rosenberg Hoffman, a Budapest-born consultant on labor problems who had worked with a number of government agencies during and after the war. Respected and admired for her intellect and capabilities, she was an intimate friend of the

Laskers, with whom she often vacationed. Rosenberg Hoffman would be an important asset to Mary Lasker's and Florence Mahoney's activities.[22]

Another benefaction that took root in those years reflected Mary's other passion — flowers, which predominated as subjects of the Laskers' art collection. She embarked on an effort to bring floral beauty to urban landscapes beginning in 1941, when she decided to honor the memory of her mother with a massive display of colorful blooms in the heart of New York City. In 1948 she and Albert gave the city park department 40,000 tulip bulbs from Holland, which were planted at Central Park Place and on islands dividing Park Avenue, spurring city leaders to plant twenty-two blocks that would bloom each spring. A *New York Times* columnist in 1953 fondly dubbed Mary "Annie Appleseed." She would go on to underwrite major plantings in and around the nation's capital as part of an initiative led by First Lady Mrs. Lyndon B. Johnson.[23]

A fruitful meeting of minds

Albert had brought Mary to Florida soon after they met, where she was introduced to Florence and Dan Mahoney.

"I'd never seen her before in my life until she came to visit me with Albert," Mahoney said of first meeting Mary in Miami Beach. While the men talked about things that consumed them, Florence and Mary became acquainted.

There was an immediate rapport "because I liked anybody who was intelligent," Mahoney said, and Lasker was. Most social friends "were not interested in anything that *I* was interested in. Mary was at least interested — very interested in flowers, and she had been interested in birth control, too, and she knew quite a lot about psychiatry." She also knew and greatly admired Margaret Sanger, to whose Birth Control Federation Albert and his sisters had given money in the 1930s (notably for demonstration projects to benefit African-Americans in the South), and with whom Mary shared a desire for more research on contraception.[24]

It was not long before Mary Lasker and Florence Mahoney found that they, too, had a lot in common.

Initially, said Mahoney, "we didn't think of backing 'causes' at all — we were just talking about things we were interested in," like the mental-health facilities that Mahoney had been pushing in several states before she met Lasker. Their time together became consumed with medical subjects — "boringly so," as Mahoney recalled. "Albert wouldn't let us discuss it — around him we had to be quiet." They also perceived the importance of close ties to politicians, something Mahoney had understood in her successful effort to fund mental-health clinics in Florida. An opportunity arose to exploit such connections at the national level.

"President Truman was coming down to Florida and invited [Dan] Mahoney to a fish fry for a Democratic fundraiser. Anyway, Mahoney wouldn't dream of going," Florence laughed, "so I talked to Mary and we decided it would be fun to go — so we went. A lot of Democrats were there and the president — we shook hands with him. I don't remember any glowing conversation."

Within three years the two women found themselves taking active positions on issues of concern — not in a formal "committee" or structured way. "We were babes in the woods," Mahoney conceded.

"It was just like topsy," she said, describing the evolution of their activism. "One thing led to another. And I think neither one of us could have done it alone. It took cooperation — and ideas," she said of their early results.

They found themselves going to medical meetings and talking to acknowledged experts. "Once we got interested in something, we went around to all the places to see what was going on. When we heard of something unusual, we would go see" the people involved.

Florence and Mary corresponded regularly when far apart, as they frequently were.

In the World War II summer of 1942, Mahoney was at the Idaho ranch with the boys, where they found the place sadly in need of repairs, which they were making themselves. "We do all the irrigating and wood and horses and ice, etc.... The country is so beautiful and the mountains still filled with snow," she wrote the Laskers, urging them to visit Sun

Valley, only sixty miles away. "Am longing for you to see the boys for they have grown up so and are such fun . . . . [They] have their cattle and horses to be looked after this summer." She added, "have a lot of new books, and am reading Kiplinger's *Washington is like that* and *Men of Bataan*. My conscience hurts me no end spending so much effort out here when it is in no way helping the war effort."[25]

Mary replied that they would come in August. "You sound full of health," she wrote. She and Albert had been entertaining all summer — "we have had everyone [including] the King of Greece for dinner, it seems to me. I need a little outdoor exercise very badly . . . . I look forward to a really good visit with you."[26]

"Albert wasn't exactly the ranch type, to put it mildly," Mahoney laughed of the urbane man in the wilds of the West, "but he was a good sport about it."

The next summer Lasker congratulated Mahoney on her success with mental-health funding. "I was happy to hear you got the bill passed that you wanted to in Florida, and also that the Women's Rights bill passed the State Legislature. I was thrilled you have been able to start work on the financial committee for the Planned Parenthood state organization. You are a wonder, and I know your help will do a great good. Isn't it great that Mahoney finally got around to understanding it? It makes me so happy that you had a good talk and that he is sympathetic." she added, referring to Dan. "I saw Mrs. Roosevelt for lunch the other day," she continued, "and she was sweet. Do you know her? I know you would like her."[27]

In time Mahoney and Lasker would buy a ranch together near Kirkland, Arizona — about ninety miles northwest of Phoenix — motivated in part to benefit Albert's health and as a possible safe retreat in case of an atomic bomb attack, the fear of which, as Mahoney noted, "was prevalent in those years." Called the "Z Triangle Ranch," it had a "big old house with a wonderful view."

The Arizona ranch became a center for activity that Mahoney would be involved in throughout her life — encouraging young people to enter public service. She often invited medical students whom she was helping as guests. One young man on whom she had a lifelong impact was Bruce Babbitt, who knew the Kirkland property as "the old Swift family ranch. It had a huge, rambling adobe mansion built in a horseshoe around a central courtyard." He was invited to join Mahoney's "extraordinary inventory of acquaintances" who gathered there. On one occasion she and Babbit "had been across the border to Mexico. On the way back," Babbitt recalled, "we stopped at a kind of roadside tavern where we were eating dinner. We got going in this discussion about running for political office," said Babbitt. "I wasn't sure that I was cut out for it. Suddenly Florence got up and said, 'It's easy — I'm going to show you, let's work this room.' She took me around to all these cowboys and truck drivers, and said, 'This is a man who is going to run for public office. He can do a lot for your state.' I was astounded. We sat down and she said, 'See, it's easy,'" even though one man responded, "Yeah, and what do *I* care?" Babbitt would go on to become Governor of Arizona (1978–87) and Secretary of Interior during the administration of President Bill Clinton (1993–2000) — a career that he frankly said resulted from Mahoney's influence.[28]

Albert Lasker and James Cox, meanwhile, maintained a lively correspondence and friendship. At the outset of World War II (shortly after Germany's invasion of Poland), in September 1939, Cox wrote a thoughtful letter to Lasker, who continued in poor health and had gone to Arizona for respite. Cox hoped that the visit would come off, "born of the hospitality of the desert and the sands and cactus [that] do something to one's better nature." He asked Lasker to "Please have your nurse write me at least once a week if you are not up to the task of handling the pen as I want to know just how you are getting along." He went on to say,

Albert, I can't convince myself that this is to be a long war. It is just inconceivable to me that Germany can carry on very long economically or that the people, as repressed and restricted as they are, will give support. I again repeat what I said at your dinner, out of this will come a spiritual awakening, tolerance, more human kindness, concern for the vicissitudes of others, etc., etc.[29]

After the war, when Cox in 1945 apparently turned down a proffered appointment to the U. S. Senate (he was then seventy-five years old), Lasker wrote revealingly of himself, "I was much impressed . . . with your refusal to accept the appointment . . . . That is the only job I ever envied in my whole life. I would rather be a United States Senator than President. I was arguing your decision . . . last evening but I understand your views and felt you had done right by yourself. None-the-less, it is a swell and deserved recognition."[30]

Lasker was about to enter the hospital for a prostate operation, "positive that what has been troubling me is about to be cleared up and as a result I feel like a boy who is certain his severance from the Army is coming through and is awaiting going home." Florence was visiting the Laskers at the time. "We always enjoy having her," Lasker told Cox, "but I am particularly glad she will be here with Mary while I am hospitalized."[31]

Just before Christmas in 1951, when he was eighty-one and Lasker seventy-one, Cox wrote a long letter to "My dear Albert" reflecting on their curious but strong friendship, one that had engendered a new and meaningful relationship between Mary Lasker and Florence Mahoney. Cox began by reminiscing about Lasker's Mill Road Farm, now broken up for development:

> . . . I knew of nothing in the country that was quite like them [the gatherings there] . . . . Time makes many changes and I don't even like to think of the dismemberment of your beautiful estate. However, nothing can destroy the recollections of the great days we had together there.[32]

Lasker in return sent Christmas greetings by telegram care of the *Atlanta Journal,* which Cox had just bought. "Dear Governor," it read, "One of the rich assets of my life has been our longstanding friendship. In the spirit of that friendship I wish you and yours at this holiday season all the good that can come to anyone. Mary joins in affectionate greetings . . . "[33]

It would be one of the last communications between the two unlikely friends. Lasker would be gone by late spring (1952) and Cox five years later (1957).

Albert Lasker, in a sad irony, died of colon cancer. He first complained of stomach trouble in December 1949 and was extensively examined and x-rayed, but no evidence of cancer was found. It was an example of what improved diagnosis and treatment of the kind that he and Mary were advocating might have done: If the cancer had been detected in early stages, Lasker might have survived longer than he did. His biographer wrote that Lasker was not told he had the disease. Lasker admittedly "would not thank anybody to tell me anything bad about myself." After rallying from several major operations, he died May 30, 1952, a month after his seventy-third birthday, leaving half of his more than $11-million estate to his widow and half to the foundation. Mary with Albert's three children donated 250 flowering cherry trees and some 50,000 daffodils to be planted at the United Nations building in his memory.[34]

Formation of the National Committee on Mental Health

By the time of Albert's death, Mary Lasker had turned her attention fully to the subject that consumed her: improving the quality of health through research. And in Florence Mahoney she had a strong co-worker.

The two women toward the end of the war had decided to form an organization, the National Committee on Mental Health, which they co-chaired, "to use as a going-off spot for various things we wanted to publicize," as Mahoney put it. The committee's loosely defined mission was to "carry on a broad educational program" that was not confined to mental health, although that was a focus of its principals. Prominent on the committee were forty-six state governors as honorary chairmen, reflecting Mahoney's recognition of their importance to public health programs. The committee had an office in Washington but no full-time staff to coordinate the women's activities and keep track of the many bills they began following. It was more than the two could handle alone, and it would be a shame, they realized, if promising legislation fell through the cracks and was not enacted for lack of organized support. Lasker proposed that they hire a full-time lobbyist to follow the issues. The committee agreed if she would pay for it. She did and the committee's first lobbyist was hired in 1945.[35]

The committee was to have a long and productive history as the fulcrum for Florence Mahoney's and Mary Lasker's advocacy.

4

Reaping Peacetime Benefits
from Wartime Research

◆————————

ORLD WAR II HAD MOBILIZED a concerted government ef-fort
— unprecedented to date — in applying research to practical
use, not the least of which were the inventions of radar and the atomic
bomb. "Government-supported research" had proven what could be
accomplished when an organized effort was made.

Mahoney and Lasker, now a team, wanted to capitalize on that success.

To address the health needs of military men, a presidentially mandated
Office of Scientific Research and Development (OSRD) had overseen
fast-track development of drugs to combat diseases. Its work was conducted in utmost secrecy and carried on without public recognition.

Mahoney noted in one of her many memoranda that some "$10–15
million had been spent on diseases connected with servicemen, e.g., malaria, etc., from '41–'44 by the Committee for Medical Research of the
OSRD" while only $2 million had been spent "for everything else in the
U.S. Public Health Service."[1]

More importantly, she and Lasker learned, a number of impressive
breakthroughs in biomedicine had resulted from the coordinated war

effort, notably, development of the antibiotic penicillin to fight staphy-lococcic infections; sulfonamide (sulfa) drugs to treat wounds and burns; blood derivatives like gamma globulin to combat such things as measles and hepatitis; adrenal steroids; cortisone; the synthetic for qui-nine, atabrine, to cure malaria; vaccines against typhus and yellow fever; and DDT insecticide powder, which had a "wonderful effect" in keeping soldiers and their clothing deloused for several months. Credited with saving hundreds of thousands of lives during the war, the new treat-ments now could be applied to civilian populations.[2]

The question was, how could the nation profit from the remarkable lessons learned in war? Should the federal government continue a role in managing research on new medicines and technologies? Many scientists, now back at university or commercial laboratories, opposed government involvement that would in any way impinge on their freedoms. The ad-vantages of a government agency's prodding and management, how-ever, were not lost on those who recognized what had been accomplished in a short time — including then-Senator Harry S. Truman.[3]

At the time, scientific research in the United States was small in scale by subsequent standards: It was conducted at universities, by for-profit companies or at nonprofit institutes with nominal support. There was no long-range government commitment to address medical problems with goals like those set by corporations. The few disease-related organi-zations that existed provided care and education, not research toward cures.[4]

Enter Florence Mahoney and Mary Lasker. They increasingly were aware that the existing modus operandi would not produce the kinds of results they envisioned. The private sector could not do it alone, and government programs were limited, officials content with the funds they had and the narrow scope of work underway.

The two women were in uncharted territory. No consensus existed about how to change the status quo for the betterment of humankind. It could not be accomplished simply by throwing money at the problem, as Albert Lasker's approach implied. Not only was funding scarce, but there also was a lack of qualified scientists interested in working on disease problems. Mahoney and the Laskers began to think that a new agency, free of an entrenched bureaucracy, might be the way to go.[5]

They must have been heartened by a *New York Times* editorial in 1944, following a National Conference on the Problems of Medical Care, that asked why a national medical foundation "should not plan long-run programs in the same manner" as corporations:

"It is little short of a disgrace that virtually nothing is known about arthritis, that the conquest of cancer is still far off.... If we had only the haphazard grant-in-aid system [then used for government support of medical research], the chances are that we would not yet have electron tubes ... and television would still only be a dream. No industrial laboratory would think of conducting research as it is now conducted in medicine."[6]

Not everyone shared Mahoney's and Lasker's vision. Some in positions of influence and respect outright opposed it or at least demurred on the need for expanding federal programs. Dr. Frank B. Jewett, president of the National Academy of Sciences and head of Bell Telephone Laboratories, one of four men called in by President Roosevelt to develop the wartime research effort, thought that "a large infusion of funds would dilute the quality of American science." Leave it to private philanthropy and industry, he said.[7]

Mary Lasker began collecting statistics on job absenteeism from illness, which Albert helped dramatize by putting in human perspectives: Only 3.5 percent of the national budget was being spent on medical care. And while a nominal sum was spent on cancer research, nothing was applied to heart disease although millions in agricultural research were allocated to creating disease-resistant crops and animals. Why not do the same for human beings, the women wondered? Meanwhile, they learned that the OSRD was about to be abolished.[8]

Mary raised the subject with Anna Rosenberg, who offered to take a memorandum to President Roosevelt suggesting that he pay attention to medical matters in conversion policies. Roosevelt in July 1944 asked OSRD director Doctor Vannevar Bush to prepare recommendations for the future relationship between government and the research community, notably how to wage "the war of science against disease." Roosevelt's letter might have been quoting Florence Mahoney and Mary Lasker when it stated: "The fact that the annual deaths in this country from one or two diseases alone are far in excess of the total number of lives lost by us in battle during this war should make us conscious of the duty we owe future generations."[9]

Another step taken in 1944 was to give the Public Health Service (PHS) similar authority as the OSRD to pay for research performed by nongovernmental scientists in the form of grants. In the new law, the word "cancer" was changed to "medical" research, a seemingly minor but important change with long-range ramifications. The federal Budget Bureau, however, was reluctant to open its coffers and pay for PHS grants.[10]

"Citizen Petitioners" — the Pepper hearings

Mahoney now became central to the fledgling effort. Her first ally was her friend and neighbor, Senator Claude Pepper, who in 1943 was made chairman of a special committee dealing with peacetime research and education. She and Lasker went to see him to explore the idea of his holding hearings on government-supported research.[11]

Lasker also began giving Pepper troubling statistics that she was uncovering about sickness and death from various diseases. A particularly shocking fact stood out: Nearly one of three draftees examined by the Selective Service for military induction had been rejected as physically or mentally unfit in what was thought to be the world's healthiest nation.[12]

Pepper, who was running for reelection, was well aware that he needed the continued political endorsement of the local Cox newspaper. While that was a strong motivation, the compelling information that he was receiving was more than enough to convince him to hold hearings and explore the concept of an expanded government role in research. "Congress was not much interested in legislation that did not directly affect the war effort," he said in his autobiography, "but I argued that this situation did — it represented a severe drain on our manpower." For fourteen months he would conduct hearings before the Select Subcommittee on Wartime Health and Education within the Committee on Education and Labor.[13]

It was a pivotal moment in the nation's history, which Florence Mahoney and Mary Lasker perceived. These would be the first congressional hearings ever held to review government-supported research. The women recognized that they could influence the conduct and content of the hearings, thus legitimizing their ideas in a public forum. The hearings would be a springboard for virtually all of their future activities (with the exception of birth control), addressing research on diseases, mental health, and aging.

It is hard to realize, with the perspective of many years hence, how important and unique the hearings were just as world war was winding down and the nation was coming out of economic depression, at a time when poor health often was accepted as fate and health care not yet considered a "right" for all Americans.

Pepper sent two subcommittee staff members to New York to review what Lasker was compiling about the economic impact of diseases. In addition, she and Mahoney offered to help line up witnesses who could tell the subcommittee what was in the best interests of the nation — distinguished scientists and physicians who advocated continuing the government program and giving it money to foster work on a grander scale than ever before undertaken. It was the beginning of a pattern that the women would follow for many years — "citizen petitioners," they termed themselves.[14]

The witnesses whom they put forward had impressive credentials, people such as leading cancer researcher Dr. Cornelius P. (Dusty) Rhoads, who had taken leave as director of New York's Memorial Hospital (later Memorial Sloan-Kettering Cancer Center) to head the Army's Chemical Warfare Medical Division.[15]

"At first everybody — all the doctors — were against using any federal money for research, as *he* was in the beginning," said Mahoney of Rhoads. "But we told him why we thought it a good idea and what would come of it. He finally admitted that he thought he could solve the cancer problem in five years if he had the proper money for research. He had been in the service and looked very thin — as if he had ulcers. But he did come to testify before Pepper. He was the first person we got to testify."

Mahoney's 1944 calendar noted that on "March 26, Mary visiting us in Miami. Saw Pepper. He was running for reelection in November. September 17, 18 and 20, 1944, Mary and I went to Washington for hearings in Committee on Wartime Health and Education. Spoke to Pepper re: Medical Research bill. Saw Dr. Rhoads. Had Pepper and Rhoads and Baehr and Truslow for lunch Sept. 20th. Dec. 14–16, hearings in Washington under Pepper on need of funds for medical research."[16]

"Talked to Pepper last night," Mahoney wrote Lasker prior to the December round, "and he said the Pres. is interested in the research bill and they are trying to get it drafted before the hearings. Said they might be about the 16th of Dec. Do let me know as soon as you find out for it is hard to get reservations" to travel to Washington from Florida.[17]

The hearings

At the time of Pepper's hearings, there was only one federal research Institute of Health, created in 1930 and moved in 1938 to a donated private estate in Bethesda, Maryland, a suburb of Washington, D. C. Of the institute's total budget, less than one third went to research grants, and the Public Health Service traditionally did not ask for budget increases, cautioning against "growth of a mushroom type."[18]

In a statement opening one set of hearings, Pepper said, "We are fully aware of the practically unlimited possibilities for health which modern medical and public health science offers. We must see to it that this science is put to use for the benefit of all people. Health is a prerequisite to the pursuit of happiness, and therefore, in a democracy, all people must share equally in the opportunity to health . . . . I believe we have been sluggards in our thinking about the reconversion," he concluded, noting that "Germany may be defeated this summer or fall." That was in July 1944.[19]

Convening the hearings specifically on medical research December 14 to 16, 1944, Pepper emphasized the successes developed during the war by the OSRD. "Can we maintain the momentum . . . or must we see a dwindling of the funds and opportunities . . . to make continued progress against diseases which take a heavy toll of civilian health?" he asked.[20]

While Mahoney and Lasker, sitting in the hearing room, would not actually have heard Pepper's words that day because he was not present to speak them (his statement was entered into the record when he was called to another meeting), they already knew what he would say. They had told him the sum and substance of what they believed the hearings should accomplish and were confident that he would echo their views. He did.

The hearings were not widely covered by newspapers (the *Washington Evening Star* and *Post* carried brief articles on back pages). Mahoney and Lasker would have to rely on the printed record, an excellent source of data that they could quote to skeptics of their mission.

They did not miss a day of the December hearings. Among others, they heard the OSRD's medical chairman, Dr. A. N. Richards, explain how a large infusion of money in three years had hastened the discovery of blood substitutes to fight infections and accelerated penicillin's development so that it now was available in quantity. "We know of no private sources of funds which could have financed the work." That was the kind of assertion Mahoney and Lasker wanted Congress to hear.

Richards' next remarks also would have caught their attention:

If the concerted efforts of medical investigators which have yielded so much of value during the war are to be continued on any comparable scale during the peace, the conclusion is inescapable that they must be supported by government.[21]

Noting one witness' profession as an investment banker, Pepper pointedly asked David M. Heyman, board president of New York City's

Public Health Research Institute, if he thought there was anything "improper" in having the government support private-sector research. It was a "necessary function of government," Heyman replied, and would not adversely affect profit-making companies engaged in research, reinforcing Pepper's point.[22]

Research without interference

The researchers tempered their enthusiasm somewhat when contemplating government's role, cognizant of the Nazis' purges of scientists and centralized management of laboratories. "Can government control, so understanding and so flexible, be created so that the imaginations and the scientific passions of investigators will not be inhibited?" Richards wondered. Furthermore, how was money to be allocated and who would make decisions over the merits of research to be supported? No precedent for peacetime research support had ever been tried on a large scale. Richards concluded that "the administration of federal aid to research must be as free from political influence as is humanly possible."[23]

Scientist after scientist repeated the same caution. The task that Mahoney and Lasker had set about would not be easy, they understood, unless scientists were allowed freedom in investigative practices.

Most scientists, though, at least those selected to testify, were enthusiastic about government's support of their work. Pepper at one point made it clear that the medical and scientific communities should not feel threatened by government interference, targeting his remarks to the American Medical Association (AMA):

"We have tried to work in harmony and accord with the medical profession. When we first began our inquiries, there were some who thought that they might be aimed at a program and policy which might be in opposition to the profession's interest and there might have been something said that gave rise to that impression. It was an unintentional utterance if one was made.

" . . . But we are as *eager as can be to be guided in our course by those who know the way we should go. We are not, as I have reportedly said, advocating socialized medicine* [emphasis added] . . .

"I really believe that if the medical profession will come and help us open-mindedly and point out our own errors, if we commit them, there is a possibility for progress generally in the field."[24]

At one point, Pepper interrupted a witness discussing cancer research and raised a prescient point. Mahoney must have perked up her ears.

"Doctor, I don't want to divert you from your train of thought, but I noticed on the program here that you were mentioned in connection with the study of diseases of old age. Have you anything to say about what should be done in that field?" Pepper asked.

"The things that can be done in the field of aging are so many that it is difficult for me to try to gather them together and give them to you in a pack," the witness answered. A subsequent witness also raised the subject: "I am not referring to the matter of keeping senile individuals alive for a longer period, but rather the understanding of the process, so that we may be able to delay the onset of senility."[25]

Another witness called attention to one of Mahoney's and Lasker's particular interests: "The problem of mental health is a very special one," he said. "It has more ramifications than any other aspect of medicine" but "is the most important area of neglect in medicine today. There are few adequately staffed or adequately endowed research or training in-stitutes" or investigators in the field. "This deficit constitutes a national emergency" that only a "federal center for research and teaching" could help alleviate. His testimony was fodder for something the women were contemplating and soon would act on.

"Am I correct in the impression I have that more hospital beds are devoted to mental cases in the country than are available for all other classes of illness?" a well-primed Pepper asked. That was true, the doctor said.[26]

Another witness friendly to the Mahoney-Lasker position was Henry S. Simms, Ph.D. from Columbia University College of Physicians and Surgeons, who said there was "unanimous agreement . . . that support of peacetime medical research is woefully inadequate." Simms was not timid about asking for money: If funding were "increased progressively until $50 million is available in 1953 and each year thereafter, I believe this could be profitably spent for important research on urgent medical problems."

Simms' figures — which he publicly attributed to Mrs. Albert D. Lasker — were startling: Heart and artery diseases accounted for 536,745 deaths in 1940, but the amount of private foundation funding for research in the field amounted to only 17 cents per death. Kidney diseases received the equivalent of only 38 cents per death. Cancer and infectious diseases fared slightly better; polio research had the highest rate of expenditure. Simms recommended apportioning federal funds "according to the number of yearly deaths in the United States from diseases or disabling conditions" — a view that Mahoney and Lasker espoused.[27]

A fundamental question from the outset was what kinds of research should be underwritten. Lasker for her part was a strong advocate of *applying* discoveries to treatment at the earliest possible time. Mahoney, on the other hand, had confidence in the long-term benefits of *basic* research, which did not always produce instant cures and whose advantages seemed remote and mysterious to laymen.

Official recalcitrance

Despite the enthusiasm of most witnesses, however, many legislators, reflecting public opinion at the time, felt that it was not the government's role to underwrite medical research, that it was being done adequately by foundations and commercial drug companies. Government witnesses were cautious and reluctant to expand their agencies' roles, and Congress was blamed by some witnesses for a lack of understanding.[28]

Even OSRD director Bush believed that the medical research budget should be raised only modestly — not to exceed $5 million in 1945, although he conceded that $20 million might be "spent effectively" if programs proved their merit.[29]

The director of the National Institute of Health, Dr. R. E. Dyer, argued that the government already was financing "a great deal of medical research," albeit principally in the military and agriculture departments. Cutting off government funds nevertheless would cause many universities and researchers to suffer financially, he admitted, and "much of the investment made in present projects . . . would be lost," to say nothing of failing to utilize "the best young research brains in the country."

If, on the contrary, the government were to continue in a role similar to the OSRD, Dyer favored putting the new authority in the existing Public Health Service, guided by the National Academy of Sciences and its National Research Council.[30]

"By the way, who makes up the National Advisory Health Council?" the reviewing body for NIH grants, Pepper asked, with a purpose that would become evident later. The council's fourteen members were largely scientists, Dyer replied.

"Are there any members of the council other than professional men — any businessmen or people from other research organizations?" Pepper continued. If so, Dyer said, they were "research men themselves, not businessmen."

Pepper honed in on another point. The total appropriation for the NIH was about $3 million, Dyer said, and grants for cancer research for the past three years amounted to $91,000 a year. "You mean the only federal funds now being appropriated for aid in cancer research are about $91,000?" Pepper asked incredulously.

Yes, Dyer said, in grants to nongovernmental institutions; the entire Cancer Institute budget was about $560,000 a year, a good deal of which went to maintenance of its building.

Pepper pressed on. "Has the National Institute of Health, or the Public Health Service, asked for more funds from the Congress for medical research, and if so, has it been receiving it?" he asked.

"One of the most pleasant duties" that he had each year, Dyer responded, was to go before the budget bureau and Congress "and ask for money. I don't recall a single instance in which a request of ours has been turned down," he stated proudly. "Our trouble is in finding ideas and the men to carry them out."

That was like a red flag to Pepper. Hadn't Dyer heard previous witnesses describe how research was going begging for lack of sufficient money, "that profitable research could be undertaken in many other fields" and that "personnel was available for cancer research?"

Dyer continued to demur. "It is very difficult, at the present time, Senator Pepper. It is hard to get men or find men to work in the cancer field particularly, on account of the war emergency."

"What about funds for hospitals and laboratories?" Pepper asked. Dyer admitted that they "could be expanded greatly."

Pepper had gotten what he wanted. "That is the kind of thing we generally have in mind, I would say, Doctor," and he dismissed him.[31]

Cornelius (Dusty) Rhoads, a well-respected pathologist, was an important witness to Mahoney and Lasker. "We simply do not know enough to prevent or cure arthritis, mental disease, high blood pressure . . . arteriosclerosis or cancer," he stated. "These disorders fill most of the hospital beds and almost all the graves . . . . The conclusion is that if we want to stay out of the hospital, to maintain normal activity and to postpone death, continued support for medical research must be provided . . . . *Where can medical research turn for support if not to the people through their established organization, the federal government* [emphasis added]?"[32]

Lasker's and Mahoney's theme could not have been better stated.

"It is my belief that health is quite as important as the preparation of plastics or of improved and speedier and more dangerous motor cars," Rhoads concluded.[33]

"That is a splendid statement," Pepper exclaimed.

Pepper wanted to know if other nations were doing what he envisioned. Yes, said one witness, Great Britain and the Soviet Union had set up research councils to administer government funds, and the latter was spending "a larger proportion of the annual budget for scientific work than any other civilized country."

"That may have some relationship to the remarkable progress in science and the other advances which that country made in such a short time," Pepper commented. The remarks, unfortunately, would work against him when it came to Congress' approving an "independent" research agency, which smacked too much of Soviet-like government "control."[34]

The hearings, he hoped in closing them, would "enable us to formulate a program by which the federal government can be really helpful . . .

[I]f we can save lives by the expenditure of money, I wouldn't think that people who have a decent respect for the dignity of mankind would prefer to save money and lose lives."[35]

Reinforcing what Mahoney and Lasker were advocating, he hoped that "some proper national research agency" would be established "through which may be channeled federal funds for the encouragement of research in the medical field." He then introduced a bill to create a National Medical Research Foundation, but it immediately met with controversy over whether the government might interfere with private-sector activities.[36]

Mahoney and Lasker liked the idea of a separate entity along the lines of Pepper's foundation, skeptical that existing agencies like the PHS were up to the job that the women had in mind. Bureaucrats whom they encountered were largely unimaginative and unaggressive, they felt — in short, lacking in vision. Ultimately Pepper merged his concept with other versions of the foundation idea, to which Mahoney and Lasker, desperate to get some form of research legislation passed, lent their support.[37]

First Mental Health Act

Mental health also began getting Congress' attention at that time, thanks in large part to Mahoney's and Lasker's Committee on Mental Health.

"Mental health was not at all popular then," Mahoney pointed out, and they had difficulty getting Congress to listen to facts about the need for more research and treatment of mental problems. "One time in the Senate, when we were going around to see people, one senator told us he wanted to hear nothing about mental health. 'Don't talk to us about *crazy people*,'" he said. It took the tragic suicide of one senator's son to convince him and other colleagues to become more interested in mental-health issues. Mahoney realized that "the kinds of things that happened to Members or their families played a very important role in what they were interested in."[38]

The high percentage of draftee rejections for psychiatric reasons had prompted the PHS in 1944 to propose a system of community mental-health programs. At the same time, the women's committee issued statistics pointing to the need for more trained psychiatrists, then in shorter supply than other medical personnel. Democratic Representative Percy Priest of Tennessee, chairman of the House Interstate and Foreign Commerce Committee, agreed to introduce a bill, drafted with the help of Mahoney's and Lasker's committee, to beef up the PHS' mental-health division, establish an advisory council of experts to oversee its grant program, and provide money to train more psychiatrists. "Mrs. Mahoney and I had gotten quite a few people to testify and to urge passage of the bill," Lasker later said. The extent of the problem was graphically dramatized by a Marine who asked to speak extemporaneously at hearings on the bill. His story of the mental breakdown he had suffered from his war experiences raised sympathy among congressmen.[39]

Mahoney and Lasker offered to help rally support for the bill. Their first move was to approach Senator Pepper, who promptly introduced the measure in the Senate. Mahoney made sure that the Cox newspapers ran stories about it and the *Miami Daily News* editorialized for it. *Washington Post* publisher Eugene Meyer also took an interest and did the same. Within a year, the first National Mental Health Act was enacted, on July 3, 1946, which both Mahoney and Lasker attributed in large part to having a lobbyist working on the bill.[40]

Flush with success, they thought the job was finished. But someone asked how much had been appropriated for the program. Seventeen million dollars was in the bill, they said. That was only the *authorization*, they were informed. Once a program had been authorized, Congress then had to *appropriate* funds to implement it. That was the critical next step in the legislative process.

"We were so dumb, we didn't know we also had to get appropriations!" Mahoney laughed in retrospect with the wisdom of many years' experience. But their naiveté had taught them a valuable lesson.[41]

Governor Cox complimented Lasker for her work on the bill, citing particularly her desire not to be publicly identified as a factor in its passage — something that she would come to be in time. "In too many instances, the architect of a great structure, whether it be a fine building or a humanitarian project, gets scant credit for what is done," Cox wrote her. "We are very proud of you, Mary, and I am sorry that you haven't permitted your identification with the movement to be known to others. God bless you in all your good works."[42]

Lasker was quick to respond, telling him, "Florence has been a great help, and has interested and inspired many people in the health field, as you know."[43]

Mahoney still hoped to set up a staffed mental health clinic in Atlanta now that the Cox-backed gubernatorial candidate had been elected, and she continued to have an ally in Margaret Mitchell. "The Governor [Ellis G. Arnall] said he would produce the money for a Dr. for Georgia for 6 or 9 months," she wrote Lasker in 1944. "Think it is really settled. Atlanta is the most fascinating place with all of the citizens so enlightened and all giving masses of money for psychiatric clinics and hospitals and medical centers . . . . Am loving the book, 'Drs. of the Mind'," she went on, "Have you read it? . . . Had several hours with Margaret Mitchell . . . and she is mostly interested in getting psychiatric help for civilians."

The new governor, Mahoney added, "is completely sold on the health angle so you can talk to him about the cancer program any time now. He was so pleased to find all of his business friends in Atlanta so interested in public health — and it was good we had already educated him." She also wanted Lasker's secretary to request a copy of an editorial in the AMA journal on false advertising. "I am writing to Western Reserve Medical school for the results they had on tests on vitamins and the misleading copy that advertises them. This one clipping is pertaining to such copy and expenditure and was in all our papers on the editorial page — not that anyone would know what they were talking about," she added.[44]

Both women shared information on a regular basis. "Thanks a lot for the books from the brief psychotherapy council, they were fascinating," Mahoney wrote Lasker soon after they had formed their committee. "I have studied the entire summer and read all of the publications of the Mental Hygiene Committee [a different organization from their's that had existed for more than thirty years] and the cancer literature and the lit. from the Social Hygiene [Foundation?], etc. Have got the superintendent of schools in the town near us interested in taking and reading all of the literature about children so she can help the teachers. I think the Mental Hygiene Committee has done the most outstanding work and I am delighted you are the new Sec[retary]. I have lots of clippings for you but will bring them . . . . Everyone must be very excited about the war," she added, referring to its ending. "What do you think of the chances for R[oosevelt]'s being reelected?"[45]

Mahoney cultivated a particularly useful member of Congress in those days, Frank Keefe, Republican of Wisconsin, who was chairman of the Labor-Federal Security Appropriations Subcommittee from which all medical research money flowed. Keefe was a believer in the cause and even told Mahoney that he gave only one speech whenever he was campaigning — on what the government should do to advance medical research. It helped elect him to five terms in Congress (1935–51).[46]

The fruits of Lasker's and Mahoney's labors were now ripening. With its new statutory authority to issue grants and contracts, the National Institute of Health appropriation had jumped ten-fold since 1941. The institute was now something to be reckoned with. Fifty projects had been transferred from the OSRD to the NIH. Most research was conducted at universities with funds provided by either government *grants* (which supported primarily *basic* research) or *contracts* for specific work (*applied*, or *targeted*, research). But the debate first raised in the Pepper hearings now took on critical importance and would continue over the years: Should the new-found riches be directed primarily to *applied* research, transferring findings from laboratories to doctor's offices and patients? Or should they enhance *basic* research to reveal the elusive secrets of biomedical mechanisms? To calm researchers' fears, an NIH spokesman said that it was the intention of "those who established the program" to give scientists "freedom to experiment" with the caveat that "Congress imposes a degree of control and direction when it appropriates funds earmarked for research on a designated disease or specific organ." Those were prescient words about the future of the young institute.[47]

President Truman and national health insurance

When Harry Truman succeeded to the presidency (in April 1945), Mahoney and Lasker had another, even more powerful ally than Senator Pepper. Both women knew the Trumans and supported his policies. Mahoney had met him in Florida because of her association with Democratic activists: "Dan Mahoney and the Governor [Cox] knew him, of course. All the Democrats knew each other, more or less. I knew all the people around the president well. When he began having the winter White House down in Key West, all those people were in and out of Miami Beach a lot. I knew them informally, and that's why they were always so helpful. I was able to talk to Mr. Truman [directly] about things, too. Even then, I was always trying to get my work done, not just being social."

With Truman in the White House, Mahoney and Lasker hoped that their proposals would be heard and backed from the highest office in the land.

Mahoney built close relationships with the president, his wife Bess, and his daughter Margaret during his administration (1945–52). She began to send him personal notes and information as well as encouragement for his programs and dined at the White House in small family gatherings.

"The first time I met him in his office, he walked up and down — he was a tower of energy. He referred to the 'pin-heads up on the Hill who are against my four-point plan'" to export American knowledge overseas. "He certainly had no hesitation speaking his mind," she said. But she realized that he needed help in building support for his legislative ideas.[48]

"Mother and Dad both liked Florence very much and admired what she was doing," according to Margaret Truman Daniel. Her mother, who was "very sympathetic" to Mahoney's causes, considered her a friend.

Lasker, too, took advantage of her personal contacts with the White House. One month after Truman became president, she went to see the man who had married her, Judge Samuel Rosenman, now counsel to the president. Truman had asked him to identify what issues on Roosevelt's agenda had not been acted upon, one of which was a presidential health message to Congress. Truman directed Rosenman to prepare such a message, a draft of which he shared with Lasker. She pointed out that it made no reference to the need for more mental-health activity, which he added.[49]

Mahoney and Lasker bombarded the president and his aides with suggestions from the outset. One of them was forwarded through Senator Brien McMahon, Connecticut Democrat and chairman of the Joint Committee on Atomic Energy, whom Mahoney had gotten to know in Florida. Timed to coincide with the very day that atom bombs were being dropped by American planes on Nagasaki, Japan (August 9, 1945), the senator sent Truman a memo expressing McMahon's, Mahoney's, and Lasker's sentiments: The president should marshal the same kinds of scientific forces that had produced the atom bomb to "discover causes and cures for the deadly diseases of mankind . . . which have up to now baffled scientific effort."[50]

A month later, on September 6, 1945, four days after victory over Japan was declared, Truman sent Congress a 21-point, 16,000-word message — the longest since one from President Theodore Roosevelt — that focused on post-war economic issues and contained a promised health-insurance proposal. Ultimately he would send Congress three messages that included requests for national health-insurance legislation, something even Roosevelt had been silent on, correctly fearing the outcry against it as "socialized medicine."[51]

The insurance proposal was introduced by Democratic Senator James E. Murray of Montana, one of the wealthiest and most reform-minded men in the Senate (who had been appalled, as a young man working in a Butte copper mine, by the ravages of silicosis [black lung] on workers and their inability to pay for treatment) and by labor sympathizers and liberal Democrats Senator Robert F. Wagner of New York, Congressman John Dingell of Michigan, and Congressman Andrew Biemiller of Wisconsin. It immediately became the target of "organized medicine," led by the AMA.[52]

Rosenman suggested that it would be helpful if a group of citizens publicly lent their support to Truman's message in principle to diffuse opposition to the national health-insurance idea. Lasker promptly organized such a group, the nucleus of the Committee for the Nation's Health, whose first goal was to place an announcement in leading newspapers, stating its position. The Laskers and other endorsers of Truman's "health plan" paid for a statement that ran in the *New York Times, Washington Post,* and *Washington Star* in early December 1945. Of the Mahoney-Lasker team, however, only Albert Lasker's name appeared on a list of nearly 200 well-known people signing the message, including Eleanor Roosevelt; General David Sarnoff, president of Radio Corporation of America; Gardner Cowles, publisher of Cowles newspapers; members of organized labor; just-retired New York mayor Fiorello La-Guardia; and musician Leonard Bernstein among numerous artistic people. The "thoroughly American plan," the statement read, was emphatically "not 'socialized' medicine" and "would increase productivity, reduce disease and save lives."[53]

A message on health

Equally important to Mahoney and Lasker was Truman's decision to issue a separate presidential message on health. They believed that research and health care through a national insurance plan were inextricably linked. Frustrated that Congress was not moving on his legislative agenda, Truman decided to accelerate release of the health message, which daily was going through revisions under the guidance of Rosenman, among others. Each morning Truman returned drafts to staff with his pencil notes in the margins. Finally, on the 16th of November, Truman approved the message, and it was sent to the printers. It was released three days later, on November 19, 1945.[54]

"In my message to the Congress of September 6, 1945," Truman stated, "I made various recommendations for a general federal research program. Medical research — dealing with the broad fields of physical and mental illnesses — should be made effective in part through that general program and in part through specific provisions within the scope of a national health program .... Federal aid ... for medical research and education is also an essential part of any national health program."[55]

Mahoney accepted credit, with Lasker, for prevailing on Truman to issue the first health message to Congress and the American people. "We got him to do it," Mahoney said. "No president had ever issued a health memorandum before, ever."

"Florence Mahoney and I were constantly going to see him about it," Lasker recounted in an oral history some years later. "Truman would agree with us, and we'd try to get Clark Clifford to write more about health insurance in Truman's speeches. And every once in a while he would say something about it but he never put his heart into it, in his speeches. He agreed with us privately, but either Clifford was worried about it as a political thing or Truman . . . didn't know quite how to express himself about it except privately. He said, 'It's ridiculous, of course we should have it.' But then he never publicly espoused it until 1948. And then the AMA got so organized and were so threatening that it looked as if [Truman might be defeated] — Truman wasn't having too easy a time, anyway, in '48."[56]

Mahoney and Lasker kept up their pressure on Truman staff and the president himself whenever they could. His reasons for not speaking out on the insurance plan, Mahoney believed, were based on a desire not to give opponents opportunities to attack it. And the opposition was mobilizing a formidable force.[57]

Fighting the American Medical Association

"Florence and I became alarmed by the violence of the AMA opposition and the lack of general national understanding or organized support," according to Lasker. "The AMA was spending between $2 and $4 million, and our side had very few spokesmen and very *little* money."[58]

Hoping to push Congress to at least hold hearings on the insurance bill, Lasker, following her meeting with Truman, sent Cox a summary, asking that he use his "great influence with Senator [Walter] George [Democrat of Georgia, chairman of the Senate Finance Committee] to urge him to have hearings before his committee, promptly.... The other version of this bill was pigeon-holed in his committee for two years .... It is most important to get influential citizens to show their interest in the over-all health and social security situation as it is covered in the bill in order that Senator George may realize that there is real desire for action in this field, and so that the public may learn the true facts in the controversy."[59]

To bypass the reluctant Senator George and his committee, another version was introduced, changing the tax-related financing mechanism so the bill would be referred to committees where it had sponsors and might receive favorable attention. But the AMA raised a multi-million-dollar war chest to defeat it and any other health program the organization "thought political in nature," as Mahoney remembered. Among them were Truman's proposals for aid to medical education.[60]

The AMA even sponsored a "contest," using what Senator Murray called "an undercover instrument," a National Physicians' Committee that offered prizes for cartoons attacking national health insurance. Murray exposed the "contest" as "a subtle bribe to cartoonists to support or oppose certain political beliefs," and the *Washington Post* dubbed it "a form of malpractice which the doctors can best cure by excising its source."[61]

Mahoney, then still in Miami, wrote an interesting letter in 1947 that shed light on how she worked, cultivating and discussing issues with those in positions to help her while not being dogmatic or forceful. In most cases, people at least found themselves reexamining their views after she had planted her ideas in their minds. "Have been very busy and hectic," she told Lasker, "and hope it will not last much longer. Everyone seems to descend upon Miami at one moment. Have so much to tell you."

> Philip Wylie's new book is just out, and spent all day yesterday trying to get him and Sen. McMahon together. The Demo. dinner being down here, had them all for Sat. lunch and racing and then on Sun. McMahon came for breakfast at 11 and then lunch with several others.
>
> Mr. [Leslie] Biffle, who was the Sec[retary] of the Senate and is very close to the Pres., became my very dear friend and may be

helpful to us. He said the Pres. is going through with all of the health legislation and will press it, said we were to come to him whenever in Wash.

I told him of your visit to the Pres. and how much you have done and what it means to the administration to accomplish something. McMahon is not for the Murray-Wagner-Dingell bill, has two brothers who are doctors. I told him he sounded just like Mr. [Morris] Fishbein [editor of the AMA journal]. Same arguments, etc. He laughed and I honestly believe will look into it further. Is nice and is devoted to you and Albert.

Pepper here just for a minute, saw Gov. [Millad] Caldwell [of Florida] for quite a visit. He is going to beautify the highways and talked about mass planting in the different towns . . . .

Am at office and have to go for it is late . . . ."[62]

Mahoney's careful groundwork paid off — at the highest level. She and Lasker met with Truman on April 24, 1947, reminding him that "Mr. Republican," Senator Robert A. Taft of Ohio, now chairman of the Labor and Public Welfare Committee — and a potential GOP presidential candidate in 1948 — was about to hold hearings on his so-called "voluntary" or "welfare" health bill. Truman did not miss the women's point — that *he* should take the initiative on health, thwarting Taft's bid to be a national leader on the issue. White House staff member John Steelman was ordered to put together another health message in a hurry.[63]

"You will be charmed to learn that as a result of your making the appointment with the President, we are going to have a Presidential Message on Health next Monday — the day that the new National Health Insurance Bill will be introduced," Lasker wrote Mahoney triumphantly on May 13, 1947. "I talked to Sam Rosenman about the matter on Saturday, and he saw the President yesterday and what with one thing and another it is arranged — thanks entirely to your original initiative! . . . The Message is highly confidential at the moment, but I expect that the Cox papers will do the maximum on Monday in honor of your efforts? . . . . Wire me what your plans are! Much love, darling."[64]

Mahoney and Lasker devoted much of their time that year to pushing for the insurance bill, trying to counter the skillful tactics of the AMA. Mahoney was always at work, even when at the western ranches. From Idaho later that year she told Lasker,

> I did a lot of work on Sen. [William] Fulbright [Democrat of Arkansas] and also on his wife, who is very nice and intelligent. We must get together with them . . . . Fulbright likes Taft. Also the Drs. in Arkansas have him in their power. He wants to be re-elected, and bad . . . .
>
> Heard indistinctly last night on the radio that some foreign Dr. was going to give a paper on the fact that cancer may be related to leprosy. Radio always difficult here in mountains to understand. That would be awful considering so many people have been afraid of [cancer] anyway as being contagious, etc., but perhaps all have been educated since the past few campaigns. Wish we were going to the cancer meetings in St. Louis. Do get all of the papers . . . .
>
> "There is a polio epidemic in Idaho — so sad . . . ."[65]

While in Arizona she contacted one of its senators, Democrat Carl T. Hayden, identifying herself as a "potential constituent." She urged him to back some form of the insurance bill and enclosed a "Health Fact Sheet compiled by Mary Woodward Lasker . . . privately," adding, "Mrs. Lasker and I own the above ranch here at Kirkland and have been working together for several years to obtain more money for medical research and better distribution of medical care. The big problem now is to make health and medical care more readily accessible to all people in all income groups, without its being the form of charity that the Taft bill proposes," she wrote.[66]

"I think it would be wonderful if you would wire [Florida Representative George] Smathers," Lasker suggested, "urging him not to do anything" about a House committee report that was unfavorable to the insurance plan. "This is trying to prevent even the discussion of National Health Insurance by employees of government agencies and is a direct

AMA move which Fishbein told me was going to happen when I saw him in Atlantic City. They really work awfully hard against man's interests, don't they?"[67]

Lasker had jaundice that summer. "It is a boring disease," she wrote Dan Mahoney with thanks for mangos that he had sent her, "and, believe it or not, no research to speak of has ever been done on the subject. In spite of this lack, I feel the National Science Foundation bill which Florence and I started agitating for two and a half years ago with Pepper is going to pass the House today. So you can see that maybe something will be done on research — if not on jaundice, on other things. The $14,000,000 cancer appropriation was pretty good. Don't you think so?" she added.[68]

Unhappily for the pro-Truman side, Taft padded his hearings with witnesses favorable to his bill and hostile to the Murray-Wagner-Dingell bill. He also deftly included a representative of a known Commmunist group, the International Workers Order, which tainted the Democratic bill by its support. The hearings turned into an inquisition of people who backed Truman's bill, even Albert Lasker, whose attendance at a Com-mittee for the Nation's Health dinner a senator hinted was un-American. Lasker joked that he was happy to discuss "the whole dark conspiracy, right in the limelight." But the situation was not funny. The hearings were crafted to doom the health security bill. One senator wanted details about the Health Committee's members, which its director snapped sounded like an "implied indictment." Another blow to the Committee's credibility was an accusation that it had supplied, albeit unwittingly, a Communist-front organization with material used in a filmstrip advo-cating national health insurance. The Health Committee reacted by resolving not to provide information to organizations associated with the Communist Party. But it was too late to save the bill.[69]

"Albert was delighted with your letter on his testimony," Lasker wrote Mahoney in July 1947. "I think we should try to get him on the air in a debate with Senator Taft, don't you?" Commenting on their success with the cancer bill, she displayed her astuteness at follow-up strategies:

The [American Cancer] Society will raise nearly $12,000,000 so we have really got this thing started, especially as the Atomic Energy Commission will have some more money for cancer . . . .

Pepper got the Heart Research deficiency appropriations heard by the Senate Saturday and we are hoping for the best this week. It certainly would be divine if it can be put over. If that happens, I will relax until January, I think. Pepper really has been marvelous about all this.

You know, of course, that the National Science Foundation bill has passed the House and Senate and has gone to the President. Now it's a question of whom we get on the Board of the Foundation and on the Cancer and Heart Commissions. We will have to hope for the best.

I think if Biffle would give a luncheon of Democratic and Republican Senators in the beginning of the next session, Albert could really move them so that we can get some place on Health Insurance. He is really hot on it and has certainly developed a wonderful "story line."[70]

The National Science Foundation bill was vetoed, however, and the health-insurance bill died in the 1947 Congress, a victim of the Republican "do-nothing Congress," as Truman called it. But it gave him good material for his 1948 presidential campaign. "Is it un-American to visit the sick, aid the afflicted, or comfort the dying?" he recanted in a 1948 campaign speech broadcast over national radio. "Does cancer care about political parties? Does infantile paralysis concern itself with income? Of course it doesn't," he said, reminding voters that if they returned a Republican majority to Congress, it would continue to block passage of a national health bill.[71]

Truman's campaign received direct input from Mahoney and Lasker through their friendship with Clark Clifford. The three often dined together, making up what Clifford jokingly called "our exclusive club." By then he had replaced Rosenman as the president's special counsel.

Mahoney and Lasker continually sent him material from the Nation's Health Committee, facts that he could use in speeches for the president.[72]

Mahoney grew increasingly disparaging of the physicians' organization. "I heard the AMA broadcast from San Francisco and it was pretty bad — never heard so much nonsense," she told Federal Security Administrator Oscar Ewing, whose agency was to manage health insurance under Truman's plan. Ewing was the target of AMA derision as a government "tsar."[73]

Mahoney kept hoping that the AMA would commit political "suicide" by its "propaganda," orchestrated by San Francisco public-relations firm Whitaker and Baxter. To Truman aide and speech writer Charles S. Murphy Mahoney wrote,

> We had Mike Gorman come from the coast to help us for he has long been a writer in the health field. He told me how Baxter and Whitaker had tried to get him to come to work for them and what a campaign they were planning. Having always worked for the president's health program, I was distressed and more so because of the political implications. As you will agree, our present predicament is precarious enough . . . . I personally don't think the people will fall for such a lot of nonsense and they may be making it simple for you and the president to use their propaganda against them to great advantage . . . .
>
> I shall be in Washington again early October and hope I may have a chance for a few minutes with you and can tell you any ideas I have to help offset their mischief.[74]

Murphy circulated the information from Mahoney to top White House aides.

What Whitaker and Baxter had offered Gorman, then freelancing, was "an expense-paid trip to England to do an 'impartial' job on British socialized medicine," as he put it. Instead he took a temporary job with the Democratic National Committee (DNC) and prepared a press release with "salient facts" that the Committee for the Nation's Health could use against the AMA. Titled "Lobbying against Human Needs," the 1950 statement read: "Organized medicine and its allies — big business, insurance and real estate lobbies — averaged close to $10,000 a day every day from January 1st to March 31st of this year fighting President Truman's Fair Deal Program." The money came from a compulsory assessment of $25 on AMA members, making it "the best-financed lobby in the country," but "not a cent of this money went to medical research, scholarships for qualified would-be doctors or nurses, or the furthering of scientific progress to end needless suffering," the release charged.[75]

The pro-Truman group, through Gorman's spies, got information from inside the AMA at its annual meetings and used quotes from its leaders to highlight its negative positions and tactics. One of its strategies was "to locate the personal physician of every Congressman and U. S. Senator" to whom doctors could write personal letters expressing the AMA position. Senator Pepper was a major target in his 1950 reelection bid.

Gorman sent Matt Connelly an analysis with "some amazing, authentic data on the power the doctors wielded," saying "Mrs. Florence Mahoney suggested I buck a copy to you. In the face of this fact, how can anyone deny that the Democratic Party must come up with some kind of campaign to counteract this vicious campaigning by the doctors? I know you are frightfully busy, but Mrs. Mahoney and I are in hopes you may find time to call the enclosed data to the attention of the President."[76]

AMA leaders bragged after the 1950 elections that, "An impressive percentage of candidates who favored government health insurance were beaten." The doctors were becoming savvy in their campaign strategies: In Miami, for example, they had persuaded funeral directors to organize an election-day motorcade, using ambulances and hearses to transport bedridden patients to polls. Such tactics had helped defeat liberal members of Congress like Biemiller of Milwaukee; Helen Gahagan Douglas, who lost to Richard Nixon in California; and Claude Pepper, who had bluntly told doctors that he was sticking by the Truman health plan, regardless of the 2,000 physician votes in Florida. That had galvanized the "docs" to rally behind his opponent George Smathers. At Tallahassee City Hospital they handed out "Can Pepper!" cards to indigent patients until complaints were raised before the city's governing body. In other Florida communities, they accosted patients as they entered polling booths. The AMA president-elect warned that the organization had to guard against another "virulent outbreak of Ewingism."[77]

Truman renewed his call for national health insurance in three messages to Congress in January 1950. But even Murray's subcommittee was turning its attention to a *study* of the existing system, and Southern Democrats, angry at Truman's pro–civil rights position, made enactment of a Social Security–based program unrealistic.

Mahoney and Lasker by then had decided to concentrate their energies on issues on which they were having success. The Committee on the Nation's Health was divided and close to shutting down because principal backers like the Laskers wanted it to address less controversial health programs. When the committee refused to do that in 1950, the Laskers withdrew their support and resigned.

It would be another fifteen years before a reduced form of Truman's national health-insurance proposal — covering senior citizens under a program called "Medicare" — would be enacted into law. In a historic gesture, then-President Lyndon B. Johnson took the bill to Truman's library in Independence, Missouri, and with the former president at his side, signed it into law on July 30, 1965. The eighty-one-year-old Truman, smiling with Bess standing behind him, told the gathering that he was glad he had lived to see it. Mahoney was not there to witness it, but with many others she had been in the forefront of the long drive to that achievement. Clark Clifford, who was there, told her that Truman was so touched that he could hardly hold back tears. "C.C. said it was a very gracious thing for Johnson to do," Mahoney wrote a friend.[78]

"It was as comprehensive a plan as Congress would ever consider again," Mahoney reflected half a century later.[79]

Mahoney and Lasker had learned one important lesson during the effort to enact national health insurance: Avoid direct conflict with the AMA. It did not escape them, though, that the medical lobby was so preoccupied with fighting the insurance bill that it had not lobbied against government involvement in scientific research. That was becoming increasingly popular with congressmen, who could back it without alienating the AMA. Mahoney and Lasker and their allies made the case that government-backed research was not a threat to the "American way" — in fact, the opposite. They realized that they had to devise a neutral approach to substantiate their position.[80]

Health Needs of the Nation

"Mary at this time was trying to get the National Democratic Committee to organize a committee to combat the AMA's opposition to Mr. Truman's health program," Mahoney recalled of their strategy reassessment. "The public relations team of Whitaker and Baxter were real demons and always making trouble, lobbying the legislators against any health bill and working against any liberal candidates, boasting of" their successes. "They also were doing their best to discredit President Truman. Since Mary and I had worked so hard to get Mr. Truman interested in a health program and the national health insurance bill, we had to get citizen support, as it was becoming embarrassing to the Democratic Party because the AMA was making an issue of it."[81]

The result, according to Lasker, was that "Florence and I urged the President to appoint a commission — the first presidential commission on health, believe it or not."[82]

"It was difficult for Mr. Truman to believe that the AMA had such a strong lobby," according to Mahoney. "But when he finally realized it, after seeing a printed plan that it had to defeat a congressman from Pennsylvania because of his presumed support for the idea of national health insurance," he ordered David Stowe, his assistant on health matters, to write a presidential statement calling for the commission. "It was good for the president politically, too — it gave him something to fall back on."[83]

The President's Commission on Health Needs of the Nation (not to be confused with the private advocacy group for national health insurance) was set up in December 1951 with the backing of Truman's health adviser and Mahoney friend, Howard Rusk. By then Rusk had gained a reputation as a pioneer in rehabilitation at a clinic associated with New York University. He also was from Truman's home state of Missouri and wrote a column in the *New York Times*.

"The commission was to consider the whole picture of health in the United States and make recommendations," Mahoney said. "Howard Rusk — who had done such good work with the medical division of the veterans — was consulted about a chairman and suggested Dr. Paul Magnuson, an orthopedic surgeon [and conservative Republican] from Chicago. He was very strong-minded and independent and knew nothing about the overall picture of the medical problem. He also was a friend of the AMA board of trustees."[84]

What had seemed to be a good idea now looked questionable for Mahoney's and Lasker's ends. "It all seemed very 'iffy' so we thought it would be a good idea to have Mike Gorman there, who knew all the problems, to help in some way," Mahoney said. "I got Gorman and Magnuson and Rusk together at my house. Magnuson and Mike got on well and he hired him to do public relations. The commission finally got off to a good start, largely due to Dr. Russel Lee," progressive-minded founder of a prepaid clinic in Palo Alto, California. "Hearings were held in various places throughout the United States, and the report was held up until after the presidential election in November, 1952 so it would not be considered political. The AMA, not certain how to react to the commission, thought it would be a disaster, but it was difficult for the doctors to use the cry of 'socialized medicine' during the campaign. It did have both Taft and Eisenhower," the rival GOP candidates, "in its pocket," she noted.[85]

Gorman's presence on the commission was essential and came about largely because of Mahoney, who had kept in touch with him since his series of articles and their successful work together on mental-health legislation in Florida. Knowing that Lasker had been paying a staff assistant to help her, Mahoney suggested that "if she were paying someone, for God's sake, get somebody good. So she got Mike Gorman." He had received a Lasker Foundation award in 1948 for his crusading series on mental institutions, and Lasker had paid his salary for work that he had done for the Democratic National Committee on national health insurance.

Gorman subsequently had written an article on national health insurance, which "Mr. Truman thought well of," according to Mahoney. As Gorman remembered it, "Somebody on the White House staff asked me to talk with the president." It was Matt Connelly who called Gorman in California, where he was working as a roving correspondent for *Reader's Digest,* and asked if he would come to Washington. Gorman initially said that he was not interested in going there, considering it "kind of a country town." Would he come, at least as a courtesy, to see the president? Yes, Gorman said, he admired Truman and was in favor of national health insurance. His wife warned that he would be seduced to take what he was offered as a "chance to promote something . . . that you are deeply interested in." She was right.

Gorman agreed to be the commission's chief staff writer and director of public hearings and was allowed to operate "pretty much on my own, which was delightful. I would come to the staff meetings at the White House to report on what was going on."[86]

The commission's charge was broad: to study long-range health conditions and needs of the postwar population; whether the supplies of medical personnel, facilities, and insurance were adequate; financing of care; and how to accelerate research — "a mighty large order," chairman Magnuson called it. "We will not come up with any device to prevent death," he stated, "but I hope we can suggest ways and means of making life more free of troubles."[87]

The intent, according to Mahoney, was to have "all these influential people *advise* what should be done — not to *complain.*" Fifteen commissioners ultimately were "decided upon between Magnuson and David Stowe (after many vetoes and other suggestions by me without Magnuson's knowledge)," she later recorded.[88]

Magnuson insisted that the commission was entirely apolitical. "No one in the White House ever raised a question as to whether an appointee was a Democrat or a Republican, or whether he was in favor of the president's plan or not," he said in a speech. Its members, after all, in addition to medical school deans and distinguished physicians with conservative political views, included liberal labor leaders like the United Auto Workers' Walter Reuther; Albert J. Hayes, president of the International Association of Machinists; and representatives of consumer, farm, and nursing organizations. But the AMA was wary.[89]

"I agree with the *Washington Post*," Magnuson went on in words strikingly like those used by Gorman, who probably had written the speech, "that, in this bitter dispute between a large government agency and the country's largest medical organization, the forgotten man has been the citizen in need of more and better medical care .... [T]hings have reached a sorry pass when the health and well-being of the American people is made the football for an obscene and vulgar battle between publicists throwing nasty adjectives at each other at twenty paces .... I don't think the average American doctor needs a $100,000-a-year public relations firm to keep the American people from biting him in the leg."[90]

The non-partisan report, completed in 1952, was a five-volume survey of health care in the nation, a "primer" that "fills a big gap," said Magnuson, giving Gorman "most of the credit for the success of these hearings. His great faith in the voice of the people and his infectious enthusiasm for the workings of democracy inspired both the Commission and the participants in the field." The results were a "tribute" to Gorman's "tremendous drive and irrepressible zeal."[91]

The report, which Gorman edited in his characteristic punchy style, emphasized opportunities not to be missed:

> Perhaps no field of human endeavor offers more in the way of possibilities for human betterment than that of medical research .... Many of the diseases that claimed their victims with dramatic speed in 1900 — typhoid fever, scarlet fever, whooping cough, measles, diphtheria, smallpox and malaria — have now become much less frequent causes of death ....
>
> In the short time from 1937 to 1949, the death rate has declined 14 per cent ....
>
> [W]e conclude that the American people are aware of the

enormous dividends to be reaped from intensified medical research. They desire to see it extended.

More importantly, he pointed out, the declining death rate meant more tax revenues to the federal coffers. Not only did people want more research, they could afford to pay for tax-supported government programs. But public policy was not following public will. In 1951, government medical-research expenditures amounted to $180 million — only three tenths of 1 percent of the national defense budget — "less than the amount spent on monuments and tombstones," Gorman sniffed.[92]

Mahoney, through Bess, sent Truman Magnuson's summary of the Commission's findings. "This is the copy of the speech I told you about," she wrote Mrs. Truman in 1952, enclosing Magnuson's remarks to the Lasker Awards presentation for medical journalism. "Know you will enjoy it. Do tell the president about it, too. The Commission may not cause legislation to happen," she added, "but it has upset the AMA's propaganda line and the AMA . . . . Hope to see you soon. P. S. Heard from many of the Senate ladies that you looked very special at your party yesterday and so pretty."[93]

"Mrs. Truman handed me your note with the clipping and the copy of the speech by Dr. Magnuson," Truman told Mahoney in a personal note dated June 4, 1952, saying that he "was highly pleased" with the speech. "When people begin to get the facts on the health situation in this country and know how difficult it is for the ordinary person to get medical and hospital care, they will all begin to wake up and find out that something ought to be done about it." Acknowledging that Mahoney had sent him the speech, Truman told Magnuson that it was "certainly a grand statement of the facts."[94]

Unfortunately, the report got little publicity at the time of its release and was "suppressed" by the incoming Republican administration and soon forgotten, according to commission study director and public-health leader Dr. Lester Breslow. But it provided solid facts and findings for future use by advocates of public-health programs.

The tactic of producing a well-reasoned report, backed by solid data, would become a practice of Gorman's to advance positions that he, Mahoney, and Lasker advocated. Gorman called it "the white-paper device." "You develop the facts, you involve a great number of organizations previously not interested, and you hopefully create a militant consensus in support of the findings," he said publicly. Such studies were "an obvious answer to the familiar myriad of charges raised by hostile legislators that 'you didn't study the problem long enough, your conclusions were hastily drawn, you didn't consult a broad enough segment of professional groups or of the American people' and so on."[95]

But Gorman was out of a job when the commission ended. As one historical account of Mahoney and Lasker stated, "When the job *for* the government was done, that left the job to be done *on* the government. Mary Lasker and Florence Mahoney thought nobody could do it better than Mike Gorman."[96]

Mike Gorman joins the team

By his own admission, Gorman "was kind of in limbo." He had "had a desk" at the Democratic National Committee where, "since October, 1950, with Mary Lasker paying his salary, [he] has been of inestimable help to us and the White House on all matters pertaining to health legislation, etc.," as India Edwards, who headed the DNC's Women's Division, wrote the chairman early in 1952. "He is one of the keenest men I know and it occurs to me that he would be a good person to be in our Publicity Department." But Gorman was not destined for a job with the DNC.[97]

"It was Howard Rusk who saved me because he had a special committee on mobilization of manpower, or something like that, and it had been set up for the Korean War. So I finished up there," Gorman told an interviewer.

Gorman at first was not sure whether he "wanted to get into the whole Lasker set." Mary, in turn, "was a little scared" of the intimidating Gorman, according to Mahoney. But "Florence was the one who bugged Mary to get me to go to work for the Lasker Foundation," Gorman admitted. "I told Florence I really didn't want to do it, and she said, 'But you don't really know Mrs. Lasker.'"[98]

"I had won the Lasker Award in 1948, but I didn't know her. She seemed quite distant to me, and I wanted to keep writing and find out what I really wanted to do. I didn't know what a foundation mechanism was or what use I could be. It would be legislative, I knew, trying to influence Congress. Nevertheless, Florence was persistent, and thought of a really shrewd gambit: She said, 'You ought to talk to Albert Lasker.' Now, Albert is one of the most charismatic figures of all time. He was madly in love with Mary, his third wife . . . . I liked Albert from the beginning. He was tough, and kind of brusque in looking me over. I said to him, 'Mr. Lasker, one thing I'd like to do is ask you to stop looking me over. This is not a beef contest. I'm not looking for anything. Florence Mahoney has asked me to talk to you, and I don't know why, because Mrs. Lasker seems to be the one who is interested in [me]. She is president of the foundation and I presume you are supplying most of the money because you're the one who earned it.' And Albert laughed and said, 'Well, why don't you do it? . . . . Mary is never going to raise enough money unless she gets the federal government involved.' He was tough in all his dealings, and tight with a buck in a sense."[99]

But Gorman was intrigued by the challenge. "The [research] institutes [at that time] were minuscule . . . . They had very small budgets . . . and they just couldn't do much . . . . [Albert Lasker] said they needed someone in Washington badly and that it would be a very challenging job. At that first meeting, I left still carrying reservations about taking the position." While Gorman was working for Rusk's panel, Albert asked to see him again. "He was not well, and in fact died in May of that year of cancer, and he asked me if I had considered the position with the Lasker Foundation. He really persuaded me, so finally I said I would try it for a year . . . and [besides] I didn't want to be constantly on the road like an evangelist. But Florence was the real initiator; she got me vis-a-vis Mary and Albert to do it. She knew what she was doing; it was that elemental shrewdness she's always used for good purposes."[100]

Gorman and his wife had previously visited the Idaho ranch en route across the country "and stayed a week," Mahoney wrote Lasker. "We had fun and he is really something. Hope you enjoyed his meeting with you.

He was fascinated by Albert and his working knowledge of the health problem. I gave him a packet (the one for speakers) with all of the Nat[ional] H[ealth] Ins[urance] facts, etc. He will be a good recruit, for he is certainly articulate . . . ."[101]

He ultimately decided to take the job as executive director of Mahoney's and Lasker's National Mental Health Committee in 1953. It was the beginning of a long partnership, and Gorman went to work with a vengeance.

He became the group's Don Quixote, challenging, prodding, using his acerbic and colorful "pen" to castigate and expose while trying to rely on documentation rather than his personal feelings, he said, but it was hard, "since my whole impulse was to write from the heart and let the hot adjectives fall where they might." He would find those skills useful in arguing for changes in many areas of health policy.[102]

Cancer and heart research

Mahoney and Lasker by then already had been involved in a precedent-setting bill to increase funds for cancer research that set an example for other ventures that followed. Representative Matthew M. Neely, Democratic former Governor of West Virginia, in 1946 introduced the measure calling for $100 million to be available until spent for the most promising work possible under the direction of a panel of world experts — independent of the Public Health Service. It was an unusual approach for the cancer program, which had existed since 1937 with nominal funding.

Pepper, a co-sponsor of the bill, again held hearings, at which NIH director Dyer was less than enthusiastic. Cancer research could not effectively use an additional $1 million, let alone an infusion of $100 million, he said. "That led our small lobby to fight for the Neely bill *outside* the jurisdiction of the Surgeon General," an early biographical draft of Mahoney and Lasker stated. The bill that Congress approved nevertheless put the cancer effort back into the PHS. Still, the women considered it a victory although the funding level was less than originally sought — only $8 million. All was not lost, however. Public sentiment in favor of the program convinced the PHS the next year to ask Congress for $14 million for cancer research — the first time substantial sums had been requested for such work. Impatient to keep up momentum, Mahoney and Lakser shifted their position in favor of building up the existing Public Health Service rather than setting up separate entities.[103]

They then realized that no federal funds were being applied to study the number-one cause of death in the United States — heart disease. They approached Pepper about doing the same thing for heart research that Congress had done for cancer, and he introduced a bill in early 1947. Mahoney and Lasker, as for all their causes, sought editorials in its favor to rally public support.[104]

"It is the first time any proposal for such a dynamic and comprehensive attack has been made for medical research in this group of diseases," Lasker wrote Governor Cox. "Don't you agree that this proposal deserves widespread discussion and support, in principle? Won't you give it editorial support and letter space?"[105]

Cox acted promptly and sent her a copy of the papers' favorable editorials. "Florida's Senator Pepper has introduced a bill which should appeal to those who believe in putting first things first," one began. "Heart diseases now cause one out of three deaths among our people .... [L]esser ills to which flesh is heir came to the attention of Congress long ago while the dreadest enemy lurked in the very shadows of Capitol Hill ... [and] overworked congressmen were stricken and rushed off to the Naval Hospital, Bethesda, Md. They were victims of the No.-1 killer."[106]

One of those, as chance would have it, was the new chairman of the Senate Appropriations Committee, Republican Styles Bridges of New Hampshire, who recently had suffered a heart attack. Congress by then had changed leadership, and Pepper no longer was a chairman. So when Mahoney and Lasker went to Washington in April 1947 to see what was being done about hearings on the heart bill, Pepper took them to meet Bridges, who was glad to hold hearings. The bill was authorized later that same year but had not gotten an appropriation. The lesson learned with the mental-health bill was still vivid in Mahoney's and Lasker's memory.[107]

"It was quite late in the session when we got the heart bill through, close to when Congress was to adjourn," explained Mahoney. "President Truman was in San Francisco, campaigning. I was at Governor Cox's house in Dayton, and I called Clark Clifford, who was with the Truman campaign, and asked him, 'If we send the bill out there, can you get Mr. Truman to sign it so we can get it back in time to get appropriations?' He said to send it.

"So I got the bill sent out on a White House courier plane. There were three hours difference in time from the West Coast to Ohio, and I kept Governor Cox and the valet awake all night with phone calls — they rang in different rooms all the time — trying to get through to San Francisco" to confirm that Clifford had been successful in his mission, Mahoney remembered with amusement. "The Governor complained about being awakened all night. I told him, 'Never mind — that bill might save your life one day.'"

Clifford succeeded and the bill was signed June 16, 1948. The NIH now was plural.

It had been another lesson in the legislative process, the nuances of which Mahoney recognized many people did not fully comprehend because of the intricacies of government — presidents recommended budget levels but Congress allocated the funds to run programs, and congressional approval had to pass through labyrinths in two separate bodies.

"I thought it was a matter of educating people," she said. "It's very hard to understand how the whole thing works," that bills must go through both the House and Senate, then to conference, and finally to the president for signature or veto. She and Lasker were learning fast — "We had to."

Sharpening lobbying skills

Mahoney and Lasker daily were gaining experience in massaging and persuading Congress. They considered themselves representatives of "citizen committees," and in that role they brought allies and "citizen" witnesses to testify before congressional committees. Well-known author and Lasker friend John Gunther, for example, generated sympathy for cancer research by testifying on the tragic death of his seventeen-year-old son from the disease, which he had related in a widely read book, *Death Be Not Proud*.[108]

Albert Lasker himself had testified before a Senate committee in 1946 in favor of federal spending on cancer research. When a senator asked, "But whom do you represent, Mr. Lasker?" he replied, "Forty million sufferers." Mahoney wrote Mary from Idaho, "Tell Albert his testimony makes me green with envy I was not there to hear it, and know they had great fun, too, for the repartee [was] unbelieveable."[109]

Mahoney's calendar between 1945 and 1949 reflected a wide range of activities. She traveled a good deal, frequently attending meetings and conferences of health organizations like the AMA, advocates for world government and the Committee for the Nation's Health, and sometimes wrote about them in her newspaper column. "Readers who are not interested in health had better sign off here," she began one piece about a National Health Assembly in Washington in 1948. Convened by Truman's Federal Security Administrator Oscar Ewing as a tactical effort to try and mute opposition to national health insurance by focusing on health programs, it brought together representatives of the medical public health, and social services professions. Truman had challenged the group to outline a ten-year plan for the nation. The consensus of the 800 delegates, Mahoney wrote, was that "1 - Our potential for good health and medical services is the best in the world but people fail to make the best use of it; 2 - there is a great disparity between the medical treatment available in different parts of the country; 3 - everywhere there is an appalling waste of human life and health because known methods of fighting disease are not adequately supplied." She added that a "noted authority on old-age problems told a true story about a Danish sailor who lived for 146 years and said there is no reason why science cannot make it possible for people to live that long."[110]

Mahoney had become well acquainted with Ewing, a key figure in the Truman administration, and regularly communicated with him, enclosing copies of editorials and columns favorable to the president's plans, particularly during Truman's election campaign against Thomas E. Dewey in 1948.

"I hope you have recovered from all the doctors," she joked following the assembly and enclosing her column, which "I thought might amuse you. I do it incognito for the Sunday paper and try to get in as much propaganda as possible since it is in [the] society [section], for it seems more people read there than otherwise."

Mahoney by then had learned to use the press to good advantage. "We had good editorials in all the papers," she wrote Ewing, referring to a speech at the assembly that she had sent to all the Cox newspapers. "It received much favorable comment [and] got responses from all of the local medical societies, critically of course." She sent one editorial "with a letter to 33 Democratic Senators whom I knew, hoping it would offset some of their fears" about the insurance bill. She felt that the AMA would indict itself in its own words, which she also circulated to the media. "In the current issue of the American Medical Association *Journal*, our friend," she said derisively, "Dr. Fishbein's editorial will interest you. Have someone get it for you, as I have sent mine to the paper."[111]

Truman officials, in turn, sent Mahoney materials that they hoped she would give newspapers for favorable comment. "Thank you for my copy of the report," Mahoney wrote Ewing in October 1948, just before the election. "Mr. Locke [*Miami Daily News* columnist] ... is studying it and will then write about it. He is so good." Truman was "unbelievable the way he continues to go," she added, "and I am delighted he is not discouraged. I still think the trend can change."[112]

The night of Truman's surprise victory (November 3), she and Lasker sent a congratulatory telegram to Matt Connelly at Truman's headquarters in Kansas City, Missouri, saying, "Mary and I wish we could celebrate with you."[113]

A few days later, on November 7, Mahoney had delivered to the White House by Clark Clifford's chauffeur a picnic basket for the Trumans with small bottles of champagne and assorted cheese. "Although I am a little late in thanking you for that delicious treat," Truman replied, "I do want you to know that the family and I are nonetheless grateful for your kind thought. Indeed, Mrs. Truman and Margaret join with us in this expression of thanks and good wishes."[114]

Mahoney was one of the few people confident that Truman would be elected in 1948. She had gotten an inkling of Dewey's personality — and political prospects — while he was campaigning in Florida. "The very young mayor of Miami Beach — he couldn't have been more than thirty — said to me, 'I'm so excited, this is the first time I have ever met a Yankee!' It was true, too, because he'd lived in Florida all his life. I sat next to Dewey at dinner and I told him that story because I thought he'd be amused, and he said, 'That's the most ridiculous thing I ever heard.' Not an *iota* of humor — and he was so rude, too. I knew from that moment he would never be president," she said. "And I won a lot of money on that election! Everybody owed me money." One of those who did was Republican Albert Lasker. "He bet me a thousand to one. But I never got the money!"

Clark Clifford, in a memo to Connelly a month after the election, made a personal request: "I know that you are acquainted with both Mary Lasker and Florence Mahoney. They were loyal to the President during the campaign and each rendered a real service to him. I would appreciate it very much if I could send to each of them a personally autographed picture of the President."[115]

"What a delightful surprise and pleasure I had when Clark Clifford handed your autographed photograph to me last Friday!" a thrilled Lasker scribbled to the president on Boca Raton Club note paper ten days later. "I shall treasure this picture always! . . . May the New Year see your wonderful legislative program, especially health insurance, in action!"[116]

After Truman's inaugural address in January 1949 Mahoney wired him from Florida, "It was a wonderful and inspiring message to the Congress and you know we loved the health part." "The President was deeply gratified by [your] expressions of approval," Truman aide William D. Hassett told her.[117] It was important to take advantage of having Truman in the White House, she knew, to get measures through Congress that they both backed. Her 1949 diary revealed her own efforts to those ends:

> April 26, 1949 – Went from Florida to Washington, to Senate floor in p.m. Dinner, p.m., Pepper, Miller, Kilgore, Reidy, Murray and David Niles.
>
> April 27 – called Senators all morning re: cancer and heart. Lunch, Senate Dining Room. Hearings all afternoon on amendments for heart and cancer appropriations. Amendments passed. Saw and talked to during the day, Senators Wherry, Hayden, [Representative] Biemiller, Murray, Neely, Chavez, Langer, Humphrey, Kefauver, Russell, McMahon, Milliken, Brannan and Johnson. Missed meeting of Comm. for Nation's Health for floor meeting.
>
> April 28 – lunch . . . Senate Dining Room with Mary & Pepper. Talked to Russell, Maybank, Magnuson, Bricker, Holland, Taylor, Miller, Hill, Fulbright, Myers and Douglas. Dinner with the Peppers out, then Dr. Rusk [came] by after dinner.
>
> April 29 – lunch in the House Dining Room. Jake [?], George S. [Smathers?] and Mary. Saw during the day [named thirteen members of Congress]. Spoke on telephone to [eight members of Congress]. Dinner, p.m., just Mary and I, F Street Club . . .
>
> Went next day, May 4, to the White House for coffee and to see the President, Connelly, Clifford, Ewing, then to the Senate Floor. Lunch with McLowery, [McNeil Lowery, Cox] news bureau chief, D. C., and later . . . to plan [how to use press] . . .
>
> Mrs. Truman and White House dinner with Adlai. M. M. [Michael Mahoney?] and I dined last p.m. at White House.[118]

"That's quite a lot of senators to see in one afternoon," Mahoney commented of one day's work when she visited more than a dozen. "We never seemed to have to wait very long" to be ushered in. "Somebody in the office always seemed to know who we were, or sometimes saw us in the halls. We would often go to the Senate dining room for lunch, and to hearings all afternoon on amendments on heart and cancer appropriations."

Teamwork

Mahoney's and Lasker's letters demonstrated their teamwork in trying to influence politicians and decision makers. Mahoney's characteristically were typewritten in a stream-of-consciousness style with abbreviated sentences separated by dots and recounted a good deal of political information. In one in 1949 she reported on efforts to get Senator Richard Russell of Georgia, a member of the appropriations committee, to back higher funding levels than the committee had approved.

> Russell wrote back most friendly about the cut in the heart-cancer appropriations in the conference and how I had heard he had not *been able* to get there.... Write and tell me... what to write to enlighten him.
>
> I had also sent him an article from *Colliers* on heart, 'The Richest Man in the Cemetary,' which I hoped would terrify him and had underlined all the gruesome facts. You know, he told me he had been terrified of heart [disease] .... You can see *quel* type humor I have.[119]

Another example of how Mahoney worked was evident in a note to Lasker from Florida.

> Am trying to do my column and all piles up. Was going to lunch with Murray Sanders [medical researcher affiliated with University of Miami] and then Leslie Biffle called and wanted me to lunch with him. He just got in last p.m. so am taking Sanders ....
>
> Biffle is off to Puerto Rico for opening of that huge new hotel there this weekend. [Eastern Airlines president Eddie] Rickenbacker had asked me to go so now I am, and will get good chance to see Hilton (the hotel man who is building the $3-mil. hotel at new air terminal here) and to see P. R. and will make Leslie tell me about all

of the Rules Comm. and the others we have to know about. Leaving tomorrow a.m. and back Sunday.

A revealing part of the same letter described the perceptions that others, including Dan Mahoney, had of the women at work in those early years, a source of mixed pride and amusement to Florence. The references were to Truman aide Clark Clifford, "Mr. C.," and Dan Mahoney Sr., "Father M."

> When Mr. C. stopped at house, Father M. was speaking of you and me in Wash. and Mr. C. said in firm voice, "I want you to know that they have the reputation of getting what ever they go after there and rightfully so." Then Father M. said we wanted to get things done too fast, and Mr. C. said, "That is a very admirable trait for there are so many people to educate who are pleased with the *status quo* that unless it is done by someone like us (in a hurry), that it would never get done." It was really the most amusing conversation and Michael [Mahoney] was fascinated and went over it all later, and said, "You know, Daddy thinks the only reason they pay any attention to you girls in Wash. is because of the paper [Cox newspaper]." Anyway we seem to have a staunch supporter under all circumstances. Mr. C. was fine and we had a lot of fun. Will tell you of conversation when me meet.[120]

Disease of the month

By 1949, with the National Institutes of Health growing in size and stature each year, new disease-related organizations began to spring up, which, like Mahoney's and Lasker's committee, attracted public, and consequently congressional, advocates. Congress' reaction to such pressure was the genesis of what would come to be called "disease-of-the-month-club" legislating. It was not the way scientists ideally would have organized their programs or allocated money (they would have preferred lump sums and grouping by scientific disciplines rather than disease categories), but it was politically popular, and even NIH officials realized that larger appropriations were generated by focusing on diseases with which public-interest groups could identify. In the spring of that year, for example, bills were introduced promoting research on multiple sclerosis, cerebral palsy, and epilepsy, and Wisconsin Representative Biemiller introduced one calling for an Institute on Blindness.[121]

"The Senate was confused about what to do with all these bills," Mahoney recalled, and the Public Health Service was less than enthusiastic about expanding its charges. "Doctor Norman Topping of NIH was opposed to any additional health institutes, saying that the administration [of them] was too complicated."[122]

Congress proposed putting all the bills together into one omnibus measure that included research on many diseases as well as the health-insurance program. "6-billion Health Bill Introduced in Congress," a front-page *Washington Evening Star* headline blared April 25, 1949. "The bill calls for payroll-tax insurance to provide medical, hospital and dental care for about 120,000,000 Americans . . . . The measure also would put into effect all the other phases of Mr. Truman's program. Those include federal support for medical education, hospital construction, public health services and research." Mahoney went to work rounding up witnesses to testify in favor of the bill.[123]

Congress in 1950 did approve an omnibus research bill that created two new institutes: one for arthritis and metabolic diseases and another for neurological diseases and blindness — "the first time the Public Health Service had any money for neurological diseases and more than half a million in the whole field of arthritis," Mahoney boasted with justifiable pride.[124]

Especially important was a single line in the Omnibus Medical Research Act: It gave the Surgeon General authority to establish more institutes as he determined the need to "conduct and support research and research training relating to other diseases and groups of diseases."[125]

On the day that the full Senate voted on appropriations for the bills, Mahoney watched from the gallery as Senator Pepper conferred with Senator Magnuson on figures. "Neely was very dramatic about needs for cancer research," she wrote in her diary. "Senator [Kenneth S.] Wherry [of Nebraska, Senate Republican leader] opposed the increases. . . . Bridges agreed to a compromise . . . Mental health failed. Senator [Tom] Connolly [Democrat of Texas], originally voted for it, but when he realized it was for mental health, he changed his vote. Senator Taft moved to recommit the bill."

"Biffle helped turn around Taft's move," Mahoney recorded. "The first of June the Senate voted to keep the original figures plus the amendment. The conference with the House was very important and [House Appropriations Committee Chairman, Democrat Clarence] Cannon [of Missouri] very difficult to talk to; he even said he hoped he himself would die of heart disease." But her position prevailed. "In the conference, it was settled for $8 million more," part of which went to the first construction money ever allocated for research facilities off the NIH campus.[126]

The battle was not yet won, however. There was danger that anti-expansionist forces within the Budget Bureau might persuade Truman not to sign the bill. To one of Mahoney's pleadings, Truman replied, "Thanks very much for your good letter of the 26th with the attached brief on Heart Diseases, Cancer and Arthritis. I will discuss the matter with the Budget [Bureau] and we will see what can be done. Our main difficulty in these things is that the Congress is against almost anything that has to do with public health, but that doesn't prevent us from still trying to get what is right."[127]

Mahoney had to marshall her best resources. "Matthew Connelly was helpful during this time," she said. "The President would not sign the bill as the Budget Bureau had attached a memorandum saying the bill was all right but the method of establishing more institutes was bad. We talked to Clifford and through various contacts, got the Budget's [memo] detached and President Truman signed it."[128]

With the legislation permitting open-ended expansion of the NIH, many of Mahoney's and Lasker's dreams were fulfilled. Now they wanted to ensure that the money was spent to the best advantage. Both would play important roles in that process.

Lay people on advisory councils

A singular, seemingly small clause in the Heart Institute bill had significant ramifications for research policymaking: It required that all National Institutes of Health have lay members as well as professional scientists and physicians on the advisory councils that oversaw the handing out of funds — something that Pepper had addressed in his hearings. "We got that passed," Mahoney said of the subtle but important provision, which reflected the experience they had had with the Cancer Society.[129]

Although the women did not have confidence in many bureaucrats to carry out their mission, one PHS officer, Dr. Leonard Scheele, whom Truman named Surgeon General in 1948, manifested a kinship with the Mahoney-Lasker mode of thinking. He perceived the value of having lay people on NIH advisory panels and backed the legislative change.[130]

Mahoney and Lasker, whose reputation as research advocates was now well established, were obvious candidates to be among the first lay people to serve on the prestigious panels. For nearly twenty years beginning in 1950 Mahoney would serve almost continuously on various institute councils, with the exception of a period during Eisenhower's presidency. Her first appointment was to the Mental Health panel (1950–54); she subsequently served on the Arthritis and Metabolic Diseases council (1959–63), Child Health and Human Development council (1963–67), and National Institute on Aging council (1974–78). Lasker served for eighteen years on Cancer and Heart Institute councils. Mike Gorman and Lasker's sister Alice Fordyce also served on councils.[131]

One NIH official, John Foord Sherman, remembered his first encounter with Mahoney on the arthritis advisory council. A scientist (pharmacologist), he and his colleagues were skeptical of the advantages that someone like Mahoney could bring to the deliberations. "None of us knew exactly why she was appointed to that council," Sherman recalled. He nevertheless was assigned to greet her at a Sunday afternoon orientation session for new members. "I was waiting by the door of the institute when up pulled a battered old sedan whose driver was a slightly built woman who carried a big paper bag and thermos jug. It was Florence, who in typical fashion, without pretensions, said that she had borrowed the car from a New York senator. Frankly, we all thought she was a real light-weight at first because she gave us a few non sequitors, but after a meeting or two, it became clear to us that she knew her business. She was very impressive. Florence stayed on the council for the full term, four years. On all committees and councils on which she served, that I knew about," he added, "she attended meetings whenever possible and did her home-work."[132]

Mahoney, who noted that she always drove herself without the luxury of a chauffeur, was not certain whose car she had borrowed but thought it probably was New York Republican Senator Kenneth Keating's, a neighbor with whom she had a close rapport. Of the brown paper bag she said it contained her lunch because she disliked the "big, heavy sand-wiches" that were served — "I was always on some kind of a diet and wanted certain food" — and the thermos, tea, a refreshing drink that she favored.

Lay members like Mahoney had different perspectives and objectives from the scientists and immediately began to cause trouble for the pro-fessional reviewers, accustomed to acting without such input. Mahoney remembered her sense of frustration during her early years of partici-pation. "The doctors controlled *everything* in the beginning. They would want a certain kind of research, not any other kind, and they would make a big deal over a grant of a few hundred dollars. When lay people got on the councils, the doctors and scientists began to think in bigger terms."

"The enthusiasm of the lay members is very hard to keep up with," Scheele had to admit after a few years. "We medical people are very conservative. These people constantly stimulate us and remind us of our responsibilities."[133]

Endings and beginnings

Mahoney and Lasker were not always victorious in their quests. Another controversial issue was whether or not the nation had sufficient scientific and medical manpower to carry out the growing number of government tasks that Congress was approving. Pepper in 1949 had introduced a bill providing federal aid to medical education, for the first time giving medical schools money to train doctors to staff Public Health Service facilities.

Again, the AMA opposed the concept. "We were all working on the bill," Mahoney remembered. "But by 1950 the AMA was well organized and against any aid to medical education. It thought that private enterprise would do it. Some of the [medical school] deans who previously had been in favor of the bill now were unwilling to do anything for it, so no bill was passed. The Pepper bill lost by one vote." It would be more than a decade before the issue was raised again.[134]

Several other measures that Mahoney and Lasker backed in those years also did not succeed. A bill introduced by Senator Murray would have provided up-to-date information on national illness statistics, the first such survey since 1937. It failed in part, Mahoney believed, because "they got Senator Bridges confused about it all when the hearings were held." A bill in 1950 calling for research on childhood diseases met Catholic opposition, led by Washington educator John O'Grady. "The Senate decided they could not report out any bill that Monseigneur O'Grady was opposed to," Mahoney said. That issue also did not receive congressional attention for another decade.[135]

Heady with success, nevertheless, the women pushed in 1950 for a whopping $64 million in appropriations for the now five existing National Institutes, which many senators supported. The funding levels were not approved, however, to their astonishment. Some in Congress were beginning to feel that the institutes were getting too fat too quickly.

"An enormous amount of work had been done with the senators," said Mahoney, who at the time was still living in Florida. "I was in Washington for six weeks with Mike Gorman (Mary was in New York as Albert had been ill)," lobbying for the huge increase in appropriations. But one of her key allies, Senator Pepper, to whom she had remained loyal despite accusations of his having Communist leanings and Communists on his staff, "had lost some of his prestige, as he had been defeated in the primaries in Florida in the spring of 1950, which was the same as losing an election. So his leverage in the Senate was not so strong. It was hard to convince people that research was the economic way to keep people in good health so they could work and give money to the federal treasury," Mahoney reflected of many frustrating meetings with Budget Bureau directors and doubting congressmen.[136]

Even during the Truman administration it sometimes was hard to get federal funding for the NIH. When Truman requested some $3 million for mental-health programs one year, "somebody came along and took it out," Mahoney learned. "I went and complained to Mr. Truman, and he said, 'Well, go and tell the director of the Bureau of the Budget. I don't do the details of the budget.' 'But you're the *boss*,' I said. He insisted that I talk to the then-director of the Budget Bureau — and I did. He said he was going to Princeton that weekend. My son was at Princeton, but I hadn't planned to go there. Nevertheless I told him, 'Well, strangely enough, I'm going to be there too, by chance. I'll come and see you *there*.' So I met him at the hotel in Princeton. And he put the $3 million *back*" in the budget.

Anticipating opposition when Republicans took over the White House, Mahoney and Lasker, in Truman's last year as president, made a concerted fight for big increases, especially construction money for the still-small Bethesda campus. At a meeting with Truman in June 1952, they gave him their wish-list budget that included $40 million for construction.[137]

"Truman smiled and said, 'You will see improvement,'" Mahoney recalled. Lasker remembered that he "asked his secretary for a letter which he had written to the Budget Bureau . . . evidently drafted by General [Wallace] Graham [the president's physician] . . . [with] figures requesting substantial increases for the various institutes. 'Has this letter gone?'" Truman asked. His secretary was uncertain.[138]

"We decided we had better call General Graham to be sure that he understood it and would remind the president of his promise to do something," according to Mahoney. "When I got him on the phone, he said, 'Well, you have given me a fine job, haven't you? The president has dumped all the stuff you brought him yesterday on *my* desk, and I'm to take the matter up with the budget boys.' He went on to say, 'Actually I am not such a good one to do that, as I have already gotten after them too much on things I am interested in.' This was a tip-off that it was all in Graham's hands — a charming man but a surgeon and not at all involved in research ideas."[139]

"This encouraged us somewhat," Lasker remembered, "but knowing the resistance of the budget boys to any increases in funds for the institutes, around the first of October I asked Lynn Adams, who was working for the National Mental Health Committee, to see if he could find out from the Budget Bureau directly if any increases had been allowed for the Mental Health Institute, which had replaced the Division of Mental Hygiene. He saw one of the key budget people who said to him cautiously that 'he wouldn't count on it if he were Lynn Adams.' That was the tip-off that nothing had been done. I immediately got in touch with Florence who decided the only way now was to get it through Mrs. Truman."[140]

The end result, as Mahoney concluded the story, "was that Mrs. Truman took up the matter of additional funds for the Institutes of Health with the president and he, in turn, took it up with our friend David Stowe." Not long afterward, Surgeon General Scheele "was calling us asking how we would like the money distributed by the institutes." The women had won an increase, although less than they had hoped — "an additional $25 million over and above what had been voted by the Congress for fiscal year 1953. It had been a tough struggle and God knows what the new administration would do with it." That would prove to be their next challenge.[141]

Mahoney's and Lasker's hard work through the 1940s, however, had paid off handsomely. Between 1941 and 1951, federal spending for medical research had risen from less than $3 million to $76 million for the five research institutes in place by the end of the decade.[142]

But it also was the end of an era for Mahoney and Lasker when Truman chose not to run for reelection, opening the way for Republican Dwight D. Eisenhower to defeat Democrat Adlai Stevenson for president. Mahoney's friendship with the Trumans had deepened over their White House years, affording her easy entrée not only to his staff but to the president and his immediate family.[143]

She and Lasker had sent the president a coin clip with "Valentine's Greetings and all our admiration for your warm-hearted support of health legislation" in February 1949. Following his message to Congress reiterating support for national health insurance in April, Mahoney had wired him, "Far greater progress has been made than we dared hope for in '45, due to your vision and courage."[144]

When Mahoney could not reach the president, she contacted his closest aides. "Clark Clifford knew *what* to do. Although I knew the president's secretary, Connelly, he wasn't involved in health things. There were two or three people at the White House who were involved in health issues, and because I'd known them all in Florida, they always got us in to see the president if we had anything to say. There was always somebody you could go to to get help." Truman aides, on their part, often contacted Mahoney and expressed a desire to visit with her, as Oscar Ewing did in February 1950, when she still lived in Miami Beach.[145]

Mahoney sometimes got her clippings passed on to the White House by high-ranking messengers such as Supreme Court Justice William O. Douglas, and she personally corresponded with cabinet members like Secretary of State Dean Acheson. As Douglas was leaving for Oregon in 1950, he sent over a *Chicago Daily Tribune* editorial with a note saying it was one "which Mrs. Florence Mahoney gave the Justice to read and requested that he pass it on to you," meaning Matt Connelly. When Acheson was the subject of controversy over his "cold-war" policies, she sent him a note along with supportive clippings and a cartoon. Acheson appreciated the gesture.[146]

On one occasion, Truman personally wrote to Dan Mahoney, expressing his views about "newspapermen." "I find in my dealings with distinguished newspapermen," Truman said, "that they are all thin-skinned — they like to give a public man hell but when he comes back a little, they find it hard to take. Nothing personal was intended in my letter," he added, "I only wanted to express my opinion. Thanks a lot for your good letter and *don't be distressed*," he underscored.[147]

Mahoney also socialized with Margaret Truman, whom she recognized was "very smart." When she went to Florida that month, Mahoney let her know, through Matt Connelly, that she wanted "to offer hospitality" and could "arrange for very quiet and private quarters at the Surf Club if Miss Margaret desires." White House arrangements for Margaret, however, had been made "some time ago," she wired back, sorry not to be able to "accept Mrs. Mahoney's kind invitation."[148]

"Before anyone knew they were even engaged, Margaret and Clifton Daniel [subsequently managing editor of the *New York Times*], came to Washington and stayed with me," Mahoney remembered. The couple confided in her, but no one else at a small dinner party that weekend knew of the betrothal. One of the guests was Dean Acheson's widow, who was misled into thinking that the visiting Daniel was a beau of Mahoney's until reading about the engagement later in a newspaper. It was a measure of Mahoney's trustworthiness — only she and Margaret's closest friend were privy to the secret.[149]

When Daniel was assigned to the Washington bureau, he stayed at Mahoney's house before Margaret, who remained in New York with their two sons while they finished the school year, joined him. One night Daniel returned from a weekend at home and did not recognize Mahoney's house when his taxi pulled up, telling the driver that he had the wrong place. No, it was the right address — but it had been transformed over the weekend by a film crew for a scene from *The Exorcist*![150]

Margaret Truman reflected that Mahoney's interests, aside from her sons, were all-consuming: "She was always working on a cause, and medicine was it." In many meetings that she had with Mahoney over the years, Margaret marveled that "it was hard to say who was whose contemporary, to realize that she was older."

Bess Truman on occasion invited Mahoney to dinner at the White House quite spontaneously, once calling to ask, "Would you come for dinner tonight? It would just be us." "I said, 'Mary's expected here tonight. Can I bring her?' And she said, 'I don't know any extra men,'" to balance the seating arrangement. "I thought it was so funny — she didn't know any extra men! But we did go, and there were only four or five of us — Adlai Stevenson, Mary, the Trumans, and me — and we had fun. Adlai was a little bit late getting there, and when he walked up, Mr. Truman was sitting outside the doorway, and the first thing Adlai said was, 'I must say, you don't look any worse for' — some kind of great catastrophe! I used to have wonderful conversations with them," she added.

Bess she considered "a great lady" who, while "very quiet," had a wonderful sense of humor (Margaret called it "wicked"). Mahoney laughed at the recollection of Mrs. Truman's forthright pragmatism, never so evident as in the much-told story about Truman's coming home to their Independence house to find Bess burning his letters to her. "You know, you're burning history," he remarked. "That's what I had in mind," she retorted.

Visiting them in Independence once, after they had left the White House, Mahoney was delighted with the former president's homey lack of pretension. "Harry set the table" with full place settings, just as Bess liked.

In the final year of the Truman presidency, Michael Mahoney, between graduation from Princeton and beginning air force training at an officers' candidate school, visited the White House several times with Florence. But it was the intimate gathering to which they were invited on the very last night of the Trumans' residency (in January 1953) that left a searing impression on Michael.[151]

All of them were aware that things would never be the same. "I remember being astounded at the fact that *tonight* Truman was president, and tomorrow at noon, he would return to being a private citizen," Michael reflected. "Two things that Truman remarked on" also were memorable: "*deep* regret that Adlai Stevenson had lost to Eisenhower, and *great* relief, as he put it, that now he would not have to decide the fate of the Rosenbergs (whether to let them be executed or not) and that 'Ike' would have to make that decision."[152]

Michael and his mother were part of a small group of friends who went to Union Station the next day "and saw the Trumans off to Missouri while the Navy band slowly and mournfully played the *Missouri*

Waltz as the train moved away. Many people had tears in their eyes," he remembered.

Truman, according to Lasker biographer John Gunther, called Mahoney and Lasker "the most tireless, consistent and effective crusaders" he had ever known.[153]

"He thought they were doing a good thing — and they got what they wanted!," Margaret Truman Daniel said of the two women's persuasiveness. "Believe me, they were very good. Sometimes there wasn't as much money as they would have liked" from budgets that the president and his treasury secretary rigorously, and proudly, balanced for three years. "It was not all the time that Dad could say 'yes' to their requests."

Still, she laughed at the recollection, "Whenever Dad saw Florence and Mary Lasker coming through the door, he would say, 'There goes another million dollars!'"[154]

5

Glorious Adversity
in a Golden Era

◆

*W*HAT CAME TO BE KNOWN AS THE "GOLDEN ERA OF NIH" was
well underway by the 1950s, a result of the unusual symbiotic
relationship between the "citizen" advocates, Congress, and government
officials, of which Mahoney and Lasker were a vital part.[1]

At the time, the two did not fully comprehend "the significance of
what we were doing," Mahoney recollected with the perspective of time.
"To tell you the truth, it was just a day-to-day operation. We were very
innocent."

And for many years it was not easy to win over members of Congress.
"Oh, they complained *bitterly* — especially a lot of senators," Mahoney
said of early opposition and skeptics. "But we didn't pay any attention to
them. We were on the right side so why bother?"

In the course of their efforts, they would become familiar figures in
the halls of Congress, accustomed to its consistently raising the NIH
budget each year, not only above previous years' funding levels but
above what presidents requested for research.[2]

The election of Eisenhower in 1952, however, posed an unknown future for Mahoney's and Lasker's efforts. Their coup in getting the Truman budget beefed up as a hedge against Republican cuts was short-lived. Eisenhower removed all construction funds from his first budget request, plus an additional $10 million that Truman had proposed for NIH. "We were back to where we were with the 1953 budget," Lasker noted in an early biographical memorandum. "How much would they have cut off if we hadn't gotten that additional money from Truman?" she asked an Eisenhower official. "God knows!" the man replied.

"This meant that we had to start over to make a drive for construction funds and for additional funds across the board," she said. "It was very hard in the House, as the new [member] of the [appropriations committee Republican Fred] Busbey of Chicago, who proudly called himself a 'reactionary' and was certainly friendly with the AMA, would undoubtedly be against any increases."[3]

Mahoney and Lasker had learned the intricacies of how government worked, but their momentum and successes would be tried as never before in the forthcoming decade.

Uniqueness of the citizen lobby

What made these two women continue to boldly approach presidents, members of Congress, and heads of medical-research units, believing that they could convince them to make radical changes in research funding? The women's impact and savvy were especially remarkable given their lack of scientific and medical credentials. Neither they nor Gorman had a degree or expertise in the fields they spoke about so convincingly. Professionals were anything but supportive of what they were trying to do.

"Every time we agitated for an expansion of the federal effort," Gorman related at the time, "we were told we didn't understand the complexities of the research process and [that there weren't enough] researchers anyway" to handle a greatly expanded program. "They accused us of a lack of appreciation of the subtleties of the research mind, of the intricacies of medical education, of the tenuous nature of the therapeutic process," Gorman said. "I accused them of living in a cream-puff world of fantasy."[4]

Despite what might have been considered a shortcoming in expertise, the impact of the Mahoney-Lasker "citizen lobby" on medical-research policy could not be denied. It was unlike any other advocacy, so unique in the history of lobbying and legislation that it became the subject of extensive analyses by political scientists and health writers. For nearly forty years the women operated independently, not associated with any organization other than their own purposeful committee.

"Except for the Army Corps of Engineers," former Department of Health, Education and Welfare (HEW) Assistant Secretary for Administration Rufus E. Miles wrote in a history of the department, "there is probably no better example . . . of the power of a triangular political force than that exhibited by NIH, with the support of Congress and outside pressure groups," notably Mahoney and Lasker.

"With the help of an old friend, Florence Mahoney, and an ex-newspaperman turned promoter of the cause of mental health, Mike Gorman," Miles wrote, they "developed a technique that was successfully used year after year to get Congress to overbid the president's budget request for NIH, usually by scores of millions of dollars." In a back-handed tribute, he recorded, "The repetitive pattern . . . sent Budget Bureau officials, White House staff and even presidents into a frenzy of annoyed frustration, and precipitated unprintable comments."[5]

As the group's successes mounted, though, professional groups themselves began to change their tack from being passive "mendicants" to Congress with their "hands out in supplication," as Gorman put it, to active backers of federal funding. "They have taken courage from the example of a few outspoken laymen who come before the Congress each session and give their representatives a real working-over," he wrote in 1956. He cited as an example Alabama lumberman Ben May, who treated congressmen to lunch every year. "After [they] have consumed the thick steaks, Ben gets off his haunches and . . . takes them to task for the way they are spending his and the other taxpayers' money." Echoing the Mahoney-Lasker-Gorman line, May would expound his theory that "research pays off, that new discoveries create new wealth."[6]

Some called it a "noble conspiracy" with Mahoney and Lasker as "its chief architects." Although Lasker referred to them as "self-employed health lobbyists," their detractors were not so kind. *U. S. News & World Report* once referred to the coterie as "Mary and her 'Little Lambs,' a circle of socialites, congressmen and doctors." Such derogation maligned Mahoney's and Lasker's serious intent and profound influence.[7]

The combination of politics with serious science also was unique. "It was no minor accomplishment to guide such a scientific effort on the one hand while simultaneously engaging in the complementary political game," a former NIH director of research planning remarked. "The pressures were often diametrically opposed." He characterized the "politically-oriented" lobbying group as relying on "speed . . . action, flashy public appeal and the glamor of public figures." Those qualities, combined with NIH Director James A. Shannon's scientific moderation, made for successful results. Each side had a "ferocity" to prevail, a dynamic that pushed the effort ahead faster and more effectively than ever before.[8]

Shannon, who was named NIH Director in 1955 and was liked and respected in both Congress and the scientific community, recognized that Mahoney and Lasker could help him build up the NIH. In a rare talent for a scientist, he also knew how to negotiate the legislative maze with subtle skill and to make convincing cases for money for his agency. "A tall man with the rumpled, informal demeanor of a small-town general practitioner," a *Washington Post* account said of him, "Shannon presides over an unruly informal constituency of volunteer 'lay' organizations, each with its own political connection on Capitol Hill." Shannon also was close personally and professionally to Surgeon General Scheele, both of whom shared views on the future development of the NIH.[9]

One way to counter skeptics wondering how all that money was being spent was to set up a valid, respected process for reviewing grant applications to NIH. The "peer-review" system was established at the behest of Dr. C. J. Van Slyke, head of NIH's research grants division, who with others created a system in which scientific peers rather than government bureaucrats examined and rated applications. Rigorous, and over many decades considered the most equitable review system, it assuaged the concerns of academicians and others in the private sector at a time when government control or interference still was feared. Of Van Slyke and Sheele, Mahoney said, "they understood everything we were trying to do."[10]

Different styles

Mahoney and Lasker had different lobbying styles, reflecting the differences in their personalities, and although their objectives were the same for many years, their differences complemented one another and worked to mutual advantage. The result was an effective team. Where Lasker was aggressive, Mahoney was gentle in her lobbying. She had a "simultaneously cheerful and calming presence," as health-policy historian Stephen Strickland put it. Another health writer, Natalie Davis Spingarn, called Mahoney "an astute lady with a talent for advocacy." If outwardly gentle, disagreeing with her nevertheless could sometimes be "fatal," one NIH official remarked of his experience. "There were two possibilities: right, if you agreed with her, wrong, if you didn't," he joked.[11]

Gorman characterized the women succinctly. After many years in the lobbying arena and observing famous people — like actresses Jennifer Jones Simon (speaking on behalf of cerebral palsy), Irene Dunne, and other notables who testified before Congress — he concluded that there were not "many of Mary and Florence's caliber. Mary Lasker and Florence Mahoney were a terrific combination. They made me a feminist!"

"As we worked . . . to build up the institutes and organize the congressional hearings," Gorman related, "Mary was the imperious one as to calling the major shots, and, in her own way, without being beguiling, she could get people like Mike DeBakey and Sidney Farber and others to come and testify, even though they had never done so before. Many [professionals] regarded it as a vulgar exercise to go before a congressional committee and explain yourself, but she was able to get them to do it."

Gorman recognized that Lasker did not like the kind of "cozying up, chit chatting, softening up" that was necessary to get what she wanted. "Instead she always carried charts around. I for one never used a chart with a senator. If I'm talking to someone directly, I don't need to pull out a chart. But Mary thought the charts were absolute magic. She would have one showing that the population in mental hospitals could be dropped by a certain figure, or another showing the effect [of research] on cancer [patients]." She also had "a little book that she could pull out wide, like an accordian, with facts and figures on everything. She had the NIH budget from the very beginning as well as all the institute budgets. This fat little book would come out with all its statistics and figures, and it was effective. So Mary was the factual one, and got a heck of a lot done," using that technique. She also "always put up an impossible monetary figure at about three times the current appropriation" for the NIH. "She was right up front."[12]

Mahoney, too, was succinct when talking to members of Congress. "She didn't mess around with a lot of niceities; she might chat a little but she went right to the point, well armed with information, and sent articles and information to people," a Senate staff aide remembered. "She was a delight to work with, I liked her energy, she had a lot of savvy."[13]

She also had "a superb political sense," John Sherman quickly recognized, and "knew exactly which buttons needed to be pushed, how and when. She worked hard and was well informed. Sure, she would slip up with the facts on occasion, but that didn't undermine the overall impression of someone who was knowledgeable and committed. In small groups she was a particularly effective spokesperson."[14]

Mahoney also worked independently, without the organizational backup and resources that Lasker had. She "did things so quietly and effectively that people *trusted* her," Strickland noticed.

The key senator who chaired both the health authorizing and appropriations committees, Democrat Lister Hill of Alabama, was "the best barometer of" the women's differences, Gorman said in an interview, quoting Hill: "'Mary Lasker comes in and she's all primed for what she wants — a new institute or new piece of legislation,' and he would call her 'Queen Mary.' He liked her in a way, but . . . he always felt that she was a bit too calculating."

"Now Senator Hill was a very proper guy in public, being an Alabaman, but in private his language could get pretty rough. He would call me up sometimes after Mary had gone to see him on her own, and she would have been raving on for about an hour about how he could have been a doctor but [instead] had done more than a thousand, ten thousand doctors could have done. He didn't like that kind of talk at all. He was a modest man. I would come in to see him and he'd be kind of irritated still and say, 'Madam Queen was down here again.' And I sometimes wouldn't have been notified so I'd say, 'I didn't know that.' And he would say, 'Yes, and she layed it on thick.' He had a salty way of de-scribing her at times. And she always had the charts with statistics on mice studies, and that annoyed the heck out of him. He'd ask me, 'Mike, do you ever do any of those charts?' And I said, 'No way, I stay away from those charts.' He said, 'Well, I'll tell you something: As far as I'm concerned, those charts are not worth a pinch of monkey crap.' I told Florence that story. But at the same time, Senator Hill respected Mary as a citizen who could have been spending her time doing a number of other things but she was coming down to try to get help for these issues.

"Florence, on the other hand, would come up unprepared and just talk. Lister Hill was very fond of Florence, and he referred to her as 'Lady Scatterbrain' who had no charts. 'But somehow,' he would say, 'she has a way of vamping me and making me think about what she's saying. She's very appreciative of my time and has a great sense of humor.'"

Gorman said of Hill's perspective, "He liked that kind of thing because for the most part, a senator has a pretty boring day. So he always felt that she had a personal effectiveness."

"I don't know how effective she was from one issue to the next," Gorman mused, "because she had very little patience with facts and got them fouled up sometimes. But in the long run it didn't really matter. If I said 4.2 and she turned it around to 2.4, it didn't really make a difference.

The point was, would certain legislation get support, or an appropriation be raised for something?"

Unlike the direct and insistent Lasker, "Florence played her part in more of a background way, with dinners and visits with these people who would become really devoted to her — Republicans and Democrats. I remember [Republican] Senator [Kenneth] Keating from New York, whom I had a lot of difficulty with over mental-health policies. I told Florence, and the next thing you know, I was sitting opposite Ken Keating at the dinner table at Florence's. Keating liked her and he felt very relaxed."

"She had a lot of congressmen over for dinner and was much more social in a personal way than Mary was. Mary was a great New York socialite, and didn't read a lot, and Florence knew this. I once sent Mary a monograph of some kind which I thought was very important, and when I asked her what she thought of it, she said, 'I ran through it.' You couldn't have just run through something like that. Florence's remark was that Mary never read anything thoroughly. She read the first few paragraphs, then she got the doctors in to listen to her. She was wonderful at getting all kinds of doctors together and asking them questions. Mary had a very quick mind." Heart specialist Dr. Michael DeBakey agreed, saying Lasker also had "an ability to focus on the central issues and to sense what combination of talents must be brought together to solve a problem."[15]

Mahoney, though, felt that "Mary was very congenial. I never noticed that she was intimidating to politicians. If she was, it may have been because she had access to presidents."[16]

"Mary was more shy than I was and did not like as much give-and-take with other people. She was probably more intelligent, probably got her lessons better when she was young. But I knew much more about medicine," Mahoney conceded. "Mary had studied the same things I had, but she thought that money would solve anything. Of course, it does solve a lot of things," Mahoney agreed with a smile, "but I never thought that money was everything that was needed. It certainly was needed in the first place, there's no question about it, and Mary was really great at getting it. She had different methods, she would always give some money to people who were running" for office.

Lasker was in a financial position to make sizeable contributions to congressional candidates although the extent of her campaign donations could not be known. Mahoney was not in such a position. Her donations generally were small, $25 to $100 was the norm (most recipients were those on the health authorizing and appropriations committees), and she did not rely on contributions to gain access to members of Congress. Neither did Lasker, for that matter. "It had nothing to do with that," Mahoney said. "I think everybody should contribute to candidates of their choice. It's not bribery."[17]

Lasker's strategy was to use the Lasker Foundation to promote her positions through its awards and annual "fact sheets" on health subjects that her National Health Education Committee published on deaths, disabilities, and loss of income from illness, which she used to justify her positions. (Mahoney was a sponsoring member of the committee.) The fact sheets also garnered publicity, like an item in *Newsweek* magazine in the late 1950s remarking humorously that the "committee's over-eager publicists underscored the certainty of death and the uncertainty of taxes. 'If 212,570 people who died of hardening of the arteries and high blood pressure in one year had lived and worked for another year,' the release read, 'they could have paid another $151,774,980 in income taxes.'" Lasker herself often pointed out that twice as many Americans were killed by diseases than in the armed services during World War II, and her facts emphasized how biomedical research was lengthening Americans' lifespans. That reminded even the most doubting congressmen of their own mortality.[18]

"Research is economy" was Lasker's theme, clearly evident in a telegram that she sent Congressman John Fogarty, chairman of the House Appropriations subcommittee on health, during congressional debate in March 1951. "The citizen budget for heart, cancer, mental health and the two new Institutes are peanuts compared with what could be saved in lives, productivity and tax-paying ability within a few years if they will fight for these increases. The discovery of penicillin and sulfa have cut

pneumonia and syphilis deaths by fifty percent in four years and tuberculosis deaths have been reduced by thirty percent with streptomycin
.... Wire me collect what happens. The telephone is almost hopeless."[19]

Lasker also could take advantage of other assets, particularly her art
collection. David Bell, appointed director of the Budget Bureau in 1962,
was impressed when Lasker and Mahoney first called on him. "She
(Lasker) looked at the walls of my office and remarked that they looked
sort of bare. She asked me, why not have some art on them? I agreed that
would be nice, and she asked me what I would like. I said Georgia
O'Keeffe. 'You know, I've been meaning to buy some O'Keeffe,'" Lasker
said. Sometime later, she had "two beautiful paintings delivered" to
Bell's office on loan. "One was a beautiful red autumn leaf, the other a
tree bursting in yellow leaves. It always made me think very warmly of
her," Bell said many years later, wondering how subsequent strict rules
on ethics would cause him to react, "as a high government official, receiving something like that from a prominent lobbyist." Undoubtedly
he would not have accepted it. But at the time, it was seen as a generous
and thoughtful act that Lasker, he understood, had done for others.[20]

Lasker later sold some art work to fund testing for the drug interferon,
believing it to be a cancer cure. Her hopes were not entirely realized
although the drug came to be used to treat certain kinds of cancer.[21]

The Laskers' art collection on one occasion suffered because of Mary's
intense involvement with matters medical. Albert had determined to
acquire several important Van Goghs: one entitled *Zouave* and the other
White Roses, the latter of which had been painted twice. He had bought
the *Zouave* in Paris, successfully beating a Brazilian collector to the gem.
One version of the *White Roses* he knew belonged to Averell Harriman,
but the location of the other was a mystery. Lasker put Mary on the
chase. Through a friend they tracked it down to a bank vault in New
York. Lasker called Mary from California and asked her to buy it at once.
She was leaving, however, to attend a meeting of the National Heart
Advisory Council in Washington. It would be safe where it was, she told
him, until she returned a few days later. Lasker implored her to buy the
painting first, but she prevailed. On her return, she found to her amaze-

ment that the painting had been sold to a dealer for $100,000. Albert, furious, began negotiations with the dealer to get the picture and succeeded — paying $135,000 for it. Mary's trip to Washington had cost him $35,000, or about $7,000 an hour, he told people good-naturedly, as the painting's value was rising rapidly to many times its purchase price.[22]

Undaunted by accusations that she was single-minded, Lasker nevertheless was fully aware of her status as a non-scientist. An article in *Medical World News*, whose editor ironically was former AMA "enemy" Morris Fishbein, described her as being "acutely sensitive to the prejudice that she is only a lay woman in a world of men and scientists." She made up for it with a "fierce passion" that caused her to say things like, "I am opposed to heart attacks, cancer and stroke the way I am opposed to sin." She also was impatient with delays in what she thought could be accomplished more quickly than bureaucratic or scientific caution permitted. Upset by what she considered unnecessary slowness in the medical profession's acceptance of the anti-tubercular drug isoniazid, Lasker exclaimed to Howard Rusk, trying to reassure her that it was moving forward, "But people are dying while we're talking, people who don't need to die."[23]

Rusk reflected Lasker's views in a column in 1958. "In all fields of science, one of the major problems is the time lag that exists between the discovery of new knowledge and its practical application," he wrote. "This is particularly true of the health sciences. In this field, life itself is at stake."[24]

Many in the scientific community, though, resented Lasker's pushiness and what they perceived as interference in their territory. One such person was James Shannon, NIH director from 1955 to 1968. He and Lasker had a somewhat icy relationship. She considered that his ego imposed a heavy, conservative hand over NIH. Although another NIH director and a deputy director were given Lasker Awards, Shannon was not so honored. Lasker admitted to having been in his office only once or twice and rarely talking with him, conceding that he usually won disputes with her when he wanted to proceed cautiously versus her desire to act with dispatch. She then would take her message higher up — directly to a president or friendly members of Congress, with whom her critics felt she had undue influence.[25]

Lasker friend, syndicated columnist Eppie Lederer, writing under the name "Ann Landers," agreed that Lasker was "intimidating" but also hard to resist with her engaging smile, bright blue eyes — she often wore blue, her favorite color — and her compelling facts. "Everything about her was so strong," Lederer said. The fact that she had "ideas and what might be called humanitarian concerns," according to DeBakey, led to Lasker's, "after a while, [gaining] the confidence of political leaders," even to the point of being "treated like royalty when she visited their offices."[26]

Mahoney, too, was usually greeted with warmth and respect in Congress, but for different reasons. "Florence was always outgoing, friendly, and warm," said Gorman, "while Mary was more mechanical . . . although she could be charming when she turned it on. Florence's approach was that of a background kind, a softening-up business which wasn't to be done mechanically." Still, he reflected, "I don't think they ever sat down to say, 'You take care of softening up this person and I'll take care of that one.'"[27]

"When I wanted to get things done, I started at the top," said Mahoney of how she worked. For example, "because I was friends with the governors of Florida and Arizona, when I wanted to work on birth control, I went directly to them." Her focus was almost exclusively on health-related issues. "I was never involved in women's issues with the exception of birth control. Nobody ever tried to get me involved."[28]

She, too, relied on facts but related them to human interests. A particularly valuable tool came to hand in the form of a readership poll that Cox conducted in 1950. Mahoney immediately perceived its potential for politicians. It revealed that articles on health subjects were the most popular by far of any other — close to 99 percent of readers said they always read health-related stories. That translated into public favor for Congress' spending money on medical research, and Mahoney frequently reminded members of the poll.

"I was with the governor when he read what the results were in the

Atlanta paper," she recalled. "He had drawn red marks around the subjects of high interest, and the only one that had, perhaps, 99 percent readership was *health*. He looked at me and said, 'Well, I guess you're right'" about how important health was in Americans' minds. "I told everybody about that poll from then on when we wanted them to do something, because they understood that" — the importance of the subject to average people.[29]

A tactic that both Mahoney and Lasker used was to recommend physicians and medical treatments for various ailments afflicting people whom they were courting, or their relatives. They advised where to obtain the best care and new or experimental medications that might help. Mahoney had sent Matt Connelly information about two physicians at the Mayo Clinic who had discovered a chemical compound — cortisone — to treat rheumatic disorders, which she said "might help Leslie [Connelly's wife?]." The researchers, Drs. Edward C. Kendall and Philip S. Hench, subsequently received a Lasker Award for their findings.[30]

It often helped if a member of Congress himself, or close relative, suffered from a disease for which the women were advocating research funding. Chairman Fogarty suffered a heart attack in 1953, which violently brought home to him what Mahoney and Lasker were trying to do. Senator Hill received help in obtaining the experimental drug L-dopa to treat his wife's Parkinson's disease.[31]

"We got one strange convert on the House subcommittee on appropriations," Lasker recalled of another member, "that was Judge [Christopher C.] McGrath [Democrat of New York]. Florence and I had talked to him when we had first tried to get additional funds for the Heart and Cancer Institutes in '48 and '49, but he had been very cynical and uncooperative. However, his brother-in-law, a priest, [found himself] in a research ward in Memorial Hospital and suddenly McGrath changed and actually said, 'You have been right all the time. I'm a sinner come to repentance.'"[32]

Republican Senator Styles Bridges of New Hampshire received Lasker's attentive ministrations one year when his vote was critical to a rise in appropriations. She sent him the latest drugs and special diet food for his hypertension. When she visited him, they talked about the ailment and the need for more research facilities. "General Motors can't work without equipment," she pointed out. It took a heart attack to get him to back the Heart Institute bill, but as a rule he usually voted the right way, from Mahoney's and Lasker's standpoint.[33]

Another empathetic member was George Smathers, whose father had arthritis, making him a supporter of research in that field. Democratic Senator Richard Neuberger of Oregon became an even more "passionate apostle of medical inquiry," as one columnist put it, after discovering that he had cancer. Thanks to radiation treatment, he was able to return to the Senate.[34]

Mahoney's knowledge of "how to do publicity" added to the team's assets. "My advantage over most people was that I knew a lot about newspapers. And I knew news when I saw it — more or less. Especially the kinds of news I *liked*," she laughed. She contacted the media herself whereas Lasker had a publicity woman. "I never had that. It wasn't difficult, though. It was the people I knew, and my friends in the press helped me. She didn't know anything about the press in Washington, and I certainly did. The press is desperately important, I'll tell you that, terribly important." She had learned very early in her career to help journalists by giving them information. "I planted things in the papers all the time."

The tactic changed the attitude of an important member of the Senate. "One time I said to Doris Fleeson, a hardworking newspaperwoman and syndicated columnist for the *Washington Star*, 'You know, there's one woman in the Senate, and she's never done a single thing for health — and she's a woman.' It was Margaret Chase Smith," Republican from Maine. "That hit Doris, she understood that, and she wrote a column about Smith. She was in Bangor when she read it, and it upset her so that she began to do a lot for appropriations for research. It took Doris Fleeson and her bad publicity, which may have forced her a little bit. She and Hill became great friends." During the Eisenhower years, Smith would prove to be an ally, urging fellow Republicans to back increased research funding.[35]

Lasker herself enjoyed press attention and used it to publicize her causes. On a three-week holiday to Hawaii in March 1955, she and Mahoney were interviewed and photographed as celebrities on their arrival. "Dark-haired and attractive, Mrs. Lasker is enthusiastic about recent progress in public health," the *Honolulu Star-Bulletin* reported. She was quoted as saying, "I believe that the two most exciting recent developments are the Salk vaccine for polio and the two new drugs for mental health which curb outbreaks of emotional illnesses and help untreatable-till-now mental diseases." That year she had received a *Woman's Home Companion* magazine award as one of six outstanding women in America; *Parent's Magazine* also had given her an annual medical award for outstanding service to children, as had the American Heart Association.[36]

Mahoney and Lasker had a close personal relationship that enhanced their ability to work together. "Your birthday present is here in your room," Mahoney wrote Lasker in December 1954, "so the next time you cannot be in such a hurry — there is always so much to tell you and so little time."[37]

In a self-mocking reference to travel arrangements to meet Lasker in Italy that year, Mahoney joked that she was "always reliable regardless of your deprecation of my character (re: plans and reservations)."[38]

Self-education

Mahoney, to enhance her education, frequently attended professional and scientific conferences on health subjects and socialized with eminent physicians who were leaders in their fields. "One night I went to a night club — everybody used to go to night clubs — and this young doctor, Bill Foley, was there. He was then one of the head heart doctors at a New York hospital with Dr. Irving Wright, the most famous heart doctor in New York. During the conversation, Foley said he'd just come back from prison camps in Japan, where he had been a P.O.W. He told me how interesting it was that Americans' blood vessels were hard but the Japanese whom he had seen had blood vessels that were just like babies because of their diet. That was the first time I ever heard the word 'cholesterol' mentioned" and its relationship to hardening of the arteries and heart disease. "No one ever mentioned cholesterol in those days. That's why I remember it so distinctly."

She and Lasker "followed a lead on *everything* that we ever heard about," Mahoney said, not only for new research potential but "just to know what was going on. And there was only one way to find out, and that was to see anybody whom you could get information from, even in a night club." She would make notes "on any piece of paper I could find" about what she learned "to remind myself to write it more intelligently."

Consistent with their desire to "see what was going on," she and Mary pursued the cholesterol matter by visiting Dr. [John?] Goffman in San Francisco. He had examined commercial airline pilots and noted their cholesterol levels, making predictions as to their longevity. While the women were sitting in his office, he received information that one of the pilots had died. He checked his records and found that his prediction on the man's early demise had been accurate. "That was very telling," Mahoney said of the information that she and Lasker could add to their case for more heart research. Other physicians were skeptical of the new cholesterol findings at the time, even Goffman himself, but Mahoney had perceived that "no doctor ever believes anybody *else* when something *new* is discovered."

She remembered an interesting incident at a heart conference that she attended in Princeton. "The chairman was a very well-known heart doctor. I guess there were about twenty people there. A psychiatrist was going to speak after the heart specialists, but the doctors hated the whole thought of that. He *did* speak, though, and after he finished, one of the doctors said, 'Please open the windows!' It was the middle of winter, but that was his comment — what he thought about psychiatry! He wanted to change the subject, and the air, I guess."

At another meeting, Mahoney heard a speaker "who said smoking was bad for people," a revolutionary thought at the time. "I went home and told Mahoney and thought he would use it in the paper. But he said that people would think he was *crazy* because everybody in the world was smoking. So the next time I went to a heart meeting and the doctors mentioned it, I took some conference papers home with me and gave them to Drew Pearson, and he used it the next day. He was the first person who ever mentioned in a newspaper how bad smoking was for you," she believed. "Right after that, both *Time* and *Life* magazines used it." She also felt that cigarette manufacturers "should not be allowed to advertise — that was a long time ago, when I was saying it should not be glamorized."

Another campaign centered on an anti-coagulant heart drug that had been tested on plantation workers in Hawaii. Irving Wright had been "one of the first people to use" the drug on heart patients, according to Mahoney, but like many other potentially promising treatments, it was not "being researched sufficiently. That was the whole point of trying to get money for research." Coincidentally she found out that the physician who headed Detroit's Ford Hospital, whom she met one evening in Miami Beach, had suffered several heart attacks. She "begged him" to talk to a doctor who she knew was experimenting with anti-coagulants. "I made an appointment for them to see each other because they were both at that moment in Florida. The doctor from the Ford hospital went on the drug and was very pleased with what happened. It benefitted *hundreds* of people after that and soon was a very well-known treatment." Mahoney's social contacts were serving her well. "I only knew about it because I knew one of the famous doctors in Hawaii. I was often where people were doing things like that, so I was always hearing everything."

Scientific breakthroughs sometimes helped bolster Mahoney's and Lasker's arguments. "The research of Drs. Philip Hensch and Edward Kendall of the Mayo Clinic in 1949 on the use of cortisone and adreno-corticotropic hormone (ACTH) for treatment of rheumatoid arthritis was a very important finding," Mahoney recorded. "It has been used since in many diseases. That stimulated interest in research, too, and in the whole field of adrenal cortex and steroids generally. The material was very expensive and it was important to have clinical research [proving its effectiveness]. We hoped for a line-item in the budget for those substances. $2.5 million was added to the budget for research of the two drugs. That stimulated funds all over the United States" for additional research on the substances.[39]

Dynamic duo in Congress — Hill and Fogarty

The two most important members of Congress for Mahoney's and Lasker's ends were John Fogarty and Lister Hill, chairmen of the key health committees in their respective bodies. They, too, were entirely different in style and personality. But both men were consummate politicians who had the same desire as Mahoney and Lasker to foster the growth of the federal NIH for the betterment of humanity.

John Fogarty was a straightforward, down-to-earth former Irish bricklayer and union official from Harmony, Rhode Island. He had been elected to Congress in 1941 at the age of twenty-eight and by 1949 had risen to be chairman of the House Appropriations Subcommittee on Labor-Federal Security Agency, which decided funding for federal health programs and departments. He attained the chairmanship by seniority, not for his scientific expertise. Fogarty, though, despite having only a high-school education, did his homework and learned his subject with astonishing mastery, particularly details about how taxpayers' money was being used. While he relied on Lasker's "facts" and Mahoney's up-to-date knowledge about what was going on in research fields, he also relied on the savvy NIH Director Shannon for perspectives on what promising research needed funding. *Newsweek* magazine in 1961 described Fogarty as "Mr. Public Health" — "soft-spoken and retiring (except for his bright-green bow ties) . . . immensely popular with his fellow congressmen . . . [having] what his colleagues consider a truly brilliant mind, an amazing memory, and a great motivation to help the helpless."[40]

"Fogarty was always very sensitive because he'd never been to college; he was very self-conscious about it," said Mahoney. "But he was so *smart*, he could talk back to the people who were doing the research. If it hadn't been for them," she added of Fogarty and Hill, "we never would have gotten all that money."

Lister Hill was entirely different in demeanor from Fogarty. Invariably described as a "gentleman," the Southern senator had a long family background in the health field. His father was a pioneering heart surgeon who had named his son after his mentor, Lord Joseph Lister, the discoverer of antiseptic surgery. Two brothers-in-law and five cousins of Hill's were doctors. He himself would have been one had he not discovered as a youth that he became ill at the sight of blood and open wounds. His knowledge of health subjects came naturally, though, and his name was attached to the first federal program for hospital construction, the Hill-Burton Act of 1946.[41]

Over the years he had demonstrated personal conviction and bold independence in advocating federal aid to education when most of his Southern peers opposed it as a way to force desegregation of schools. Hill, once a majority whip, had resigned that post during early civil-rights debates and regrouped his Southern partisan credentials by filibustering against such bills, but in his heart he was a "New Deal" Roosevelt Democrat, aware that the States' rights "Dixiecrats" had limited scope and popular appeal. By 1955, because of his seniority, Hill had become chairman of the Appropriations Subcommittee on Labor-Health, Education and Welfare and had the rare opportunity of chairing the corresponding authorizing Committee on Labor and Public Welfare.[42]

Mahoney, justifiably, felt a personal responsibility for this dual power base. She had gotten to know Hill through the Democratic Party and his brother, who had been stationed at Miami Beach during the war and lived near the Mahoneys. When Democrats regained control of Congress in 1954 after one term, Mahoney learned that Hill might not seek chairmanship of the Labor and Public Welfare Committee and set about convincing him to do so. One night she joined the senator and his wife for dinner at their house — just the three of them. While Mrs. Hill was cooking, Mahoney "sat for a long time, holding Senator Hill's hand" and talking with him about the chairmanship. "I didn't tell him we *needed* him as chairman. I just stressed how important it would be for him and his reputation." Lasker was backing another man for the post, but Mahoney talked with Hill about how the Eisenhower administration was not interested in supporting health legislation, especially research, and pointed out that Hill could become a national leader in the field.

"He was the most popular man in the Senate, really, and the most important. He was head of appropriations, too. He could have had anything" he wanted to chair because of his seniority and popularity. "So we sat together and I told him the story about Governor Cox's readership poll in the papers. I told him how it would be the best thing he could do, that it would make him far more famous than anything else. Well, anyway, he took it."[43]

For the next fourteen years, Hill, with his counterpart in the House, virtually controlled legislation over all government health programs. For good reason, he was called "Mr. Health," steering to enactment some sixty bills. His combined position was a fruitful one for Mahoney and Lasker. "I was very close to him," said Mahoney, "Mary related to him in a different way."[44]

Gorman's relationship with both men was another important catalyst. "He got along with Fogarty quite well, being Irish as Fogarty was, but he and Lister Hill always saw eye to eye," Mahoney related of Gorman's compatibility with the Irish bricklayer and the physician's son. "They all understood each other" even though the two members of Congress, an unlikely pair, "didn't mesh very much together."

With the help of the Mahoney-Lasker-Gorman team, Hill and Fogarty made sure that Congress, rather than presidents, kept the initiative in setting spending priorities. An example of both legislators' political strategy was their disdain for annual budgets submitted by presidents. Each year the appropriations chairmen went through the same routine with department and executive-branch officials. Knowing that NIH's budget requests — which institute directors and their advisory councils prepared — were reduced by higher-ups in the HEW Department and cut further by the Budget Bureau acting for the president, Hill and Fogarty would press NIH witnesses to reveal their original desires. Then they would blame the present White House for ruthless cuts and ultimately get their subcommittees to restore what NIH originally sought.

During one hearing in 1956, Hill reflected on a theme of Mahoney's and Lasker's: "My mind continually goes to the atomic bomb," he said. "If we had sat down and said, 'Well, now, we can't spend too much . . . we have to take this a little more slowly,' we wouldn't have gotten the bomb when we did."[45]

Fogarty in particular derided the budget bureaucrats, saying that he based his judgments on the "experts," particularly Shannon, who understood what kinds of research would benefit from funding in a given year. Fogarty also combined his growing knowledge with a personal commitment and political astuteness, choosing for emphasis medical programs that he knew his colleagues would like. His choices were reinforced by carefully chosen, well-briefed, and friendly "citizen witnesses" from the Mahoney-Lasker-Gorman stable who presented a "citizens' budget" that often bore a striking similarity to what NIH directors had originally proposed. Fogarty referred to such witnesses as "window dressing" for his purposes, unwilling to downplay his own role. But to Mahoney and her colleagues, they were essential to convincing Congress to act. The famous names also garnered good publicity whenever they appeared, which members noticed.[46]

Fogarty was overtly scornful of federal budget staff, even insulting one hapless man at a party in 1958 for retiring HEW Secretary Marion B. Folsom. It caused such a commotion that President Eisenhower was visibly startled, and Fogarty hurriedly escorted out of the room by Labor Secretary James Mitchell and Assistant HEW Secretary Elliot Richardson. Hill was even more disdainful of the "green eye-shade" accountant-bureaucrats, not bothering to have budget staff testify before his committee and maintaining that they were of no help. He, too, relied on the medical "experts" and Shannon.[47]

Both Hill and Fogarty were credited by NIH officials for giving the agency money without too many strings attached, thus allowing exploration in basic medical sciences despite pressures for attention to specific diseases and applying research to cures. "We'll get the money," Fogarty was quoted as saying, "You fellows spend it." And it was Mahoney and Lasker and their band of distinguished backers who helped "get the money."[48]

The reports that accompanied committee recommendations, laying out Congress' legislative intent, often were reviewed and augmented by Gorman as well as government officials like Shannon. Once Fogarty had convinced his committee to raise figures, he generally had no trouble getting them past the full House. The Senate then acted. Hill and his committee, as well as the full Senate, usually added to the House figures, necessitating conferences between the two bodies in which compromise figures resulted that were higher than the House's and the president's.

All of this Mahoney and her colleagues understood. They carried their message daily in private visits to congressional members, beginning with committee "mark-up" sessions and through the legislative process each year until bills finally were signed by a president.

An important tactic, though, was to make it appear that Congress had acted alone. "Originally we pretended that we weren't responsible, that it was all the senators and congressmen who were doing it," Mahoney noted. "I thought we should be very quiet and that nobody should know what we were doing at all, that the congressmen had to get credit for it themselves."

As their successes grew, the women realized that the issues had their own momentum and that they did not have to broker with politicians or government officials who balked at their objectives. "Nobody bothered us at that point; we just went ahead and did what we wanted to do," she said.

Hill and Fogarty needed Mahoney and Lasker as much as the women needed them, and all frequently socialized together. Fogarty honored Lasker at a party in June 1952. "I am having a group for dinner at my home on Wednesday next, and I hope you will be able to join us," his invitation to both women read. "The group will consist of Members of Congress and people directly concerned with the Public Health program. Dress comfortably because it will be in the nature of a barbecue and will be outdoors entirely," he added. "We will have an opportunity for some discussion before dinner if everybody arrives around that time (6:30)."[49]

Albert Lasker had just died, and Fogarty wrote Mary a touching note of condolence: "You have lost Mr. Lasker as a companion, but you will never lose the good things that live on in his name .... I hope in the years to come that we will all justify his high hopes for doing more for people and making this a little better world to live in."[50]

The following month Mahoney wrote Lasker, "Saw Fogarty who tried to get me to go out to dinner, etc., but never did get to. I told him [how] very appreciative we had been and especially you that he had taken such trouble to have the party for you. He was pleased. I told him how touched you were."[51]

Mahoney's relationship with Fogarty was so well known that she was asked to help keep him in the House of Representatives when he briefly considered running for the Senate, which, if he had won, would have meant giving up a powerful senior post in the lower body to become a junior member of the upper one.

"I was in a pool in Florida when a call came from Democrat Claiborne Pell," who said that he was considering running for the Senate from Rhode Island and wanted Mahoney's help persuading Fogarty to stay out of the race. Fogarty had been under pressure from friends to run, and Pell was aware that Mahoney knew the congressman well. She agreed to talk with him. "Fogarty really liked the House," she realized, "and decided to stay put" — as much to her advantage as Pell's, who was elected to the Senate, where he remained for thirty-six years (1961–97).

Like Fogarty, Hill had his full committee pretty much in line. A few, like Republicans Everett Dirksen of Illinois, Gordon Allott of Colorado, Roman Hruska of Nebraska, and Democrats William Proxmire of Wisconsin and Paul Douglas of Illinois, made efforts on the floor to stop the NIH bandwagon, but they rarely succeeded, prompting Hruska to quit the committee in frustration.[52]

"Charming" was another adjective used to describe Senator Hill, "so persuasive . . . so quietly indispensable, and so personally self-effacing," Douglas said, "that we want to give him everything that it is possible to give him . . . . The National Institutes of Health owe their extremely flowering condition to the Senator from Alabama," Douglas conceded before the full Senate but added with sarcasm, "They have money running out of their ears, money they do not always know what to do with."[53]

Mahoney's relationship with Hill was exceedingly warm, so much so that he did not hesitate to recommend her for another advisory council after her four years on the Mental Health Institute's ended in 1954. Mahoney wrote him from Italy, where she was traveling with Lasker, to ask him "to do what you think best about the following problem."

You know how important it is to have lay members on the various Institute Councils and people who know what is going on. Before this administration, the choice of the lay members was not political and should *not* be. Senator [Edward] Thye [chairman of the Labor-HEW appropriations subcommittee] wrote to Madam [Oveta Culp] Hobby [Eisenhower's secretary of HEW] asking to have me put on the Heart Council. He has never heard anything from her and I know she will try and not do it by saying there is no place. However, one of the members has just died . . . so that leaves one place that we know of. You would think that she might like to do what Sen. Thye wishes considering he is chairman of the subcommittee but I don't know him well enough to tell him he should make an issue of it. So . . . . [sic] I thought you might suggest me and she would be *terrified* not to pay attention to you! Mary's name was suggested for the Cancer Council by [Senator Styles] Bridges and we hear that [Hobby] thought that could not be ignored.

You know it is a lot of hard work but since we work so hard to get money for research it is important to have representation on the Councils so you can direct or help get things to happen.

I heard that [Hobby] tried to find a Republican Negro from the South for the Heart Council (this from a very high Republican friend who is on one of those presidential advisory committees).

You will know best what to do and perhaps you think you should stay out of it and if so, I shall understand.[54]

"I am sure you know Mrs. Mahoney," Hill wrote Hobby a few days later, "and are familiar with her great interest and devoted efforts in the cause of research, and prevention and cure of heart disease. I think Mrs. Mahoney would be an excellent appointee, and I strongly commend her to you." It was "a pleasure for me" to make the request, he told Mahoney. "I do not know of anyone who more richly deserves the honor or who will render finer, more devoted or more constructive services than you will."[55]

As Mahoney expected, however, she was not appointed. A polite response to Hill, signed by Acting HEW Secretary Nelson A. Rockefeller, said that although Mahoney "is well known to us," council members had been "selected for all of the vacancies for next year. However, we are happy to receive your recommendation and will keep her in mind when future appointments are made."[56]

Hill renewed his request in 1956, telling the new HEW Secretary, Marion B. Folsom, that Mahoney was "tirelessly and unselfishly serving the cause of the health of the American people," adding, "She is a very intelligent and fine lady." Again, she was rejected by the Republican administration. Hill shared the disappointment, telling her, "You may be assured that I shall continue to do everything I can in behalf of your appointment to the Advisory Council of the National Heart Institute. I so much want to see you on the Council. A million thanks for everything."[57]

Hill repeated his request with a third HEW Secretary (Arthur S. Flemming) in 1958, this time for the Cancer Council. Mahoney finally was appointed in October 1959 to the National Arthritis and Metabolic Diseases Advisory Council. Hill jotted a personal note on a letter of congratulations saying, "I rejoice over your appointment." (Following that she would serve on the National Child Health and Human Development Advisory Council beginning in 1963.)[58]

Mastering the art of lobbying

With the help and skills of Gorman, Mahoney and Lasker became masters at lobbying during the 1950s.

Part of the technique was to keep things simple, in terms that Members of Congress and the public could readily understand. For that reason, the Microbiological Institute had its name changed to Allergy and Infectious Diseases when a powerful congressman, according to legend, was said to have sniffed, "Whoever heard of anybody's dying from microbiology?"[59]

By the mid-1950s the Mahoney-Lasker team had put together a stable of "citizen" or "outside witnesses" (nongovernmental), renowned publicly as well as in their professional fields, whom they regularly called on to testify before Congress. Senator Hill "loved to have a witness whom he could call 'Doctor,'" former Senate Labor and Public Welfare Committee chief clerk Stewart McClure recalled in a biography of Hill. Rusk, Farber, and DeBakey were regulars before the congressional committees, usually testifying on behalf of professional societies or medical schools.[60]

Mahoney and Lasker themselves, as members of NIH advisory councils, were legally precluded from officially lobbying for the institutes they served. Their National Mental Health Committee, however, was not and became particularly helpful to Congress because it could gather and present more timely data than that provided by government agencies, often outdated because federal budgets were drawn up months in advance of hearings. Congressmen therefore often called on groups like Mahoney's and Lasker's, whose committee, thanks to Gorman, built a reputation for accurate, objective information. Its noted medical experts then would tell Congress which promising projects would go begging if money were not forthcoming to complete certain research.

"The President's budget was prepared at the time by men who did not have available the figures that I have been giving you on the number and cost of approved research projects," Farber, speaking as professor of pathology at Harvard Medical School, told one panel, when arguing for more cancer funds than the president's budget requested.[61]

Lay witnesses also proved to be tremendous assets to the cause. For years hearings had been dominated by medical practitioners and scientists, but it was the lay testimony that often caught the congressmen's, to say nothing of the media's and public's, attention. Senator Hill considered citizen witnesses very influential because, he was quoted as saying, "They had the knowledge, the expertise, the facts."

They also provided emotional drama. When a constituent of Fogarty's from Rhode Island, Daniel McIver, a victim of multiple sclerosis, appeared before Fogarty's committee in 1956, one congressman said, "I know I will not say anything embarrassing to you when I say how deeply I feel for the courage with which you have adjusted to this situation."

Gorman was very effective at finding such witnesses and increasingly was called upon by Hill and Fogarty to do just that. He steadily gained their respect because of his knowedge of data and his personal commitment to improving research efforts, which made up for his lack of a professional degree.

Members of Congress who had personal experience with diseases also made excellent witnesses, like Senator Charles Tobey of New Hampshire, whose daughter had died of cerebral palsy, pleading for increases in funding for that problem.

Government officials, however, accused Mahoney's and Lasker's committee of inflating their figures in hopes of restoring what the Budget Bureau had cut from NIH's wish list. Mahoney and Lasker responded to such charges by saying that their "citizen committee budgets" reflected what they believed could be effectively spent and were often compromises between high and low budget estimates. Indeed, even Shannon credited citizen groups as more helpful and far-sighted than the directors of some of his institutes in making persuasive cases for higher funding.[62]

Gorman early on perceived that it was important for his witnesses not to talk in technical terms that put congressmen to sleep or went over their heads. He absolutely forbade those whom he brought to testify to use such terms as "myocardial infarction." "I say, 'You call it a heart attack or leave the room,'" he told a reporter of how he prepared his witnesses. "That, and no smoking," he added. "Those are the two rules."

It was hard, he admitted, to find the "right combination" for witnesses — they had to be respected but able to use plain language while being passionate about their subject. Baylor University heart specialist DeBakey was "unique," Gorman said at the time. "He has the aura of the surgeon, he's articulate and enthusiastic. Most doctors are not enthusiastic, not used to the verbal give-and-take. The Rusks, Farbers, DeBakeys have evangelistic pizzazz. Put a tambourine in their hands and they go to work."[63]

Occasionally things did not go according to plan. In 1955 Farber brought to testify with him a presumed ally, University of Chicago cancer researcher Dr. Charles Huggins, like Farber a future Lasker Award winner. In response to a question, however, Huggins stunned Farber and Gorman by agreeing that a ceiling on research funds was advisable to avoid their being wasted. That was not what he was supposed to say. Fortunately for their side, Huggins was followed by the well-briefed director of the American Cancer Society, who stated that a "flood" of money to the Cancer Institute would push forward projects that otherwise would go unfunded.[64]

On another occasion, a medical expert whom Mahoney had persuaded to appear before Hill described in graphic detail every known method of birth control. In pursuit of knowledge about research innovations in reproductive biology, Mahoney had visited one of the leaders in the field, Dr. Kermit Krantz at the University of Kansas. She was so impressed with what he was finding that she asked Senator Hill to invite him to testify before his committee. Krantz, whom Mahoney had gotten to know as a fellow member of the NICHD Advisory Council, startled the senators with his avid support of family planning in any form. "You don't wait for a smallpox epidemic before you vaccinate!" he exclaimed before Hill's committee. "If I had *my* way, I'd put the [contraceptive] pill in the water supply!" he blurted out to an increasingly squirming panel of senators.[65]

"He called a spade a spade," as Mahoney put it. "Hill said to me afterward, 'Don't you *ever* do that to me again!'" she laughed of the reprimand, imitating Hill's Southern accent. "He was *so* embarrassed! You know, men used to be embarrassed if we *mentioned* birth control." One senator who was not, though, was Ernest Gruening of Alaska, who asked that Krantz's testimony be sent to a long list of people, including the secretary of HEW, India's Prime Minister Indira Nehru, other members of Congress, and influential columnists who could spread the word.[66]

By the mid-1950s Mahoney had a reputation in Washington that merited media comment. Her friend George Dixon portrayed her as "one of the nation's leading do-gooders" — "vice chairman of the National Mental Health Committee; vice president of the National Health Education Committee; a member of the [Advisory] Council of the National Mental Health Institution; and the Washington contact of Mrs. Mary Woodward Lasker of the Mary and Albert Lasker Health Research Foundation."

Mahoney, Dixon said, "had Dr. Paul Dudley White [an eminent heart surgeon and one of Eisenhower's physicians] in her corner long before Ike did. She had the now world-famous heart authority pounding the Capitol corridors with her in efforts to induce Members of Congress to vote for money for health research. It was tough going, and many were the rebuffs they endured. On one occasion they were coming out of a Senate Appropriations Committee hearing, after being virtually told they were socialized-medicine crackpots, when they bumped into the senior Senator [Republican John W. Bricker] from Ohio going in."

"We sort of bumped into each other," Mahoney said of the encounter, "and he started giving me hell; he was really quite loud about it. He was saying how his state didn't need any more research money from the federal government and how he wasn't 'influenced by the Cox papers either.' He obviously knew who I was. He started *screaming* at me — I was terrified. He really was quite rude talking to me! Just then Dr. White walked up — he'd been there to testify. And I said, 'You know who Dr. White is?' — President Eisenhower's heart doctor and before that the best-known heart doctor in the country, and such a *gentleman*. So I introduced them, 'Senator Bricker, meet Dr. Paul Dudley White.'"

Dixon was a witness to the confrontation. "I just happened to be passing," he wrote, and "had the inestimable privilege of watching my former dancing partner join with Dr. White . . . in making Senator Bricker pull in his neck . . . Bricker glared at Dr. White and began to rant. 'Don't pressure me!' the GOP stalwart bellowed. 'Stop trying to get my people in Ohio to bring influence to bear on me. I won't stand for it.'

"'Stand for what?' asked Dr. White politely.

"'You've been telling my people Ohio needs money for health research. Ohio doesn't need money.' The Boston cardiologist remained soft-spoken and courteous. 'That's strange,' he told the fuming senator. 'We have a request right here from the Medical School of Ohio State University.'

"Bricker gulped. He came down off his high horse. 'Somebody lied to me!' he apologized."

"I asked Mrs. Mahoney what keeps her working at fever pitch for health," Dixon concluded in his profile of her. "She gave me the smile that once palpitated hearts from Moose Jaw to Medicine Hat. 'I don't want to see my friends dying ahead of their time,' she replied. 'And I don't want to die ahead of schedule either!'"[67]

It also helped, Mahoney, Lasker, and Gorman knew, if witnesses were friends, constituents, or at least acquainted with members of the committees who listened to them. Gorman often arranged for that to happen, selecting witnesses from members' districts and personally setting up social opportunities for them to meet and talk informally. It was then harder for a congressman to vote against such witnesses' positions. After some years on the job, Gorman claimed to be "on a first-name basis" with 175 members of the House and able to get "a few senators on the phone" without any trouble. Many in Congress in fact often called Gorman for advice.[68]

Fogarty was good at drawing out witnesses to his ends for the legislative record — like getting the anti-research president's personal physician to justify such expenditures of taxpayer money. "So there isn't any question in your mind that this money is being well spent, that we are advancing and getting greater knowledge every year because of the amount of money we are spending on research? Is that a fair statement?" Fogarty asked Dr. White.

"The difference in the situation [from] when I was a medical student forty years ago and now . . . is the difference in night and day," White responded. "We were really in the dark ages in medicine then. The dawn is here. I don't think we are quite fully in the golden age of medicine, but we are getting there."

Fogarty put to a cancer researcher in 1958, "This budget that the president has given us is going backward. What does that mean so far as the general public is concerned?"

"It means a great impediment to progress in the field of cancer," she replied.

"I thought it was worse than that," Fogarty persisted.

"I would personally consider it catastrophic," the witness stated. That was more like it.[69]

Surviving setbacks

Coping with the Eisenhower administration posed problems that the women had not encountered before.

Mahoney had been a devoted backer of Adlai Stevenson, the 1952 Democratic presidential candidate. Her description of the Chicago nominating convention, which she attended, was full of enthusiasm for her candidate. "It was fun being right in the middle where I knew *all* from every angle," she wrote Lasker.

> It really looked as if [Vice President Alben W.] Barkley might be the one for a short time . . . . [I]t was almost 2 a.m. when Stevenson was nominated and then after that Truman and Stevenson spoke. It was very exciting and in my life have never known anything as thrilling as Stevenson's speech. I have saved it for you . . . Mrs. T[ruman] looked so pretty and both had tears in their eyes during Stevenson's speech . . . . Our editorial writers said [it was the] greatest speech since Gettysburg . . . .
>
> I feel certain after listening to Stevenson that Eisenhower hasn't a chance . . . . This will be a campaign that will change the old ideas of campaigning and no name calling of the candidates. They are killing the General with kindness.[70]

Mahoney's presidential prediction this time, though, would not be as correct as for Truman in 1948. The Republicans not only took over the White House but both Houses of Congress as well.

"At that time the atmosphere in Washington for cutting the budget was hostile to anything that had been done by Mr. Truman or the Democratic administration," she said. Her immediate reaction was to make friends with Republicans in positions of power, such as the new chairman of the appropriations subcommittee handling Public Health Service funds, Senator Edward Thye of Minnesota. "He was very interested in the NIH work," apparently because "his wife had diabetes. Anyway he was easy to work with and came to my house for dinner several times with his wife. Frank Neeley [prominent businessman], a very good friend from Atlanta, tried to help with the new director of the budget, Joseph Dodge of Detroit, whom [Neeley] had known in business. Floyd Odlum, also well known in business and in California and Republican circles, was interested in arthritis as he [was] an arthritic patient. I think he took that up with Eisenhower."[71]

Mahoney's decision to befriend Republicans had been made early in her career, when she first learned that Albert Lasker had campaigned against Governor Cox. "I decided that you couldn't let politics interfere with everything." It would be a useful philosophy and a trademark throughout her life. She now set her sights on an important figure in the Eisenhower administration.

Confronting Secretary Hobby

Mahoney and Lasker wasted no time in contacting the person who would head the new president's health department, a woman whom they initially hoped would think much as they did. Slightly more than a week after Eisenhower's inauguration, "we could no longer wait and felt we should visit with Mrs. Oveta Culp Hobby, the newly appointed Federal Security Administrator, who was soon to become the Secretary of Health, Education and Welfare (HEW)," according to Mahoney. "I had known her previously" through contacts with newspaper people.[72]

Hobby, who had served under Eisenhower during World War II as director of the Women's Army Corps in Europe, was a Texas-born politician married to the owner of the *Houston Post*. A lifelong Democrat and former parliamentarian of the Texas House of Representatives, she had switched to backing Republican Eisenhower in the 1952 race. He picked her to succeed Oscar Ewing, initially as head of the Federal Security Administration, which then merged with the newly created HEW. She was the only female member of his cabinet.[73]

"We had asked her to dine with us alone, just to get to know her," Mahoney remembered, "and she came very prettily dressed, amiable, non-committal, sympathetic but cautious. She was very pretty, sort of beguiling. I thought we should tell her what we needed in money. We did not talk about anything specific and felt friendly toward her but realized that it would be a long pull to get her to take any important forward steps in the health field as she would have to get the support of the AMA. She did say, however, that night that she did know how the AMA worked and had had great trouble with it in Houston in connection with the blood program.

"We were determined the next morning that the thing to do was to try to introduce her to Mike Gorman and Dr. Russel Lee of California, one of the outstanding members of President Truman's Commission on the Health Needs of the Nation. We met within the next ten days. We also had an appointment with Mrs. Hobby in her office. She looked small behind the big desk that Oscar Ewing had formerly occupied. She was calm and composed and very careful but cordial at the same time. We had a pleasant talk with her and she promised that the research funds in the budget would not be cut as far as she was concerned."[74]

Mahoney invited Hobby to dinner several times, at least once with Russel Lee and Howard Rusk. On such occasions, "All was very agreeable and we explained to her the importance of the research program." But it became "rather obvious that she wasn't going to make any big effort in the health field."[75]

Hobby was to prove a particular thorn in their sides. She consistently asked the Budget Bureau to cut NIH's research allocations, even when Senate Majority Leader Robert Taft, one of Eisenhower's closest advisers, died suddenly of cancer in 1953. "Many senators, especially in view of Senator Taft's tragedy, were shocked" by Hobby's budget cuts, Mahoney recalled. "They felt that medical work to find cures for these dread diseases was all important. But though Mrs. Hobby wanted medical-research funds reduced, simultaneously she wanted her own budget for her own office to be increased."[76]

Mahoney had a fortuitous opportunity to counter Hobby during a 1953 conference between House and Senate committees trying to resolve differences between respective funding figures. Hobby was observed sending a note to conferees. A friendly Senate staff aide, who saw Mahoney in the press gallery, where she often watched floor debates, slipped her

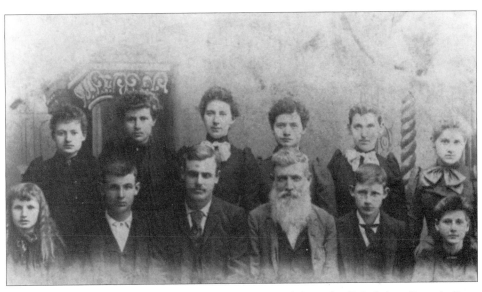

Florence's mother, Julia Tina Stephenson (upper right), and Julia's father (bearded) and brothers and sisters, circa 1892. Julia's mother was no longer living. *(Courtesy of Florence Mahoney)*

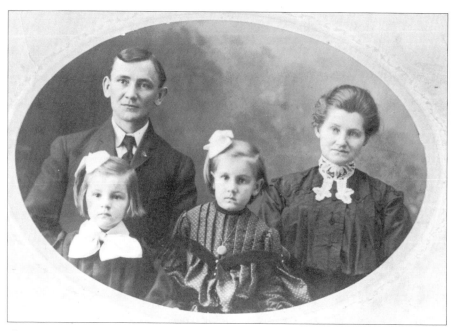

Florence (in center) with her parents and younger sister, Mildred, circa 1904. Her second sister, Mary Louise, was not yet born. *(Courtesy of J. Michael Mahoney)*

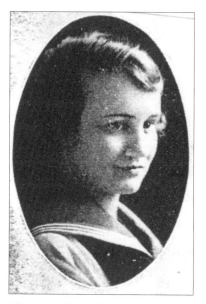

Florence Sheets in Muncie High School yearbook, 1917. *(Courtesy of Central High School)*

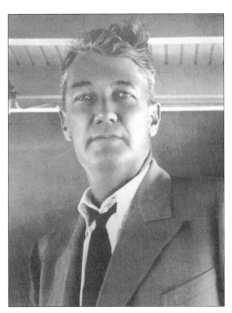

Daniel J. Mahoney, early 1930s.
(Courtesy of J. Michael Mahoney)

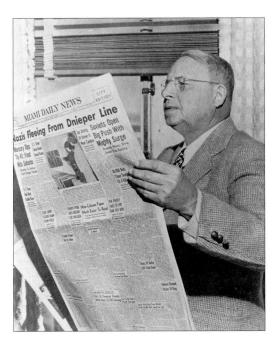

James Cox reading one of the newspapers he owned, December 1943. *(Courtesy of Cox Enterprises)*

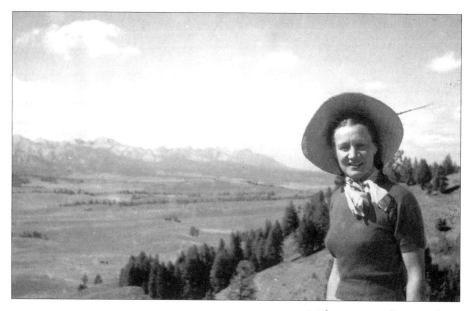

Mahoney traveling north toward her ranch near Stanley, Idaho, 1940s. The Sawtooth Mountains are in the background. *(Courtesy of J. Michael Mahoney)*

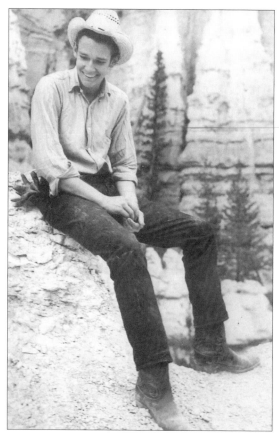

Daniel J. Mahoney, Jr., in Idaho, circa 1948. *(Courtesy of Florence Mahoney)*

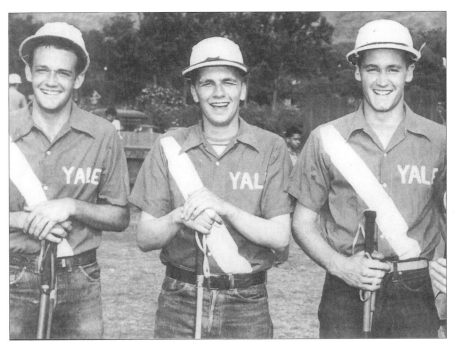

Michael (right) joins the Yale polo team of Daniel Jr. (left) and Greg Baldwin (center) for a game in Honolulu, 1950. *(Courtesy of J. Michael Mahoney)*

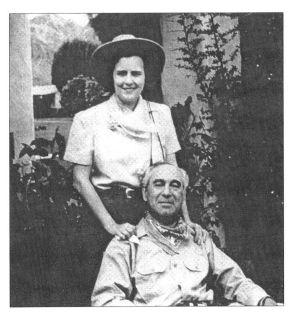

Mary and Albert Lasker, 1940s. *(From* Taken at the Flood *by John Gunther)*

Sep. 5, 1944

HYANNISPORT
MASSACHUSETTS

Dear Madam Mahoney:

I hope this reaches
you before you leave Ketchum.
I did'nt receive your letter untill
yesterday, due to that superhuman ability of the Navy to
screw up everything they touch-
even the simple delivery of a letter
frequently over-burdens this heaving
puffing war-machine of ours. God
save this country of ours from those
patriots whose war cry is " what this
country needs is to be run with
military effenciency". Anyways,
thank you very much for your thought.

Joe's loss has been a great shock
to us all. He did everything well
and with a great enthusiasm, and even
in a family as large as ours, his
place can't ever be filled, andhe
will always be missed. But thank
you for your sympathy.

In regard to the fascinating
subject of my operation, I should
naturally like to go on for several
pages on a subject of general interest
like this- but will confine myself
to saying that I think that the doc
shaould have read just one more book
before picking up the saw. It may
have to be done again. I got out
of the hospital the other day, and go
back the nineteenth. If you are in
Bosoton that day, I should love to
see you.

HYANNISPORT
MASSACHUSETTS

Otherwise you can get me on the
phone Hyannis 980.

I have read ᴃᴏᴛᴃ Mr.
Vansittart's book- I imagine that
a great deal of his force comes from
his remembrance of his son, and what
the Germans did to him. In regard to
Monsieur Menninger's Love against
Hate and Man against himself, I shall
put them on my Fall reading list,
and from the titles, I feel sure
that they will enable me to dominate
the annual meeting of the Bosꬵton
psychiatric ᴍXXXXᴍXX association.

Thanks again for writing-
please remember me to Dan and the

boys.

Affectionately

Jack

Letter from Jack Kennedy to Mahoney, 1944. *(Courtesy of Florence Mahoney)*

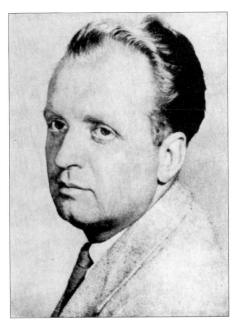

Mike Gorman, 1956. *(Courtesy of National Library of Medicine)*

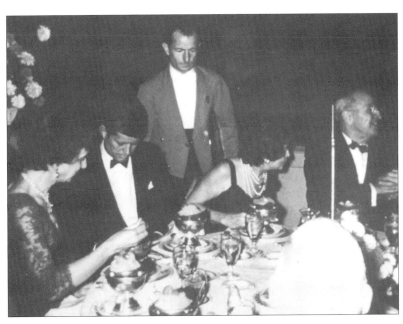

Mahoney flanked by Senator John Kennedy and former president Harry Truman at a dinner in honor of Eleanor Roosevelt, 1959. *(Courtesy of Florence Mahoney)*

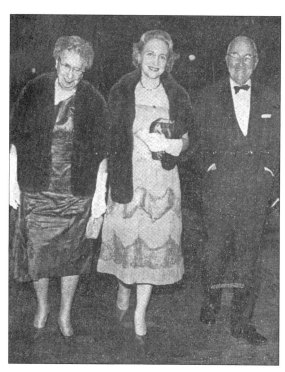

The Harry Trumans
and their daughter
Margaret as they leave
a party given for them
by Mahoney at her
Georgetown home,
January 18, 1961.
*(Photo by City News
Bureau)*

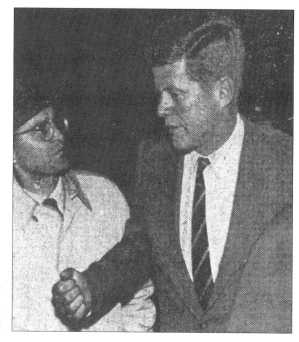

President-elect
Kennedy drops by
Mahoney's party for
the Trumans. *(Photo
by City News Bureau)*

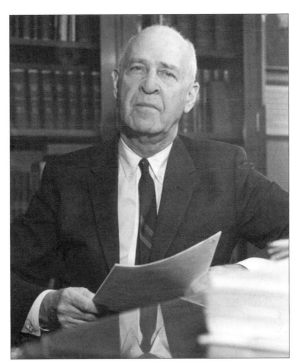

Senator Lister Hill, 1962. *(Courtesy of Library of Congress)*

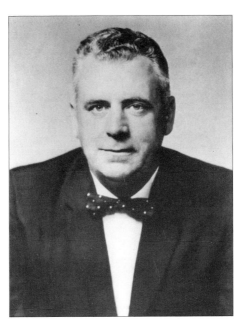

Representative John Fogarty, 1960.
(Courtesy of National Library of Medicine)

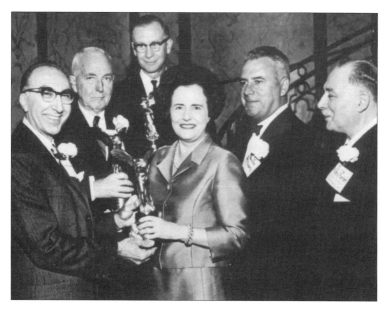

(from left to right) Michael DeBakey, Lyman Craig, Charles Huggins, Mary Lasker, John Fogarty, and Sidney Farber at 1962– 63 Lasker Foundation Awards presentation. *(Courtesy of National Library of Medicine)*

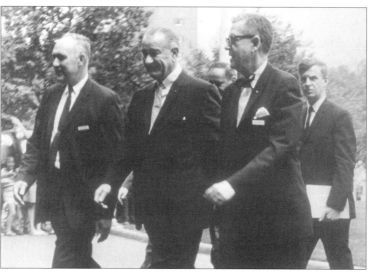

On a visit to NIH in 1967, President Johnson is accompanied by NIH Director James Shannon (right) and Surgeon General William Stewart (left). Philip Lee, carrying folder, is walking behind. *(Courtesy of NIH History Office)*

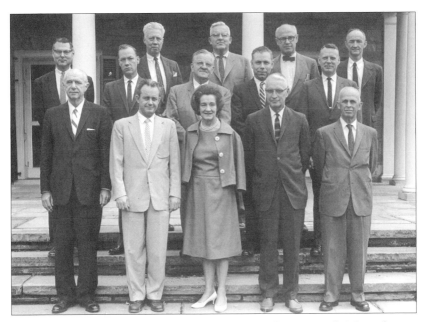

Mahoney and other members of the National Advisory Arthritis and Metabolic Diseases Council, June 1962. *(Courtesy of John F. Sherman)*

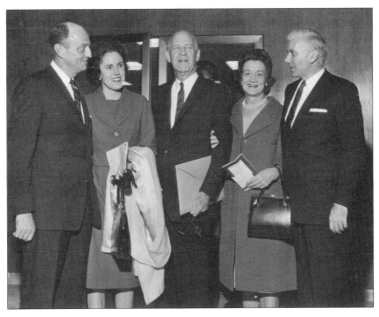

Surgeon General Luther Terry, Mrs. Boisfeuillet Jones, Senator Lister Hill, Florence Mahoney, Boisfeuillet Jones, at NIH ceremony, circa 1964. *(Courtesy of Boisfeuillet Jones)*

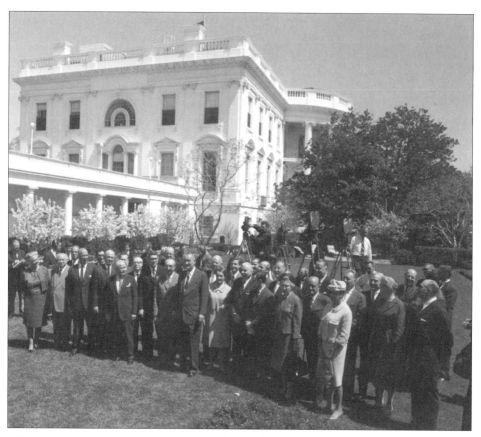

White House lawn ceremony with members of Heart, Cancer, Stroke Commission, April 1964. Mahoney is standing next to President Johnson. *(LBJ Library, photo by Cecil Stoughton)*

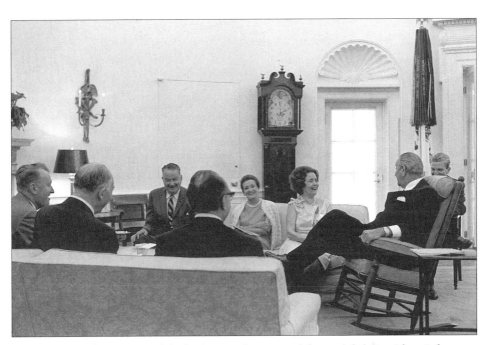

Oval Office, White House. (clockwise starting second from right) President Johnson, Douglass Cater (behind rocking chair), Michael DeBakey, Sidney Farber, Mike Gorman, Howard Rusk, Florence Mahoney, and Mary Lasker, July 1968. *(LBJ Library, photo by Yoichi Okamoto)*

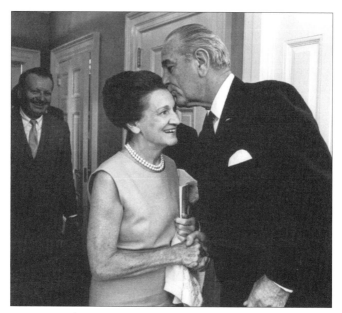

President Johnson greets Mahoney at White House, July 1968. *(LBJ Library, photo by Yoichi Okamoto)*

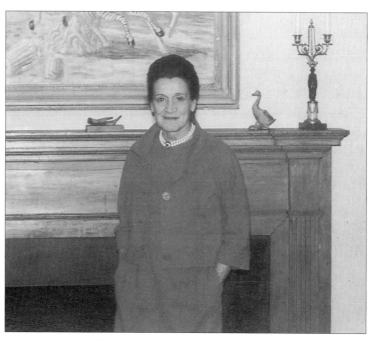

Mahoney in her living room in Georgetown, December 1968. *(Courtesy of Florence Mahoney)*

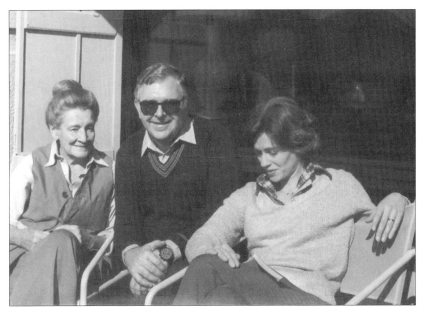

Mahoney with Joseph and Ann English, 1968. *(Courtesy of Joseph T. English)*

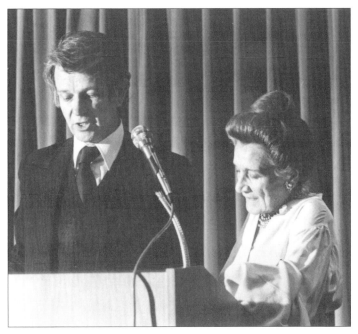

Robert N. Butler, first director of the National Institute on Aging, presenting Mahoney an award in 1978 acknowledging her service on the Institute's Advisory Council (1974–1978). *(Courtesy of Robert N. Butler)*

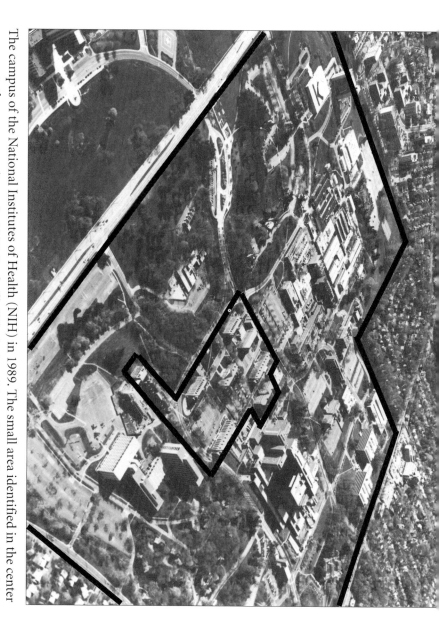

The campus of the National Institutes of Health (NIH) in 1989. The small area identified in the center represents the campus as it was in 1947. Rockville Pike is the wide road in the lower left portion of the photograph. (*Courtesy of NIH History Office*)

one of them, saying "I thought this might interest you." To her astonishment, it argued against raising NIH's budget on grounds that it would "discourage" private enterprise in the research field.

Hobby made the case that most researchers in recent years were finding adequate funds in the private sector. "While it is clearly important from the standpoint of the public interest to move ahead with medical research," the note read, "the question is one of rate of increase and of the distribution of funds . . . . [T]he great majority of scientific investigators . . . who have demonstrated promising talent have been provided the opportunity to pursue their research interests . . . . It is well to leave room for private participation in these areas," she concluded. "The larger increases [that have been] suggested might tend to discourage such participation by private or other non-federal funds."[77]

That point of view was a holdover from the days when private disease-oriented societies feared that government involvement in research would put them out of business because contributions would dry up. The contrary, however, had occurred: As government funding rose and new institutes were created, so did private contributions and the number of disease-related organizations. (Another factor was the pharmaceutical industry, which was concerned that government development of drugs threatened its investments in patentable products.)

Mahoney acted quickly to expose what she considered Hobby's outdated and unreasonable rationale. "I showed the memo to Murray Kempton," columnist for the *New York Post*. "He was appalled and wrote a column for his paper the next day saying something about how this woman must have 'ice water in her veins.' She was shaken by the column, which many other papers used."[78]

Kempton's column, under the headline "Death and the Lady," excoriated Hobby for fighting for research budget cuts "like a she-wolf for her cub."

In this case, she was in flat disagreement with the medical profession's major authorities on cancer and heart research . . . .
Mrs. Hobby told the Senate Appropriations Committee with total

absence of shame that she had cut the heart and cancer funds without talking to any experts in the field . . . [adding that] nobody "ever wants to recommend a cut" — nobody, of course, except this "Iron Maiden."[79]

When Hobby was asked by Democratic Senator A. Willis Robertson of Virginia if she would "violate the law" by refusing to spend additional funds appropriated by Congress, "She responded with manful silence." Meanwhile Republican Senator Charles Tobey of New Hampshire had died of heart disease and Taft of cancer, prompting Kempton to say derisively, "But Mrs. Hobby is unbothered by the night thoughts that afflict Senators. Whatever her weakness, the symbol of warmth is untroubled in the region of the heart."[80]

Another friend of Mahoney's, widely syndicated investigative columnist Drew Pearson, also wrote scathingly, "While Sen. Robert A. Taft was fighting for his life," Hobby was asking the Budget Bureau director to cut the federal cancer-research budget by $5 million and other medical research by $10 million. "Private fundraising for medical research has never been remotely adequate," he continued, noting that even "Walter Winchell, who has faithfully plugged for cancer research for years, has only been able to raise $5 million. In comparison, Congress has voted approximately $20 million for cancer every year . . . . With Senator Taft dying and with three other Senators out of five dead of cancer in the past three years — Kenneth Wherry of Nebraska, Arthur Vandenberg of Michigan and Brien McMahon of Connecticut — Congress, in the end, voted against Mrs. Hobby."[81]

Although no longer attached by marriage to the Cox newspapers, Mahoney maintained her productive relationship with members of the press, especially syndicated columnists. "I have asked many of the correspondents to keep asking everyone about their stand on health and research," she wrote Lasker in 1952. "The Alsops, especially Joe, and I became great friends, also Marquis Childs and a few others. I told them all how sad it was re: Brien McM's dying of cancer so young. He is the 3rd now . . . . Said what good did it do him to try and save the world from atomic bombs if he had to die of cancer? I am getting Mr. Locke [of Cox newspapers] to do one of his columns on it for he is good and then we can use them for propaganda purposes. Sent him all of the fact sheets and told him no one had approached McM.'s death from that angle."[82]

"Thank you so much for the editorial re: cancer and McMahon," Mahoney subsequently wrote Locke from London. "It is perfectly written and I will have it read in the Senate and put into the *Congressional Record* and then use it in many ways, in our nefarious maneuvers."[83]

Hobby nevertheless defended her budgets on a "Meet the Press" appearance in October 1954, touting the administration's generosity. "We have this year the greatest sum of money we have ever had to spend for direct research and for research grants — [$63 million], $10 million more than we had last year and, I believe, in '52 [when] it was $43 million. I believe we have used it wisely and intelligently."

But one panel reporter, Lawrence Spivak, quoting figures that sounded as if they came from the National Mental Health Committee, caught her out. "Isn't it true that the Eisenhower administration cut the programs as against the Truman budget on various projects — on cancer from $22 million to $15.7 million, mental health from $15.9 to $9.8 million, heart disease projects from $16.5 million to $11 million? In the line of our urgent needs in these fields, do you think these cuts were justified?"

"I believe we are spending as much money as we can spend intelligently," Hobby repeated. But Spivak pressed on: a total of $60 million for research compared to "$50 billion for arms, $500 million for one aircraft carrier alone? What do you think of this?"

Again, Hobby demurred, reiterating her theme that other entities besides the federal government contributed to the work — "states, private foundations and other groups interested in research."[84]

Polio scandal

Mahoney and her forces, however, got an unexpected break that aided their cause. In the spring of 1955, the public was informed that Dr. Jonas Salk of Pittsburgh had developed a successful anti-polio vaccine.[85]

Hobby's "real blow came after the announcement of the Salk vaccine, when Senator Hill, in a hearing, asked her — very politely — 'How are you going to distribute it?' and she said 'People can just go to their doctors and get it,'" as Mahoney put it. "I can still see Senator Hill's face turn red. A newspaper columnist called me about that." It would make sensational headlines.

The manufactured supply of the vaccine was insufficient to meet the huge demand for it, something Hobby weakly told the senators "no one could have foreseen," an oft-quoted phrase in the press that would come back to haunt her. There was such a clamor for the vaccine, and for government help for the poor who could not afford to pay for it, that Senator Hill sponsored a bill to make it free to all children between the ages of five and twenty. That smacked too much of "socialized medicine," Hobby argued. The bill was enacted over her objections.[86]

Drew Pearson wrote that Hobby "had taken the stand that polio vaccine, like cream cheese, is a commodity and ought to be distributed under a 'voluntary' system." She finally agreed to some government management after continued media attacks and an exacerbation of the problem when batches from one manufacturer actually infected 204 children with polio. Although such problems were not her fault, Hobby became the butt of cartoons by the *Washington Post*'s Herblock, calling her Secretary "of Not-Too-Much Health, Education and Welfare," something Mahoney thought apt, given Hobby's concerted efforts to cut research spending.[87]

"This is not the first time that Senators have raised the question of whether Mrs. Hobby, a woman of immense charm and proven business ability, is not miscast in her Cabinet post," Mahoney's friend Doris Fleeson wrote in the midst of the crisis. "It is almost an article of faith with most men that all women are deeply and emotionally concerned with the problems which come under HEW jurisdiction, but in the words of the song, 'It ain't necessarily so.' Mrs.Hobby is a cool conservative by conviction who moves cautiously in areas of social policy which arouse the crusader instincts in her critics." Mahoney, who marked the column "file," counted herself among the latter.[88]

Her hand was evident in another Fleeson column, in which she wrote,

"Figures have been presented to Congress and Mrs. Hobby showing that the tax return from those saved by present new [medical] techniques has far exceeded the cost of research for those techniques." The "figures" no doubt were supplied by Mahoney from the Mental Health Committee and Lasker's fact sheets.[89]

"One trouble with Mrs. Hobby," Pearson wrote in another column, "is that she's been so gun-shy of being tabbed a 'welfare state' executive that she's run away from some of her most important duties. Even [former Republican President] Herbert Hoover [in a commission report] points this out . . . . [She] is scared to death about promoting health, education and welfare . . . . Why did Mrs. Hobby want to cut medical research by 10 million dollars in 1953? When the Senate, led by Lister Hill of Alabama, opposed a budget cut in research on cancer, polio, heart disease, epilepsy, muscular dystrophy, etc., Mrs. Hobby actually wrote to the Budget director urging that her own budget for medical research be cut — even though the Hoover Commission now has urged more money for research . . . . It's almost unheard of for a Cabinet member to urge a budget cut. Yet Mrs. Hobby took a definite stand against medical research. Fortunately, Senator Hill put through the appropriation over Mrs. Hobby's protest . . . . [She] seemed afraid she might be accused of promoting socialized medicine," Pearson wrote, chiding Hobby for behaving more like a Secretary of Commerce than Health, Education and Welfare.[90]

Despite the criticism, Hobby continued her cost-cutting approach, which kept Mahoney, Lasker, and Mike Gorman busy. One Hobby scheme was to shift from individual research grants to a formula for grants-in-aid. Hobby and Nelson Rockefeller, her undersecretary, made presentations to Congress that Gorman derisively noted required "two days of rehearsals" and featured "loads of snappy charts." They "exaggerated the complexity and difficulty of the present individual grant formulas," he told Mahoney and Lasker in March 1954. Despite Rockefeller's "beautifully straight-faced job on each of the formulas, by the time he got through listing all the varying percentages and other yardsticks, he had a number of committee members laughing out loud." One chart was "fraudulent," Gorman said, and the new formula meant "very little to us." He predicted that it would die in the House appropriations health subcommittee, whose chairman, Fred Busbey, had told Doctor Sheele that he was "tired of hearing requests for general health grants. We are interested in specific diseases and we want to find out where our money goes," Gorman paraphrased Busbey as saying.[91]

That, of course, was just what Gorman and his colleagues liked to hear, that Congress was interested in "specific diseases." It was no coincidence that the two diseases that got the most money were cancer and heart because they were the leading causes of death and the most feared.

Hobby got out of the public spotlight when she resigned in 1955 to take over management of family businesses when her husband became gravely ill. Her successor, Marion Folsom, was more of an advocate for medical research on grounds that it could prevent or rehabilitate people who had chances of returning to productive work. Folsom's first budget justifications in fact used Lasker Foundation figures. He was "as forward-thinking as you could be in the Eisenhower cabinet," Hill reflected. Folsom appointed a "blue-ribbon" panel of advisors chaired by Doctor Stanhope Bayne-Jones and, on its recommendation, proposed a substantial increase for NIH in the 1958 budget. Even then, Congress exceeded the president's budget request, as it would continue to do under Folsom's successor, Arthur S. Fleming, and for many years forward, to Mahoney's and Lasker's satisfaction.[92]

Mahoney deplored an editorial in the Cox morning newspaper in Springfield, Ohio, that praised Hobby when she resigned, "not only because she brought a compassionate and conscientious mind to [HEW] but also because her stewardship during the first two years of its existence involved her in certain difficulties inseparable from pioneer ventures. She has known all the perils, but few of the rewards of trailblazing," it stated. On the clipping that she sent Lasker, Mahoney wrote, "How uninformed — I complained to him [the editor] and Cox and Dan'l." The afternoon paper, however, more accurately reflected Mahoney's views, that "The long-rumored departure of Mrs. Hobby from her Cabinet post . . . need cause no one pain." With Hobby and the polio debacle gone, Mahoney could once again turn her attention to the things that mattered most to her.[93]

Countering Eisenhower opposition

The Eisenhower administration had two friends on the House Appropriations Committee, Democrat Clarence Cannon of Missouri, chairman of the full Appropriations Committee, and Republican John Taber of New York, who did their best to hold the NIH budget down and thwart Fogarty. "Crusty budget cutters," the *Washington Post* called them at Taber's death, "prone to debate money matters at the top of their lungs in rasping voices hard to follow."[94]

They rarely succeeded because Fogarty's strategy was to promise other subcommittee chairmen that their pet measures in his appropriations bills would not be modified when they were considered by the full committee. In effect, Fogarty was able to overrule his chairman. By the time the money bills got to the floor of the House, there was little that antagonists could do but bluster and complain. It helped that a large body of fellow Irish members always rose to speak in favor of Fogarty's increases and to praise the gentleman from Rhode Island for his able leadership in the field.[95]

Fogarty's success in leading a floor fight for NIH increases in 1954 inspired Majority Leader Sam Rayburn to praise Fogarty's floor speech as "one of the most powerful and convincing . . . arguments that I have listened to since I have become a member of this House," and "I am not given to complimenting people on this floor, as everybody who has served with me knows." A Republican colleague, Representative Charles A. Wolverton of New Jersey, admitted that "The gentleman from Rhode Island leaves no doubt that he is the best informed man in Congress on all details affecting our national health program." Fogarty would have chuckled had he heard the future chairman of his committee, George Mahon of Texas, modify the praise by remarking that "The trouble with John was that he wanted to give NIH *everything* but the Capitol dome."[96]

Another unexpected, if unfortunate, benefit to the Mahoney-Lasker cause came in the form of another heart attack — this one suffered in

1955 by then-Senator Lyndon Baines Johnson at the relatively young age of 47. It offered an opportunity that Mahoney may have suggested to her friend with enormous media exposure, Drew Pearson. "The best tribute [Congressman Fogarty of Rhode Island] and other Congressmen could give to Senator Johnson stricken with heart trouble is to okay the increased appropriation for medical research that has already passed the Senate," Pearson suggested in a July 10 broadcast. "Even though Secretary Hobby says she doesn't want the money, that appropriation contains important funds to find a cure for America's number-one killer — heart disease. Passage of that bill without further delay would be a belated tribute to Lyndon Johnson."[97]

Responding to a note that Mahoney had sent the senator, "Lady Bird" Johnson told her, "It means much to him to know that others are carrying on work which he considers important even when he himself is ill and cannot take part . . . . Meanwhile, during this period of inactivity, which is so difficult to bear, he is being greatly sustained by the thought that his friends are concerned and are wishing and praying for him to be restored to health."[98]

Johnson, to whom Republican Albert Lasker had given $500 in a 1948 campaign and who also was personally acquainted with Mary, became an even more enthusiastic backer of the Mahoney-Lasker cause than he had been before his attack, always supporting increased research funds. After addressing the American Heart Association in 1958, he wrote Mahoney, "It means very much to me that you appreciated my speech . . . . It certainly was a pleasure to have an opportunity to pay tribute to you and Mary — two people who deserve a lot more credit than you have received," he added. In another note to Mahoney he said that he would "be happy to meet the head of the News Bureau just as I am happy to have such a good friend as Florence Mahoney."[99]

"I have a personal interest in research on the problem of heart disease, of course," Johnson explained to a friend in Fort Worth, "and the death by cancer of Senator Taft a few years ago and former Secretary of State Dulles this week should certainly dramatize these needs."[100]

When President Eisenhower himself was stricken by a massive heart attack a few months after Johnson, the cause of heart research was further advanced in the public mind but especially in the minds of congressmen. Senator Robertson of Virginia commented to Mahoney in October, 1955, "While I personally think that the President's attack was of sufficient severity to make it extremely hazardous for him to attempt to run for re-election, I also am convinced that he might not have been able to finish out his current term but for the splendid treatment that he has received . . . from such a man as Dr. Paul White. And, of course, his illness has emphasized the importance of heart research and you and Mary won't have to work so hard in future years to get enough funds to keep the program going."[101]

Eisenhower, though, did not change his point of view on federal funding of research. Toward the end of his presidency, in 1959, he told his cabinet that "money alone isn't going to keep [Senator Johnson] or anyone else from having a heart attack."[102]

Lasker, by then on a first-name basis with Johnson, now Senate majority leader, sought help from the masterful politician. "I know you can get anything done that *you* want," she wrote him. "I am convinced that in the area of medical research we are preeminent in the world, and we must stay preeminent. We seem to be lagging in other areas of science as compared with the Russians. More breakthroughs in medical research will give us the energy, as a Nation, to go forward and stay ahead in the other scientific fields."[103]

Johnson agreed to speak in support of a $200-million increase over Eisenhower's request for the 1956 NIH budget. The speech was written by Gorman in his punchy style and reflected Mahoney-Lasker themes. Who had not been touched by childhood diseases like diphtheria and smallpox that now were largely eliminated because of research, Johnson asked rhetorically? Cancer had recently claimed five members of the body he was addressing, and the appropriations committee had held hearings on the Cancer Institute budget on the very day that Eisenhower's Secretary of State John Foster Dulles was laid to rest. "What the Commies couldn't do to our former Secretary of State, cancer did," he said, quoting the labor magazine *Machinist*. Johnson denounced Eisenhower's strategy to balance the national budget at the expense of medical research. Nearly two million lives had been saved since World War II because of such research, he stated, providing government coffers with additional tax revenue from healthy workers. Still, he argued, disease cost the nation's economy $30 billion a year and cut "at the very core and strength of our posture in the free world." The United States faced a "medical Sputnik" because Russia, ahead in space research, also had launched a fifteen-year program to conquer heart and cancer diseases.[104]

The strategy worked and the Mahoney-Lasker forces won the day. Two years later, then Vice President Johnson was the featured speaker at the Lasker Medical Awards Luncheon.[105]

Division in the ranks

The difficulties with the Eisenhower administration's budget-cutting efforts strained the relationship between Hill and Fogarty in 1955, when Fogarty adamantly refused to go along with big increases for research. He also may have had some controversy associated with campaign contributions at the time, to which Gorman alluded in communications with Mahoney and Lasker. Fogarty kept repeating at conferences between the House and Senate that NIH did not "need the money" — an additional $23 million that the Senate had allotted above the president's budget.

One source of Fogarty's antipathy may have been the fact that Mary Lasker had not gone "to the hospital to see him when he had a slight heart attack," Mahoney speculated. "He was so mad, he wouldn't give us any money."

For six weeks conferees haggled, finally agreeing, just before Congress adjourned, to a modest increase rather than the Senate's figures. Senator Hill was furious.[106]

During the lengthy negotiations, Mahoney, Lasker, and Gorman found themselves running back and forth across Capitol Hill to mediate between the two members of Congress. Just after Congress recessed in August, Hill urgently summoned Gorman to his office late one afternoon. They had an "unusual conversation," as Gorman reported to his chairwomen, exemplifying both the influence that the National Mental Health Committee had achieved by that time and how it operated.

> After some preliminary conversation about health legislation [in the forthcoming] 1956 session, the Senator got down to what was really bothering him — John Fogarty.
>
> The Senator was very angry about Mr. Fogarty's House speech of Wednesday, July 20th, in which he said the House figures were the most that could be properly spent by the Institutes during the coming year. Fogarty also implied in the speech that the Senate obviously didn't know what it was doing in appropriating higher figures. Hill said to me in a very angry voice: 'Who the hell does Fogarty think he is?' Hill pointed out that if Fogarty had had his way during the conference, there would have been no increase over the House figures. Hill said flatly that [Representatives] Lanham [of Georgia], Fernandez [of New Mexico] and [Winfield K.] Denton [Democrat of Indiana] would have gone up to $12 or $13 million but Fogarty wouldn't let them.
>
> Hill was even more annoyed at Fogarty's action in trying to kill the paltry sum of $250,000 for the first year of the mental health survey. He said that Fogarty fought against it for two days and only gave in because Hill told him the Senate would not appropriate any money in the supplemental bill unless the mental health item was included . . . .
>
> After documenting his case, the Senator said to me: "This man Fogarty has some personal reason for this negative attitude he has taken. I tried to explain to him that we were trying to build up the health issue for the 1956 [presidential] campaign and that therefore we had to vote appropriations much higher than the [Republican] Administration had asked for. Mr. Fogarty was deaf to this plea as to all others I made to him."
>
> I don't know how much Senator Hill knows about what happened during the last election with regard to Fogarty's campaign funds. However, he had called me up for the specific purpose of

warning me that the Fogarty issue must be resolved before the 1956 session. He pointed out that the Democratic Party could not make health an issue if Mr. Fogarty persisted in his present attitude.

"What does this all add up to?" Gorman asked rhetorically of his co-chairs. "Hill is the strongest ally we have in Congress. However, he is a political realist. At one point, he said to me very directly: 'Why should we in the Senate break our backs trying to pass health legislation which has no chance in the House?' The very fact that he called me to his office right after the close of the session is indicative of how strongly he feels about this."

Gorman realized that he, Mahoney, and Lasker were being given marching orders. "Hill understands that there are only two approaches to Fogarty," Gorman continued, "either an agreement with him . . . prior to the 1956 session, or an all-out effort to expose his negativism publicly. At one point Hill said: 'If you can't make an agreement with him, you mustn't let him get away with what he is doing.'"

"I still feel that Fogarty can be made to see that he is pursuing a harmful course," Gorman concluded. "However . . . a real effort must be made to sit down at the table with him early this fall and reach an understanding on outside witnesses, research construction, appropriations, etc. I think it will be well for us to make the pilgrimage to Providence," Fogarty's Rhode Island district, "and to see Pope John in the Vatican," Gorman joked.

"In the event that Fogarty decides to continue his spiteful ways," Gorman felt, "then we ought to inform him, politely and pleasantly, that it is our duty to inform the people of his actions. For example, if he does not agree to hear outside witnesses in 1956, we can bring so much unfavorable publicity down on his head that he will have to hear those witnesses. I have never believed in skirting a basic issue."[107]

That was a pointed reference to the fact that Hill had taken testimony from friends of research like Doctors White, Farber, and Rhoads, while Fogarty had not.[108]

Another troublesome problem for Senator Hill was the fact that an old friend of Fogarty's, former Air Force Colonel Luke Quinn, had taken a part-time job with the lobby group after his retirement in 1952. Fogarty had talked Lasker into contributing funds to the American Cancer Society to retain Quinn, who had been a legislative liaison for the air force and thus was well known in Congress. Hill believed that Quinn had drafted Fogarty's negative speech and, if true, warned that "Colonel Quinn had better stay away from the Senate side."[109]

"I think this indicates that the Quinn matter ought to be resolved, too," Gorman wrote. "I have long been of the opinion that Quinn does harm rather than good to our cause. He is merely a hostile shadow of Fogarty and he reinforces Fogarty's prejudices."

"I urge you to do some thinking about it," Gorman concluded. "If it bothers Senator Hill, who has a million things on his mind, then it certainly should bother us to the point of a solution."

Fogarty was brought in line and in the end rewarded for re-joining the fight on the side of the advocates: In 1959 he was given a Special Lasker Award as was Hill for their "extraordinary public service, unique and preeminent contributions to the public health and medical research."[110]

Society and monkeys

Mahoney's style of advocacy centered on her genial way of entertaining, bringing together people who otherwise might not have spoken to one another or discussed matters thoughtfully without the benefit of relaxation and time to indulge such conversations. In that social role, Mahoney was a natural.

"It is probable that there is no one who has been important to health policy in Washington who has not dined — on, among other things, assorted tasty health foods — at Mrs. Mahoney's. They usually leave with an armload of reading material," political writer Elizabeth Drew stated in a not entirely flattering retrospective article about Mahoney and Lasker in *Atlantic Monthly*.[111]

Rather than a "socialite," although she was referred to as such in society pages, Mahoney was a master at putting people together. "I could just see they *ought* to be together," she said, "it was the chemistry of the people I invited." She scoffed at the image of herself as a salon hostess. "Not exactly that!"

She favored small groups of only six or eight people for dinner so that they could talk at the table. "Never more than that. If it were a big party, that was different, but I generally just had dinners. At first I had all these senators and people coming to my house but they didn't accomplish anything because they drank too much — as happens quite often at a party when you have cocktails first." Her goal was to educate by letting certain people make their points to the assembled group. "I generally tried to get just *one* person to talk at the table. It's the only way you can *learn* anything. You didn't want them all to talk at once." Columnist Joseph Alsop, a frequent guest, helped control the conversations. "If anybody spoke when he wasn't supposed to, he gave them hell!"

The intimate scale of her house, filled with antiques and fine art, necessitated keeping parties small. On occasions when the number exceeded the size of the dining room, they spread across the hall into a library.

George Dixon, in his autobiography, called Mahoney "one of the most effective and accomplished women in Washington . . . [who] moves robustly among the nation's great . . . . This charming, if some-times impatient, lady . . . has no time for the purely social, preferring the socially pure. She is a militant foe of 'ordeal by cocktail' as Ireland's Ambassador Thomas J. Kiernan described our civic pastime after only four months in our midst. Mrs. Mahoney holds that no party, except the Democratic, should have more than eight people." As a result, he added, "Many [Washington] hostesses have become converts to this theory. Seated dinner parties of not more than 16 are making inroads upon stand-up canapé-snatchings . . . . Chairs are replacing buffet tables. (Note to furniture manufacturers: The sofa is making a comeback.)"[112]

"Florence Mahoney hates to cook and never does," another journalist's account of her social activities stated, "but she loves to entertain influential members of the House and Senate in her elegant Georgetown house. Eventually, during one of her small dinner parties, she will bring the conversation around to what she sees as the enormous benefits of health legislation. A lobby, of sorts, social and unofficial — but often effective."

"She collects china and people," the account continued. "She eats peanut butter sandwiches at her desk at lunch and pours over medical journals. Her . . . house . . . is full of fresh-cut flowers, 18th-century Chinese pieces and an orange tree. The coffee table is piled with magazines and books from Albert Camus to Dan Greenberg. The bar is well stocked and even includes a special vermouth imported from France." Her "consuming interest is health care," and although "she is not a registered lobbyist nor is she paid, she takes advantage of every contact with every legislator she knows to get her thinking across."

"Mrs. Mahoney dresses conservatively in a simple sheath and double strand of pearls," the reporter wrote, "her reddish hair piled in a beehive. She often stops work in mid-afternoon for tea with honey and a pastry baked by her Mexican cook. Most of her friends are Democrats, although she knows and likes [a number of Republicans]. She never has more than eight for dinner. 'I invite doctors, senators and congressmen,' she says . . . . 'The Democrats are much livelier than the Republicans — that's not something I've dreamed up. You can see the difference during a Democratic rally and a Republican rally.'"[113]

Mahoney kept Lasker, who lived in New York City, informed of her social activities as they affected legislative objectives. Describing a typical weekend in the spring of 1954, Mahoney wrote:

> [Republican Senator John Sherman] Cooper [of Kentucky] was here Friday p.m., came by after dinner to introduce a friend to me
> . . .
>
> Saturday we went to the Senate for lunch with Smathers and several others and . . . saw the Senate in session. Then I asked some people for cocktails and all came and stayed for supper — very gay, some young and some old. Sen. and Mrs. [Eugene D.] Milliken [Republican of Colorado] came early, he in snappy white suit — the Mansfields, Mike Monroney, "Scoop" [Henry M. Jackson, Democrat of Washington], the Fulbrights, Russell, Sen. [Prescott S.] Bush [Republican of Connecticut] (he is Jean's [daughter-in-

law Mrs. Daniel Mahoney's?] godfather or her sister's) and Sen. Thye, the Scottie Restons, Bill White of the N. Y. Times, Doris [Fleeson?] Sr. and Jr., etc. The young stayed down in yard on terrace (it was cool for a change) and the others sat upstairs and ate off trays and on floor and discussed the week of McCarthyism. The Restons had a 1st cousin of Iphigene Sulzberger [wife of Arthur Hays Sulzberger, publisher of the *New York Times*] with them. Sen. Thye calls me Florence and seemed to have a lovely time.

Then yesterday the Drew Pearsons had a party at their country place — swimming and sit-down supper on terrace with most beautiful view in Wash., high up over the Potomac. Thurman Arnold and Justice Black and lawyer Randolph Paul plus some young at my table and the conversation very interesting. Arnold is always thus. Came to town with the Hennings [Missouri Senator] . . . . Hennings says no one can come close to Mr. S[tevenson] for the nomination in '56.[114]

The anti-Communist campaign of Wisconsin Republican Senator Joseph McCarthy in the early 1950s concerned Mahoney in great part because of its chilling effect on NIH and research scientists. When McCarthy's investigators targeted the Public Health Service as a hotbed of disloyalty, Eisenhower directed the FBI in 1953 to set up a security office to screen scientists receiving NIH grants, and Secretary Hobby began denying support to grantees on whom the FBI had derogatory information. Some thirty scientists, including Nobel Laureate Linus Pauling, were removed from their projects and a number of grants terminated. NIH advisory councils (Mahoney was not then on one) started requiring that grantees sign loyalty oaths, something that scientists deplored as irrelevant to their work and debasing of their integrity. At one point, Mahoney wrote FBI Director J. Edgar Hoover, who responded by thanking her for newspaper clippings and "remarks which were published . . . emphasizing the need for retaining the FBI solely as an investigative agency."[115]

In 1950, after the outbreak of the Korean War, Mahoney became involved in a personal campaign to acquire a large number of monkeys for a colony in Florida that NIH wanted to establish to study the long-term effects of radiation. Mahoney contacted every person she knew who might be in a position to help.[116]

"There were all these monkeys set aside in India for research at the University of Miami, but the war came along and there were no plans to pick them up. I wanted to get them to this country where they could be used for research. So I went to President Truman and he said, 'Go and see Secretary [Louis] Johnson, secretary of defense at that time. He was irate and said it was the most ridiculous thing he had ever heard, think of the negative publicity if it came out that the government was transporting monkeys. He was remembering the experience when [Elliott] Roosevelt had a dog shipped by government plane, but that was no comparison, I said. This was for medical research. 'You have the cargo planes, just bring them back on those.' I said that because I had learned that all the planes carrying cargo to the war zone were coming back empty. So there was no reason not to" transport the monkeys that way. "But anyway he wouldn't do it." So she next went to the president of Pan American Airways.[117]

"Such a day," she wrote Lasker, "have been trying to get 2,000 monkeys over from Calcutta for Sanders and all freight planes have been taken from Pan Am for the Pacific war effort, so had to call Sam Pryor [airline executive] and [Juan] Trippe [president of Pan American Airways] and now they think they can get them over on a returning plane under the defense dept., namely via my friend [Louis] Johnson again. Then a VP of Pan Am has polio and wanted to get his Dr. in touch with Sanders to see if he wouldn't try the present serum. All of this via tel. as Sanders is in Chicago. The VP is only 42 and both arms and legs paralyzed and very ill (he in N. Y.)."[118]

Another whom she contacted was Donald S. Dawson, an administrative aide on Truman's staff to whom she wrote from the Arizona ranch in August, with a delightful aside, "I hear via sonar (such a new word not even in dictionary) — (we have a dear little colony of bats in the patio here and if you are up on 'bats' they travel by sonar) — that there is a move afoot, bypassing Mr. Johnson, to bring the monkeys in through Sam Pryor via General [Laurence Sherman] Kuter [distinguished U. S. Air Force officer]. Will let you know how it comes out."[119]

She finally went to Secretary of the Air Force Stuart Symington. "I complained so strongly to him, that he said, 'I'll bring back your god damn monkeys!'"[120]

Mental health

Mental-health programs, an ongoing concern of Mahoney's, Lasker's, and Gorman's during the 1950s, fared badly compared to other health programs, receiving fewer than 5 percent of grants and contracts for all medical research. "Our knowledge of mental illness today," Gorman wrote, "is in many ways as limited as that of undefined infections in the days when we lumped them all together as 'fevers.'" In his book, *Every Other Bed*, Gorman angrily pointed out: "There is always money for more B-52s, but when those of us who testify for more psychiatric research ask the Congress for an additional million or two, the screams of 'economy' and 'where will we get the money?' can be heard over in Virginia" [where the Pentagon was located]. Yet, the equivalent of only "three-tenths of one per cent of the nation's defense budget" was spent on medical research, "less than the amount spent on monuments and tombstones," Gorman sniffed.

He was recommending changes throughout the mental-health system, which, even by 1956, he felt was "still incredibly isolated from the main stream of American medicine, a stagnant and weary tributary cut off from the bubbling river," what he called "a sorry chapter" in the nation's health history.[121]

Surgeon General Scheele, too, advocated changes such as reducing institutionalization by shortening hospital stays for mental patients and helping them return to society, thus lowering the "staggering" financial burden on state and local institutions. Such concepts were relatively untried in the 1950s but needed to be expanded, he said, along with experiments on alternative treatments like halfway houses that were community- rather than hospital-based. "An ability to assimilate new concepts, new methods and new partnerships in the solution of old health problems" was needed, he argued.[122]

Gorman himself was given credit for stimulating mental-health legislation when he testified on appropriations in 1959. He praised Chairman Fogarty for getting Congress to fund mental-health training, to which Fogarty responded, "It was *your* idea." Maybe so, Gorman said, but "I had no vote when the mark-up session came" in committee.[123]

Mahoney continued her own mental-health advocacy and served from 1950 to 1962 as a "governor" of the Menninger Foundation, a board formed to help raise funds for the clinic and research. The clinic was responding to the movement that Gorman's articles and Mahoney's early advocacy had helped start, which had grown into a popular cry for more humane treatment and care of the mentally ill than the traditional custodial hospital system and more preventive activities and community-based treatment that brought patients out of hospitals into society. It was aided at the time by the development of psychotropic drugs such as Thorazine. Mahoney took a special interest in the potential for new drugs to aid the mentally ill.[124]

"While I was on Menningers' board, it came out that a pill had been developed that might help people with depression. We were very excited about that, but we had to get [government research] money for it. We finally did, but when I went out to a board meeting, the doctors were talking about everything else but didn't mention medication for depression. They were all dead set against medication, it was so new. I told them that when I had studied in high school, we were taught to examine, explore new things. And it was hell to get the money for it." Soon afterward she left the board. "They did such good work that I didn't want to be too upsetting."

She tried to get experts in the new drugs to appear before congressional committees to make the case for medication and one day arranged for Gorman to meet the director of the National Institute of Mental Health, Dr. Robert Felix, to talk about its setting up a pharmacology testing program. But knowing of Gorman's unabashed candor and quick tongue, she exhorted him to behave. "Now Michael," she said, "we're going to have lunch with Dr. Felix. Will you promise me you'll be good? 'Yeah, yeah,' he promised he would be polite and nice. And he was absolutely fine at lunch." It was a "very cool lunch," Gorman himself remembered, "it lasted about three hours," and Felix made it clear that he did not support such a program. "He was going to find the answer to schizophrenia . . . by chasing molecules," as Gorman put it; "he would not get into the business of a practical clinical approach to mental patients." When he and Mahoney left and got into a taxi, "as soon as Mike was out of hearing, he screamed and yelled and swore and said he was so angry at the fellow," Mahoney recalled. "He talked that way all the way to the Capitol. When he got out and asked the driver, 'How much?' he said, 'Not a penny. I've never had such entertainment in all my life! I've always loved vaudeville but this was it!'" Mahoney chuckled with delight at the image.[125]

Their efforts were successful despite such setbacks; Fogarty put a provision in a bill for a psycho-pharmacology service center, which inaugurated NIMH's evaluation of promising drugs. Mahoney nevertheless continued her advocacy on behalf of mental health: "Have been trying to get a psychiatrist out of the Air Force to run psy[chiatric] dept. at Oklahoma medical school," she wrote Lasker in 1954.[126]

The lobbying group's name, a few years after its formation in 1953, was changed from National Committee on Mental Health to National Committee Against Mental Illness during the period when rabid anti-Communists hinted that psychiatric treatment smacked of "brainwashing" and might be part of a "Communist plot" against America.[127]

Birth-control advocacy

A highlight of the decade for Mahoney was a journey halfway around the world that she undertook on another mission — to support the cause of birth control with its principal advocate Margaret Sanger. "Birth control always made sense to me," Mahoney said of her life-long interest in promoting it.

Referred to politely as "child spacing," birth control had begun to get attention from federal agencies by 1941, thanks to Sanger's and Mary Lasker's urging the Roosevelt White House to take stands in favor of public-health programs that provided such services to needy women. Mahoney was aware of those efforts and sympathetic with them though not active in Sanger's private organization.[128]

Like Mahoney, Sanger put her cause in broad perspective: "If one-tenth of the money spent on the atom bomb were spent on safe and effective birth control," she stated after the war, such systems might have been developed by then. By that time she had become an international figure in support of accessible birth-control methods for women who wanted them and for contraceptive research, connecting population control to world peace, as did Mahoney. Following the war birth-control advocates became particularly alarmed over population growth rates in Third World countries. To address the problem, Sanger helped found the International Planned Parenthood Federation (IPPF) in 1952 and began working with family-planning leaders in Europe and Asia.[129]

Sanger was felled by a heart attack in 1949 (at age seventy) and suffered another in 1950, becoming addicted to the painkiller Demerol for recurrent chest pains. To cheer her, Mary Lasker in 1950 insisted on awarding Sanger a Lasker prize for pioneering work in family planning. Sanger was too weak to travel from her Tucson home to receive the award in person.[130]

Sanger had visited Japan twice, first in 1922 (with her son Grant) and most recently in 1952. Her first visit, which was opposed by the Japanese government, created so much publicity that her name became "a household word," one of her women advocates, Shidzue Ishimoto Kato, wrote in an autobiography. "Not since Commodore Perry had forced Japan to open its doors to foreign commerce, in 1852, had an American created such a sensation," Kato recorded.[131]

The second trip was no less controversial, this time opposed by the Supreme Commander of the Allied Occupation Forces, General Douglas MacArthur. Mahoney became closely involved in the matter. Sanger in 1949 had been invited by various leaders and Japan's largest newspaper, the *Yomiuri Shimbun*, whose president, in a letter begging her to come, stated that "the Japanese people who are crowded in a small country with more than 80 million people . . . are still ignorant of the real significance of sex education and scientific method of birth control which would be of great help for the reconstruction of [a] peaceful and cultured nation."[132]

Sanger sought help from her friend Mahoney, who got in touch with a newspaper publisher with contacts to MacArthur, the editor and publisher of the *Arizona Daily Star* in Tucson, William R. Mathews. He in turn contacted every high-ranking military and government official whom he knew in an effort to plead Sanger's case, referring to her by her second husband's name, Slee. MacArthur sent back word that Sanger-Slee's application was "disapproved as her presence in Japan at this time would contribute nothing to the occupation"; to the contrary, it "would necessarily carry the connotation that she was" serving an occupation objective. Furthermore, it "would have revived the birth control issue and projected the General and the Occupation right in the center of it" after MacArthur had been careful to "take [a] neutral position on the issue." The Japanese, meanwhile, in 1949 legalized abortion, making the subject even more controversial in the international arena.[133]

Sanger angrily replied, "I do not wish to embarrass the Occupation authorities, but it is scarcely a neutral position to block a request that comes directly from the Japanese people themselves." She refused to take MacArthur's "no" as final. In a separate public statement that she issued in February 1950, she noted, "This is not the first time I was told I could not visit Japan. In 1921 I was refused permission by the Imperial Japanese government. It is tragic to see that our Occupation authorities, while mouthing democratic principles, are emulating the old Japanese military regime." It was the "angry protests of the people" in 1921 that "forced the lifting of that ban," and she hoped the same would occur in 1950.[134]

Mahoney went to work, contacting Secretary of Defense Louis A. Johnson to see what could be done. "Will try to bring you up to date on my activities in your behalf," she wrote Sanger February 14, 1950, from Miami Beach, where she was still living. The letter is revealing of Mahoney's style and low-key approach.

When I was in Washington I went to see Secretary Johnson, who is a dear man and both he and his wife are friends of mine. His wife is extremely sympathetic and read all the letters and did her work on him on the weekend. He sent me to see Under-Secretary of War [Tracy S.] Vorhees. Mr. Vorhees dictated a very favorable letter in my presence, but I am not exactly certain to whom. He said it was to someone on the staff. I had expected him to send me a copy of it, but so far have not received it.

The same day I saw Secretary Johnson I stopped by to have lunch at the Army-Navy Club with Surgeon-General Scheele and two other doctors. Just by chance General Sams was there, who is a doctor in charge of the health program under MacArthur, a horrid little man whom I had met the year before in Boston. We had a stormy session when he told me it was he who had stopped your visa, and said. "We do not want Margaret Sanger barn-storming Japan. It's a newspaper racket for publicity, and birth control has nothing to do with population trends." I behaved as well as possible and was delighted the Surgeon General heard his remarks. I also told Secretary Johnson and Mr. Vorhees of the conversation. I am with you in this fight to the end.

This past weekend I went down to the Little White House in Key West as the guest of Secretary and Mrs. Johnson, who were there resting for a few days. To my surprise and delight, on Sunday night, in walked Mr. Vorhees to dine with us. Secretary Johnson asked him pointedly what he was going to do about Margaret Sanger. He answered that he hoped that he could work it out, and that if he heard nothing in the near future he would go into it personally when he goes to Japan to see MacArthur in the next two or three months. I assure you that nothing could be better than having Secretary Johnson's interest and support. Even though they all say that they hate to go over MacArthur's head, they are going on the theory that MacArthur knows nothing about it.

I have also given them the impression that it is going to create a lot of bad publicity from your newspaper friends unless they deal with it quickly. I will not return your letters for the moment in case I need some of them again. Fortunately, Mary had with her copies of the letters from the Japanese people asking you to come to Japan and they were most valuable.

I shall write to Mr. Vorhees again today and try to get a statement from him in writing on the status at this point.

She signed off saying, "It was such a joy to have my visits with you. I shall always remember our ride in the foot hills and the sunset."[135]

Sanger thanked her "for everything" in a letter February 21. "Your experience in Washington was surprising," she added. Newspaper accounts, including one apparently in the *New York Times*, also may have resulted from Mahoney's contacts. "Hundreds of letters, telegrams, etc., came from all over regarding the *Times* article," Sanger said. She blamed pressure from the Catholic Church for the ban on her visit: "The Japanese people are frightened at its growing influence over the Occupation," she told Mahoney. "Let us keep pushing on the Japan question and see what can be done. Ever my thanks, Affectionately, Margaret." A postscript suggested that "A line from you to the *Wash. Post* would be helpful."[136]

Push they did. The *Post* published an editorial, possibly prompted by Mahoney, to whom *Post* editor and publisher Philip Graham wrote April 10, "Thanks for your letter about our editorial on Mrs. Sanger. We have had quite a correspondence with MacArthur as a result of this, and I shall be interested in talking with you when you are up this way." Mahoney sent the editorial to Sanger.[137]

MacArthur, as a result of the publicity, was forced to defend his position to Charles E. Scribner, chairman of the Planned Parenthood Federation of America. Under-secretary Vorhees in March wrote Mahoney, however, that his department had concluded that MacArthur had processed Sanger's two applications in proper fashion and the denial had been made with his knowledge. "In consequence . . . I do not feel that there are any further steps which the Department of the Army may appropriately take" to help Sanger.[138]

After seeing MacArthur's letter to Scribner, Sanger told Mahoney,

. . . He has certainly gone into the subject fully and evidently bases his stand on a letter I had written to one of the Japanese officials who had invited me to come to Japan, and my answer was — "I could not plan to come . . . without an official invitation from the Japanese people." He claims also that the statements in the American press were entirely erroneous relative to Catholic pressure on him. He also claims that the birth control work in Japan is getting along on its own pressure and doing very well.

I think there is nothing further we can do about this at the moment, but the contents of a letter from a physician in Tokyo states this — "Many of our friends are indignant over . . . the refusal of your entry . . . but they are silent. Our own feelings have to be suppressed, as we have learned by experience to swallow big lumps. It is difficult for our friends in the States to understand what we are up against . . . . [T]he Potsdam Agreement forbids us from any remarks that are derogatory to the occupation policies and punishment will be severe. Our manuscripts were returned because the Press were afraid of publishing such material, and until the Peace Treaty has been signed we will not be safe to discuss on paper what is at the bottom of our hearts." . . . So, if the General seems to think that the Japanese people are not clamoring for my entry, perhaps the occupation authorities have put the curtain of fear, as this letter seems to indicate.

I am going to let the matter rest temporarily, for I am quite sure if I am here and able to be of use that I will some day receive official invitation, as soon as the Peace Treaty has been signed. Thanks again.

It was signed, "Me."[139]

Sanger subsequently wrote Mahoney that Scribner, "a mild-tempered gentleman," decided not to continue the correspondance "but rather almost congratulated the General for not allowing religious pressure to influence his decision on so important a subject . . . . I think that all of this agitation has really done some good in Japan, for now a magazine has come forth on birth control in both English and Japanese . . . the censorship was waived," she continued. "I don't feel that this ends the problem — I think we must just mark time and eventually something is going to happen, and not in the too distant future."[140]

Indeed, Sanger finally was permitted to visit Japan in 1952 and again in April 1954. Her mission was to help set up the Fifth International Planned Parenthood Conference scheduled for the following year. Mary Lasker had given her money, which Sanger told Mahoney she would use to hire a young Japanese-American girl to accompany her as secretary and helpmate. Sanger's son Stuart, a physician, "will teach her what to do for me in case I flop over or my heart pumps too fast," she wrote Mahoney before leaving.[141]

Such was the background for the trip in 1955 that Mahoney enthusiastically joined. In May Sanger requested "an official invitation" be sent to Mahoney. "I am seriously planning to go with you" to Tokyo, Mahoney immediately replied to Sanger, "and we will have a superb time . . . . Send me a note and tell me the date you have booked for sailing." In July Sanger warned, "Have you done anything about getting accommodations on the *President Cleveland* to sail with me on Sept. 17th? It is usually a popular and very crowded boat but I know that you have friendly admirers on the President Line and can doubtless get the bridal suite with a bend of your finger. Do let me know." The conference was scheduled for October 24 to 29.[142]

The trip was to lend backing to Japanese family-planning efforts led by Kato, who had been imprisoned during the war for her Socialist and pacifist positions. It would be the first national meeting of the newly chartered Family Planning Federation of Japan, which was to be taken into the International Planned Parenthood Federation.

"The Japanese loved her," Mahoney said of Sanger's reception. "They understood about birth control. We went to the international conference and also to Hong Kong," where she was shocked by the crowded living conditions. "There were people living in tin shacks, sometimes as many as twelve to fourteen in a room." Despite the interest in birth control in Japan, Mahoney noted one day that all the educational literature on the subject, which had been put on a table in the conference room for attendees to take, had mysteriously disappeared. "They took everything out," apparently at the behest of anti-birth-control interest groups.[143]

At the time, Sanger was seventy-six and in frail health. She got stronger as she traveled, however, and by the time the party reached Hong Kong, she was out of a wheelchair and on her feet. A photograph on the front page of an English-language newspaper in Tokyo November 5 showed Sanger and Mahoney, with two other Western women delegates to the conference, observing a traditional Shinto wedding ceremony. "The simpler marriages are, the longer they last," the caption quoted the American women as saying. It was "their first glimpse of a truly Japanese-style wedding — the starting point for planned parenthood," it stated.[144]

"The . . . Conference in Tokyo in 1955 provided a great impetus to the family planning movement in Japan," Kato later wrote. Sanger was the first foreigner to address the Committee of Public Welfare in the House of Councillors of the Diet — the upper house of parliament in which Mrs. Kato sat. Although Sanger's speech was rambling, she also helped organize another conference and was officially presented to Emperor Hirohito.[145]

Arranging the meeting was not easy, though, which angered Mahoney. The U. S. Ambassador, John M. Allison, initially refused to formally introduce Sanger to the emperor, who wanted to meet her. "The ambassador said he didn't have time to get dressed up and present every American who wanted to meet the emperor, and he didn't take her. I was *so* angry and raised such a fuss about it that I don't think he was there very long," she joked. "I told everybody I could think of how awful I thought it was" that the ambassador had snubbed Sanger.

She told George Dixon, for his profile of Sanger a few months after their return, that she "will go down in history as the greatest woman since Florence Nightingale."[146]

In January 1956, Sanger, feeling somewhat sorry for herself, wrote Mahoney, "Have you forgotten me? A letter from Captain Neilsen [of one of the ships they had sailed on] mentions you as my 'playmate,' so perhaps that is why I have not had one word from you since over the telephone in New York. Not that friendship or affection depends upon constant contact, but when two people travel together and end up with a friendly relationship and *more*, it is just nice to know how things are going with each other . . . . I long to hear from you and would telephone you, but am never sure where you are. You are a bird on the wing, as I am."

"You must be happy," she continued, "at the way the present government is now pushing Congress for money for research in all the fields that you and Mary have been pushing for the past several years. Now you really should get busy with Planned Parenthood." She enclosed a photograph, "although it is not flattering," of the two of them taken on the trip.[147]

Mahoney had not neglected the cause. She met with sympathizer Agnes Meyer, wife of Eugene Meyer, publisher of the *Washington Post*, "and gave her a lot of papers, clippings and personal impressions of our meeting in Japan," which Meyer used in a speech that Sanger said was "very courageous" and "hit the headlines." In addition Mahoney was "trying to get Mary's foundation to do a fact sheet on planned parenthood but I have to get all the information together first . . . . I think the Conference has created a greater national interest in population controls," she concluded, "for I seem to hear and see much more about it."[148]

Sanger fully appreciated Mahoney's skills and assets for the crusade and sent her reports on projects in which she was involved, ending one letter wistfully, "I wish you were traveling with me and had nothing else to do but just to look into the various situations from place to place to needle up activities . . . and to help the groups enlarge and expand their activities. We could remake the world in a very short time."[149]

On another occasion she asked Mahoney to advise her on approaching the Lasker Foundation for funds. "I would rather consult you first to see what you think of the possible ways of making a proper presentation to the Board to get good results. I know how much Mary thinks of you and of your opinions relative to financial matters," she said.[150]

Mahoney and Sanger remained in communication for many years after the trip to Japan, although they rarely met personally, and Sanger tried to engage Mahoney's talents whenever she could. "I wish that you, dear Florence, would get in touch with Mrs. Richard Cross of the Planned Parenthood Federation [in] Washington, D.C. and perhaps offer to help them on organizing the next International Conference to be held in May 1958," she wrote at the end of 1956. "I am sure they will be looking for someone to help them in publicity." Mahoney responded, "I will telephone Mrs. Cross after Christmas when I can get a moment to breathe." They also talked about making other overseas trips — "Let's go to China!" she exclaimed in one letter to Sanger.[151]

In 1957 Sanger agreed to a television interview with tough questioner Mike Wallace, who asked her what she thought was "sin" in light of having had extra-marital affairs herself. "Sin," Sanger sternly retorted, was having uncared for, or defective, children for lack of attention to birth control. She also was quoted as saying, in an earlier interview about how to handle aging, that people should be so involved in a cause that they have little time to think of their own problems and complaints (with which she was plagued). "All of life," she told the journalist, "you must have a vital interest in something outside yourself." It was a philosophy that Mahoney, too, would manifest in her own long and full life.[152]

Sanger was ending her role as president of the international federation in 1959 when she and Mahoney talked of going to India, although Sanger's health remained precarious. "I shall certainly plan to go to India with you in '59," Mahoney said, reassuring Sanger further, "I still work in every way for B. C. [birth control] and gave Drew Pearson yesterday a lot of info for his column re: same." In addition she was trying to help find a publisher for a Sanger book. "I have Josh Logan reading your autobiography and am still trying to get someone to do a play about your life," she wrote her in May 1959. "Am also talking here to various senators hoping we can get some *added* money for research in the fertility field." Mahoney did not go to India with her, however, writing, "I know you were a great success."[153]

Mahoney herself took an unusual initative in trying to gain some form of Catholic sanction for family planning and population control. For some years, she had tried to find a way to get scientific information to the Pope. She even had tried to get the Duke and Duchess of Windsor to help at one time. The couple had visited her while in Florida one year "and I thought I had sold the Duchess on birth control. But she never did anything" to follow up. Mahoney tried again when a wealthy man in Florida, a Papal Marquis sympathetic to birth control, had the couple to dinner one night. "I was happy to sit on the Duke's left," but nothing came of that either. Still, she kept trying. "I used to send the Papal Marquis scientific articles to send the Pope, and he did." Another hope was the Kennedy family. She tried to persuade Sanger that the potential election of a Catholic president was not worrisome: "The Kennedys are both so smart and completely in sympathy with all of our problems," she told Sanger in the fall of 1960. "Papa Joe" Kennedy was also a possibility: "One time he was out at the house and I heard him say to Mahoney, 'Every time I see Pope Pius XII, that's what he wants to talk about — birth control,'" which was unusual at the time, as Mahoney noted, because "people just didn't mention it, you couldn't talk about it."[154]

Finally she wrote directly to Pope John XXIII, who had publicly expressed concern over human misery caused by population explosion, and had a personal audience with him.

"Everybody thought I was Catholic because my name was Mahoney," she said. One Catholic whom she got to know well was the Vatican delegate to the United States, Cardinal Egidio Vagnozzi, "rather a raucus character, to tell you the truth! I was working on him and trying to get him to do something about birth control with the Pope — the *nice* Pope. He had been the Pope's secretary when he was in France, so he knew him very well. Finally he said to me one day, 'Why don't you write down what you think the Church should do?' It took me about a week to write it because I weighed every word so carefully. But anyway he sent it to the Pope, and the Pope gave me a private audience, at his summer place in Italy."

She knew that "birth control in Catholic nomenclature meant 'responsible parenthood' by the spacing of children for acceptable social and economic reasons. They already had accepted birth control when they accepted the rhythm method, and the reason for it — to benefit the health of people" in increasingly congested living conditions. What was needed, she realized, was "research to find something the Church did not disapprove of. It was as far as you could go then."

Her carefully chosen words to the Pope, contained in two paragraphs that she hoped he would publicly endorse, urged backing for research on natural birth control:

> The Church has always accepted the principle of Responsible Parenthood and in modern times has come to terms with it in practice. It is the method rather than the principle of family planning that has been controversial. The Church does not sanction artifical methods for limiting population, but will welcome any scientific advance furthering natural methods. [Those] approved by the Church are a) delayed marriage, especially beyond the very productive years of the early twenties, b) continence within marriage for a protracted period, and c) periodic continence or use of the sterile period during the woman's monthly cycle.

> The Church recognized as an *acute international problem* the excessive rate of growth of the population in underdeveloped areas and the large percentage of the population without food, clothing and shelter. The excessive population is largely a result of recent scientific research that has reduced greatly the infant and child mortality by applying new methods to the control of malaria, dysentery and cholera. Let us hope the *scientists* will now turn their attention to the problem of a (natural) control that can be morally accepted as well as applicable to all countries.[155]

"This is the result of my friendship here with the Apostolic Delegate and various people," Mahoney wrote excitedly to Sanger in October 1961. "I was in the south of France this summer with Mary, and then went to Rome for a week and while there I had an audience with the Pope. It was semi-private so I had an opportunity to talk to him. His interpreter listened to all I had to say and said he would explain it to the Pope, and I gather that the question of population problem will be one of the first things on the agenda at the coming Ecumenical Conference."[156]

Those were "the last words he said to me," she later recalled. "He seemed to understand everything perfectly. He had the most beautiful face I've ever seen and handsome big eyes. And he said that I should send him any information that I wanted to from then on. I can see why people loved him." Alas, Pope John XXIII, who convened the Second Vatican Council in October 1962, died the following year, and her hopes were unfulfilled that the leader of the Catholic world would take up the cause of overpopulation.

Mahoney had better results with Indian leaders, she recounted to Sanger. "The present Ambassador from India here, Mr. B. K. Nehru, is a very dear friend of mine and so intelligent on the problem of population in India, and I am going to some functions for [him] next week. Write to me if there is anything you would like for me to find out from him. What do you hear from our friends in Japan?" she added. "Should we go back again to visit?" She shared with Sanger what she knew, as a member of the Child Health and Human Development Advisory Council, about "all research being done at the National Institutes of Health that would have any bearing on fertility and, therefore, be useful for population control. This is not public, so will you please return it to me as I especially asked to have it [the account] done?"[157]

Mahoney carried on Sanger's work during a trip to India on a Food for Peace mission with the program's director George McGovern. "We had over two weeks in India," she wrote Sanger. "Lady Rama Rau came to see me in Bombay and we had a long visit and, naturally, talked about you. She is very well and working hard. The sterilization program in Madras and one other state is so popular they can't get enough doctors to do the operation on the men who ask for it. There is a great deal of interest and more research in this country, as you probably know," she continued. "I've been trying to get various research men in all the universities to try for grants. The Academy of Science may call a seminar this spring of the outstanding people in research to see what progress can be expected and the current status. I certainly thought about you and wished you could have been with me," she said.[158]

A year before Sanger's death (in 1966 at age eighty-seven), Mahoney read a stirring column that put Sanger's accomplishments in historical perspective. The need for birth control (a term the writer credited to Sanger), from being considered a "derided folly . . . whispered furtively in polite conversation," even obscene when she started her work virtually alone in 1912, had become generally accepted, "moved governments to action, and made us all aware of the pressures of population on the margins of poverty." More to the point, the writer continued, Sanger had led a campaign "which gave new status to women, made the raising of a family no longer a personal whim but a serious responsibility, and made a wife something more than the slave or dupe of a husband's passion." "All honor to her comrades and companions," the writer said, but the red-headed Sanger, whose "gentle spirit" was deceiving, belonged "with the great benefactors of history." There was more work to be done, he concluded, but "the debate is now being conducted in a new spirit of mutual respect . . . . Mankind does not relinquish its hold on truths that give it new dignity and new hope."[159]

Similar words might have been applied to Mahoney for her quiet but determined dedication to causes. She obviously was moved and saved the column. She herself was deeply involved in carrying on the work, playing an effective role in setting new birth-control policies for the United States and other countries. It shared her attention with mental-health issues and biomedical research. "It was *all* equally important," she felt.

Old friends

Mahoney maintained her close friendship with the Trumans after his presidency ended, writing about them in her newspaper column and corresponding with them regularly about personal and political matters.

In 1957 Mahoney wrote that she and Lasker were sorry not to be able to attend the opening of Truman's presidential library because they were "flying to Europe the end of June by way of celebration. You will be pleased to know that we got $36 million more in the Senate for research than the appropriation figures," she boasted. "This seems to be quite a victory in this year of budget altering."[160]

"It was a pleasure to receive all those clippings," Truman replied. "You furnish me with more information than I receive from anyone else in the country, and I am very grateful to you for your thoughtfulness. We expect to hear from you again" after returning from Europe, he added, writing in a postscript, "We are almost 'mad' at both of you because you won't be here Saturday for the dedication — an impossible chore accomplished, as [was the victory in] 1948."[161]

Mahoney apprized him of improvements in Missouri's mental hospitals promised by its Governor James T. Blair in 1958, reminding Truman that "the Committee against Mental Illness that Mary and I are co-chairmen of is always furthering work in the states."[162]

"I saw in the paper only yesterday that a new director for the State's Division of Mental Diseases had been appointed," Truman wrote her a week later, "so you see our good Governor was not talking through his hat."[163]

Following the 1958 congressional elections in November, he thanked Mahoney for "the neckties you sent me. Your ties are always of the sort I can wear. In fact, I had chances to wear two or three of them, and they made a hit wherever I went. I hope," he added, "that you're not too badly disappointed by the election returns."[164]

End of an era of "glorious adversity"

Indeed, it did not seem to matter to Mahoney's research cause which party dominated Washington. By 1961 federal research spending had risen dramatically despite Eisenhower, giving the National Institutes of Health more than $460 million — a 150-fold increase since 1945.[165]

The success of the unique triumvirate on its behalf — the Mahoney-Lasker team, Shannon and his scientists, and Hill and Fogarty — brought few complaints from within the institution. Thanks to them, it was growing so rapidly that in 1956 New York Times science editor, Pulitzer Prize–winner William Laurence, predicted that cancer, heart disease, and polio would be conquered within a decade.[166]

As its fortunes rose, so did applications for the money, straining NIH's resources and staff. "There was no peacetime NIH precedent, nor comparable sequel, for the growth surge that ensued upon passage of the final . . . FY 1957 appropriation on July 31, 1956. Within four years, the NIH budget ballooned from $98.5 million to $400 million," one historian wrote of that period.[167]

A worldwide epidemic of the Asian flu in 1958 furthered the cause of research and prompted Senator Hill to introduce a congressional resolution to set up a National Advisory Council for International Medical Research within HEW. He noted at the time that cancer was still killing "one American every two minutes," many between the ages of thirty and fifty, that ten million Americans suffered from heart and circulatory diseases, that cerebral palsy was on the rise in the United States and other countries, and that the number of people crippled or disabled by disease or accident each year was greater than the number who were successfully rehabilitated "and restored to active life." Such a "cooperative war against disease and disability, those historic enemies of all man and all peoples," should become "a major and vital part of American foreign policy," Hill said of the $50-million proposal. Congress approved a National Institute for International Medical Research in 1959, which the president's brother, Dr. Milton Eisenhower, backed on behalf of the administration.[168]

Howard Rusk in his column praised Hill's idea, pointing out that less than 1 percent of U.S. foreign aid went for health programs. The concept provided an opportunity for the Mahoney-Lasker forces to reiterate the advantages of research in keeping people alive and healthy longer.

Hill's "Health for Peace plan" also was a chance to link the advocates' positions to Eisenhower's own state-of-the-union proposal for an international Science for Peace program, and to challenge the president to back more money for medical research.[169]

"Although the Eisenhower Administration has been plagued more than any other in recent times by illness and death," Marquis Childs wrote in June 1959, referring to the president's own heart attack, cancer death of Secretary of State Dulles, and "the tragic plight [mental illness] of Gov. Earl Long, the Bureau of the Budget comes in with recommendations so small that each year they are raised substantially by the Senate." Only continued massive funding could push promising research to fruition, even one of Eisenhower's surgeons testified. And Sidney Farber brought news that the cure rate for cancer had risen from one in four to one in three people as a result of successful research findings.[170]

The intense pressure in favor of increasing the Eisenhower figures worked. Doris Fleeson touted Hill's getting the Senate to raise the NIH budget $32 million above the president's in 1959. It was "a triumph not only over the winds of economy which have been blowing through Congress," Fleeson said, "but over an administration [that Senator Hill] thinks has been lagging in promoting medical research."[171]

Eisenhower threatened to veto the 1961 HEW appropriations bill because of its huge increases for NIH but backed down after hearing pleas from Sidney Farber (Mary Lasker arranged for him and Jules Stein, head of the Music Corporation of America, to talk to the president on a golfing outing in Newport, Rhode Island) and Republican Representative Melvin Laird, who told him the veto would not be sustained.[172]

Advances made in heart research provided a measure of the successes that large sums of money in the "golden years" wrought. Top scientists were attracted to NIH by the promise of a supportive environment and world-class peers with whom to work and learn. They developed such new techniques as catheterization of the heart, better diagnosis and correction of valves or other defects, drugs to treat hypertension, and diagnostic methods to detect fatty substances (such as cholesterol in the blood that clogged arteries) resulting in new thoughts about diet as a prevention to heart disease. Heart-lung machines to permit open-heart surgery soon followed, as did pacemakers and other artificial parts to the body, heart monitors, and other devices to detect and repair the body's defects. Heart victims now were recovering, living longer, healthier, and pain-free lives. No taxpayers quarreled with those achievements from use of their money.

Even the AMA had come to accept that federal funding of medical research was beneficial.[173]

To counter Republicans' growing concern nevertheless over NIH's "runaway" budget, Senator Hill himself offered to direct a study of how the money was being spent and appointed the Committee of Consultants on Medical Research in 1960. It was dominated by people like DeBakey, Farber, David Sarnoff, and others considered part of the Mahoney-Lasker group. Not surprisingly, they concluded that research would benefit from a substantial increase in federal support. That justified Hill's and Fogarty's positions for the near future.

In the end, Mahoney and Lasker found that they didn't have to "pay any attention to Eisenhower at all because we always had the senators on our side." Thus they weathered the Eisenhower years, a period of what Gorman called "glorious adversity."[174]

It truly was the height of a "Golden Era" of medical research in the United States, for which more than one observer gave Mahoney and her colleagues full credit. "In weighing the importance of single persons on the course of a national policy, and in that sense on the course of history," Stephen P. Strickland wrote in his book, *Politics, Science and Dread Disease*, "perhaps it is enough to know that some are perceived as giants. In the politics of medical research, Hill, Fogarty, Lasker, Mahoney, Shannon and several others certainly are."[175]

6

Impatience with
Things as They Are

———————◆———————

WITH THE RETURN OF THE DEMOCRATIC PARTY to the White
House and control of Congress in 1960 following the election
of John F. Kennedy, Mahoney and Lasker expected sympathy toward research. Indeed, Kennedy's first budget request contained the largest increase for NIH ever proposed by a president. Even so, Fogarty and Hill
had their way and further raised biomedical research funding. But increasingly its advocates would be called on to justify their figures. By the
mid-1960s, anti-poverty and civil-rights initiatives, and an expanding war
in Southeast Asia, were laying claim to larger chunks of the federal budget.
Expenditures for medical research would be subject to growing scrutiny.[1]

Mahoney's and Lasker's personal relationships with both Presidents
Kennedy and Johnson would be crucial through those administrations
when Congress' largesse toward NIH was challenged on several fronts.

Friends of the Kennedys

Lasker's first meeting with Kennedy, she recorded in an oral history in
1966, had been "in the Capitol someplace with Florence Mahoney. She

was a friend of his. . . . She had known him since the early '40s or late '30s. She'd always liked him and, in fact, was always devoted to him. And she often talked to me about him and said that he was surely going to be president sometime. When I met him, he was this very, very skinny, very young-looking congressman, and I thought, 'Florence is a wonderful girl and I'm very fond of her, but this is a very unlikely candidate for president.' He looked incredibly young. His arms were too long for his coat, his pants were not fitting — or the bottoms were turned up. He was really a very unimpressive-looking candidate for president at that time."

"However, he was always very cheerful," she continued, "and he was often teasing Florence about being interested in birth control. Florence is very interested in birth control as a public-health problem, and so am I. And he was always saying to her, 'Well, have you any new methods?' Or, 'What is the situation?' There would always be some crack about it. And even when he'd see me alone in the halls in Congress, he'd say hello to me and, 'How is Florence, and how is she getting along with birth control?' Well, little did he realize, or did any of us realize, that later on he would be the first president to make any official kind of statement on the subject of birth control . . . . I thought Kennedy was charming, and Florence's affection was so great for him that I was influenced by her to try to help him when he was ill of malaria."[2]

When Kennedy had a spinal operation in 1954, Mahoney sent him a gift. "I can't remember if I wrote to thank you for the present you sent me in the hospital," he said on Senate note paper. "It was almost worth the operation to receive it. All the nurses wanted to take it home, but I said I would have to come with it in order to maintain it and that lessened their interest."[3]

Mahoney was delighted when Kennedy decided to run for president and was an active backer.

Mike Gorman, too, saw the advantages of having friends in high places once again. "I am sending you two copies of the basic health speech," he wrote Mahoney just before Kennedy was elected in 1960. "You might smuggle the second copy into the Kennedy camp." It was all "very conspiratorial," he jotted across the top, signing it "Comrade Mike Gorman."[4]

By then Kennedy was a different man from the skinny congressman she had first met, Lasker remarked. "His looks changed completely from what they had been four or five years before. He didn't look like the same person . . . he became very handsome."[5]

Two nights before Kennedy's inauguration, Mahoney had a preinaugural dinner at her home. "I told Kennedy that Mr. Truman was coming and these various people, so he said he'd like to come, and he did. Mr. Truman was at the table with me. Kennedy came in, and before he sat down — we were already at the table — he went right up to Mr. Truman and said, 'Mr. Truman, we just had an argument. Who is third in command if anything happens to the President?'"[6]

"Mr. Truman didn't even stop to think," Mahoney said. "'Speaker of the House — and do you know why? That's where the money comes from!'" referring to the constitutional requirement that appropriations initiate in the House of Representatives. "The fact that he said it so fast was funny!" Mahoney remembered.

"Florence's role in that period," according to Russel Lee's son, Dr. Philip R. Lee, then serving at the Agency for International Development (AID), was to facilitate meetings with people who could help one another, like White House aides and department officials. "She introduced me to Ted Sorensen, for example," Kennedy's adviser and speechwriter, "and we had a long discussion one afternoon sitting out on Florence's lawn. She basically said to Ted that she thought he ought to meet me because I was working for the president, too, although at a lower level. And when I was asked by Wilbur Cohen to come to HEW in '65, Florence arranged for me to have dinner with Senator Hill." Her affinity with Hill, Lee saw, was related to the way both operated politically — "more genteel" than Fogarty, who was "down in the trenches," Lee laughed. "In our little cluster, she was an extremely important person, facilitating, you might say, our *entry* into that political world." She seemed to intuit the connections that were beneficial, taking the initiative rather than responding to requests from people to put them together.[7]

In the middle of the Cuban missile crisis, Sorensen was engrossed at his desk on October 19, 1962, when he suddenly remembered that he had been invited to Mahoney's for dinner that night. "I had to call her and say, 'I can't make it, I have this work I have to do.' She naturally asked what it was about, and I couldn't tell her a single word. She said, 'Well, you have got to eat.'" No, he protested, he could not come. A little while later, there arrived "a whole dinner, in a covered dish, which I could eat at my desk while writing the speech that Kennedy would deliver on October 22 on national television, announcing that we had found Soviet missiles in Cuba and were determined to remove them."[8]

"She not only facilitated a smooth working relationship [between the White House and HEW] by inviting us," Lee said, "but she got the subject around to things that she was concerned with, like family planning and contraceptive research, and she would have her own input. She would substantively contribute at times, and at other times, simply facilitate" discussion. Only occasionally did she "call you up about something, if she wanted something done. She didn't do that very often, though; she didn't push an agenda."[9]

If not overt, Mahoney always had a purpose at her "genteel evenings," reflected Dr. E. Grey Dimond of those years when the medical educator and Mahoney worked together. He called her "the most skillful lady in Washington" who provided him with "a ringside seat on the Washington scene, especially . . . the health legislation field."

"With no weapon other than herself and her skill at picking an objective . . . then 'educating' Capitol Hill and the White House, she became a one-person, extraordinary lobby. 'Educating' was one of her favorite words," he realized. "In the main, she used the phone and her home to talk, explain, and cajole . . . never with the slightest personal gain involved, which, of course, was a major part of her effectiveness. No one at the table knew they were there to be manipulated — but *she* knew it!," he added. "Nothing was unplanned." Unlike Lasker, Mahoney worked "quietly, behind the scenes, but she was oh so able. Never heavy-handed — but she wasn't afraid to speak up."[10]

"So adept and thorough was Mrs. Mahoney at this particular modus operandi in the early '60s," wrote one historian, that a magazine article describing her closeness to White House insiders was entitled "Den mother to the New Frontier." (The article was killed when President Kennedy was assassinated.)[11]

She "would be busy with her food and then sweetly and cheerfully turn to" a guest such as HEW Secretary John Gardner and say, "John, tell Hubert about that wonderful paragraph in your book on how much talent is being wasted by forcing people to retire at 65," as Dimond remembered one evening that included Vice President Hubert Humphrey and *New York Times* columnist James Reston. "With that done, she serenely and enthusiastically returned to her meal. The evening was off with the thinker, Gardner, stimulating the politician, Humphrey, and the powerful columnist, Reston, getting material for several columns which would [inform] the public. All this was carried out with a single woman in the kitchen, handling the cooking and serving. The hostess' good taste in every aspect . . . made it more elegant than a dinner costing ten times as much." The food was often Latin and simple, and Mahoney provided "that useful interlude, too often forgotten, when the women are escorted upstairs and the men gathered with an after-dinner drink," providing "moments for . . . gossip and hints."[12]

Mahoney had a close association with Kennedy's wife, Jackie, extending to shared interests in politics, art, and rare Chinese procelain. They first met when Mahoney and her sons were invited to a party for Jackie at the Georgetown home of friends whose son she was then dating. "It was the first time I think I ever saw her, and I thought, I've never seen anyone with such beautiful eyes in my life! She had such taste, and humor, and was very, very smart." Mahoney was invited to her wedding in Newport, Rhode Island, but did not attend because she was at her ranch in Idaho at the time. She often visited the young bride at their home on N Street in Georgetown — "lunch in garden, just us," she recorded of one visit.[13]

Jackie took a particular interest in porcelain after seeing Mahoney's growing collection of rare pieces. "She was fascinated by the procelain and asked me about it, and the next day, she went out and bought books on it." She borrowed containers from Mahoney to hold flowers for her sister Lee's quiet wedding to Prince Radziwill, and after Jackie admired

Chinese black lacquer "nest" tables that Mahoney had, she ordered a set from Taiwan for her. After the Kennedys were in the White House, Jackie asked Mahoney if her cook would teach the White House chef how to make spun sugar. When Jackie was having trouble finding a birthday present for Jack one year, Mahoney gave her plates that she had commemorating an Italian poet that the president admired. Jackie in turn gave Mahoney a framed collage painting of her own creation. Mahoney had vivid images of the beautiful young mother waiting at her front door in Georgetown for her daughter Caroline to come home from school "so she'd be there to greet her when she opened the door."[14]

One day Jackie called Mahoney and said, "'*You* know Greta Garbo — let's get her down to dinner with Jack; he's been working so hard, he's never met her, and it will keep him from being bored,' or something like that. So I called her and she came down." Mahoney had met the famous actress in the south of France, but she had never been to Washington before. "Do you think I could wear pants?" Garbo asked. If you wish, Mahoney answered. "Mrs. Lincoln, Jack's secretary, forgot to ask one person, so we were only seven at dinner. But we had a wonderful time. We were downstairs, looking at things in Jack's office. And she stayed on another two days at my house — we had fun. She had a *wonderful* humor."

Garbo told a friend fourteen years later that the guests included "a lady who was instrumental in getting us there by hook or crook, a White House friend, a man who was a friend of the president and some other lady, I've forgotten — a princess or somebody. That's all." Besides Mahoney, the others were Jackie's sister Lee Radziwill and Kennedy's Choate school friend and adviser, K. LeMoyne ("Lem") Billings, according to a biographer of Garbo. She ended by wearing a dress and came with the husband of fashion designer Irene Galitzine, a couple with whom she was close, Mahoney said.[15]

Kennedy in 1961 appointed Mahoney to Food for Peace Council, which was set up "to help enlist support for the attack on world hunger" directed by George McGovern. It was part of the Kennedy administration effort to fight the Cold War with Russia by providing aid to underdeveloped countries worldwide. Other council members were author James H. Michener, actors Yul Brynner and Danny Kaye, Clark Clifford, Drew Pearson, Mary Lasker, and California Episcopal Bishop James A. Pike. McGovern asked Mahoney to chair a subcommittee on public information and education and to sit on the council's executive committee. "I am convinced more each day that the United States has an enormous national asset in its food-producing capacity," he wrote her. "How the Soviet world must covet this tremendous U. S. capacity!" In that role, she traveled with McGovern to India, the Near and Far East, and Africa. "I paid my own way because I didn't want to be obligated to anybody," she said.[16]

When McGovern told members that he was resigning to run for the U. S. Senate from South Dakota in 1962, he penned a personal postscript to Mahoney: "Florence, you are the most enthusiastic of all the Food for Peacers. You have been such a great friend from the first week I was in this office and especially during that long siege of illness. We must get together often."

Mahoney hosted a large reception to help McGovern's Senate candidacy, which was successful.[17]

"The proverbial soup"

On the home front, Mahoney and Lasker believed that President Kennedy was sympathetic to their research cause, evident when he had requested, while a junior senator, additional money to fund a backlog of approved grant applications. He nevertheless had called Fogarty to the White House soon after his election, hoping to prevail on a fellow Irishman and New Englander to hold the line on research budgets to what the generous president was offering. Fogarty told Kennedy he still considered the budget lacking and asked him to "reconsider."

Kennedy's Secretary of HEW, Abraham Ribicoff, soon dropped a bombshell that startled the Mahoney-Lasker forces, who thought they were safe from the kinds of budget cuts they had fought for the past eight years: He impounded $60 million of the $738 million that Congress already had voted for NIH's fiscal 1962 budget.

"We are really deep in the proverbial soup," Gorman wrote the women while they were vacationing in France in August 1961. Fogarty had "produced the surprise of the year. He read into the record letters he had written to President Kennedy and Secretary Ribicoff asking for their opinions as to the vast increases voted by the Senate" for HEW programs. It seemed that Republican Melvin Laird objected to much of the language that Gorman had written and the House committee had included in the funding bill, prompting Fogarty's action. "Fogarty, who can be very Irish and very immature, told [Luke] Quinn that he didn't give a damn what the White House did — he would take care of his business in the House." Senator Hill, though, was "on the warpath." He wanted to stop any negative response from the White House in its tracks. Gorman had been busy: "Acting upon Senator Hill's instructions," he had called HEW's special assistant Boisfeuillet "Bo" Jones, Surgeon General Luther Terry, and NIH's James Shannon, telling "all of them it was a moment of truth — they had to stand up for the Senate figure."[18]

Ribicoff (whom Mahoney considered a good secretary) was forced to be the administration's spear carrier for economy. "Some of the Secretary's fiefs are very rich, and some are poor," the *Washington Post* editorialized November 22, 1961, in favor of cutting NIH's budget. "Even the most enthusiastic supporters of the National Institutes of Health must concede that they have money pouring out of their ears, and can accommodate even a large reduction without difficulty."[19]

Mahoney turned to her friendship with media people to publicize her messages in such situations. Television nightly newscasters Chet Huntley and David Brinkley of NBC were happy to help in this case, broadcasting tidbits they received about research breakthroughs. "President Kennedy, in trying to get the government deficit down, has ordered a cut in the Department of Health, Education and Welfare, about $60 million of it to come out of medical research," Brinkley reported in November 1961. But "Today a group of cancer specialists said they were making . . . tremendous progress in treating cancer with drugs. They pleaded with the president to put the money back so they can start working full speed." Eleanor Roosevelt joined the outcry, stating in her column that

she thought it "the best example of how one should not economize . . . .
Granted we must keep a balance in military preparedness, but if our
people deteriorate in health and education, all the military preparation
in the world will not save them." Such reports were music to Mahoney's
ears.[20]

When Russel Lee joined a public-television debate on health issues,
Mahoney wrote Bess Truman, "I think David Brinkley is going to film it
and re-run parts of it nationally. Such a pity *you* are not here to help on
all this work!"[21]

In 1963, Congress, for the first time in decades, nevertheless reduced
the president's proposed research budget. Fogarty, apparently convinced
by Kennedy, told the House that the administration's figures were
"forward looking" and sufficient for the institutes' needs. More Members
of Congress now were beginning to question the high NIH budget.
Wisconsin Democrat William Proxmire, in an annual cost-cutting role,
introduced an amendment to reduce NIH appropriations, which this
time received support across party lines from both liberals and conserva-
tives. While the amendment failed, it worried Senator Hill, and he
agreed to moderation the following year in return for non-partisan
support in his committee. The NIH fiscal balloon was beginning to lose
air.[22]

Again, Mahoney and her team, especially "outside witnesses," were
called upon to make their case, disease by disease, for greater research
expenditures. Proxmire complained that opponents of such spending
were branded as "friends" of cancer or heart disease. But proponents
continued to prevail because the facts were clear — that progress against
diseases was being made.

Skeptics

Such contretemps were fodder for a growing number of skeptics about
NIH's unprecedented rapid expansion by Congress. Members who were
less successful than Fogarty and Hill "wondered aloud what the secret
weapon was" that their colleagues had. Some attributed much of it to

Hill's personal charm, but others "pointed to the powerful and ubiquitous lobby that supported and reinforced [them] in myriad ways," according to historian Strickland.[23]

By the mid-1960s, however, public pressure for better access to health care arose commensurate with anti-poverty and civil-rights initiatives that Congress, heeding President Kennedy's call for a "New Frontier," enacted. Questions began to be raised about NIH's large portion of the federal budget — could it justify its size and activities? Were people in need receiving research benefits, now widely publicized and touted? [24]

Such questions prompted Congressman Lawrence H. Fountain (Democrat of North Carolina) to begin a series of investigations on NIH management in his Government Operations Subcommittee on Intergovernmental Relations. The Fountain committee in 1961 began to scrutinize the NIH grant-making program, which represented more than three-fourths of its half-billion-dollar budget. The money went to researchers in some 400 universities and nonprofit institutions for more than 11,500 projects on many fronts. Ninety percent of the funds went to 200 universities and medical schools.

The value of the research was not in question. Fountain's concern was the quality of management by an institution that had grown rapidly and hugely, without long-range planning. Another factor was that while Congress gave NIH money for research, it held down expenses for the employees who administered the burgeoning agency.

Fountain insisted that his probe would not "impair the effectiveness" of the NIH program and that he simply wanted to help the agency address problems caused by its booming growth — in short, whether it was a "prudent expenditure of public funds." A *Washington Star* editorial that he quoted complained that NIH was being "force fed" by Congress.

Such unfavorable press must have irked Mahoney, but she was relieved when the first Fountain report, in April 1961, had little to criticize. "NIH is not adequately organized to adminster the grant programs with maximum effiectiveness," it stated, offering thirteen suggestions for improvement, most of which Shannon found "entirely acceptable." But it put the appropriations committees on notice, and, by implication, the Mahoney-Lasker team, which had been so inextricably involved in NIH's growth.

NIH friends were outspoken in defending it, especially before Fountain's committee that March. Director Shannon, perturbed at the idea of having to carry out all of the committee's recommendations beyond those he thought necessary and practicable, considered the complaints "essentially trivial in relation to" the good work that NIH was doing under rigorous criteria to avoid misuse of its funds. Fountain, Shannon felt, was nit-picking at unimportant matters. Senator Hill reportedly was furious at Shannon's effectively questioning another member of Congress' actions, although he may privately have agreed with Shannon.

The whole pro-NIH operation now had to walk on egg shells so as not to offend other congressmen and jeopardize future legislative actions. Until then only Fountain and his chief investigator (Dr. Delphis Goldberg) had been pushing the issue. Now additional committee members were offended by what they considered Shannon's arrogance, and their report (June 1962) pointedly took exception to his views, going so far as to say that Congress appeared to have been "overzealous in appropriating money for health research" and that "the pressure for spending increasingly large appropriations has kept NIH from giving adequate attention to basic management problems."

The next round of appropriations, as a result, saw NIH's funding reduced again, even below the president's request. Kennedy also requested a review of the entire federal medical-research program. His role in history was soon to be tragically cut off, however.[25]

The words that Kennedy had written Mahoney at his own brother Joe's death in 1944 echoed in her memory as the terrible news from Dallas on November 22, 1963, washed over her:

> His loss has been a great shock to us all. He did everything well and with great enthusiasm, and even in a family as ours, his place can never be filled and he will always be missed.[26]

Gazing at a signed photograph from Kennedy to her, she reflected thirty-five years later, "He had a wonderful smile."

Mahoney looked to the future, though, confident that many Kennedy advisors would carry on. "They have lost their patrol leader, but the issues are still there and they will accomplish their mission," she said in a published interview after the assassination. "They will work with Mr. Johnson," she expected, because they shared common ideals and because Kennedy had the "highest respect for what anyone could do well, tremendous respect for other human beings [and] for politicians — and all this came through." She had not seen any instances of internal friction among the Kennedy team, each of whom respected "each other's talents" and loved Kennedy for his sense of humor and fairness. His successor would be "a different kind of man," she admitted, "but that will be good for" the Kennedy aides, who she perceived wanted to stay on with the new president. [27]

Johnson administration

With the succession of Vice President Lyndon Baines Johnson to the presidency, Mahoney and Lasker knew that they had a sympathetic ally in the White House. Johnson nevertheless followed through with his predecessor's review, appointing a thirteen-person committee headed by Dr. Dean E. Woolridge to "study how NIH spends its approximately billion-dollar budget [and] to judge whether the American people are getting their money's worth." This committee differed, however, from those that had looked over NIH's shoulder previously, reinforcing the Mahoney-Lasker position. "This time there were no members of the committee who could be said to be faithful champions of the Cause," wrote Strickland.[28]

The "cause," though, and NIH, again came through largely unscathed. The Woolridge Committee reported that "the activities of the National Institutes of Health are essentially sound" and its budget "is, on the whole, being spent wisely and well in the public interest." The committee did recommend strengthening NIH's "organization and procedures" but concluded in words that heartened NIH backers like Mahoney:

We suspect that there are few, if any, one-billion-dollar segments of the federal budget that are buying more valuable services for the American people than that administered by the National Institutes of Health.[29]

Mahoney and her friends were relieved and went back to work with Hill and Fogarty on their side.

After two years of cutbacks, NIH budgets once again rose, even above President Johnson's requests. The billion dollars allocated to NIH, Senator Hill pointed out, was small compared to the $30 billion a year that Americans spent for health *services*. In addition, he noted, NIH's growth had stimulated private organizations to raise their donations for research at about the same 100-percent rate as NIH's budget was rising.[30]

Mahoney and Lasker both had close ties to the Johnsons. "He had heart," Mahoney said of the president, "and was very smart." As with the Trumans and Kennedys, her relationship with the Johnsons was warm and personal, evident in thoughtful notes between them, the Johnsons often replying the day after they received dispatches from Mahoney. She frequently visited the White House for social or ceremonial events such as bill signings and swearings-in, sent them (gifts like a pair of china plates from Andrew Jackson's administration for the Johnson Library), and acquired antique artifacts for them, such as a set of eighteenth-century marrow spoons purchased in Dublin in 1956. She invited Lady Bird to tea and sent greetings on the Johnsons' birthdays and anniversary. "You are a sweet, thoughtful lady — as I have always said — to remember me on my birthday," Johnson acknowledged in 1960. "It was nicer because you did."[31]

"The enclosed cup and saucer is for you," Mahoney said in a note to Johnson accompanying an anniversary gift. "It is quite rare and made in China about 1775. It is difficult to get pieces with the Eagle on and the initials say FMLL which stands for Florence M Loves Lyndon," she added at a time when he was becoming increasingly unpopular because of the Vietnam War. The gift was "to amuse the President," she told Mrs. Johnson, "he can always get interested in porcelain. A diversion???" Lady

Bird said in thanking her, "The nicest thing is what the FMLL stands for!"[32]

Mahoney's notes invariably tried to reinforce and cheer the beleagured president. "Do tell [him] for me that he was so good in the televised press conferences," she wrote his personal secretary in March 1964. "Florence Mahoney called to tell you how terrific you were last night," presidential assistant Jack Valenti said in a memo to Johnson following a speech in March 1965.[33]

"Thank you for thinking of me on the speech," Johnson replied, "and for doing all I know you do to support our purposes. You and Mary [Lasker] mean so much to us."[34]

Mahoney as usual also passed on medical tidbits. To George Reedy, the president's portly press secretary, she sent an article on dietary fat. "Perhaps things will slow down soon and we will be able to have a good discussion on calorie counting and the best ways to handle fat," he responded soon after the 1965 inauguration. To Mrs. Johnson she enclosed a biography of Margaret Sanger, asking if the First Lady might send her a message on the occasion of Sanger's eightieth birthday, and a copy of Mahoney's own statement to the Pope in an effort to enlist the First Lady's interest in international population control. "I appreciate your taking the time to keep me informed on the things in which I am interested," Mrs. Johnson replied to another package of information.[35]

"Florence shared a lot of values with Lady Bird," Phil Lee realized. "They were like colleagues, in a sense, more so than with Jackie [Kennedy]. With Lady Bird there was a real friendship. That was my impression." Both women were busy "activists, and they gave a damn" about issues. "With Lady Bird, I'm sure she talked about [everything from] beautification [to] highway safety [to] birth control."[36]

Dr. Joseph T. English, a former Peace Corps psychiatrist newly appointed to work on the Johnson anti-poverty program in the mid-1960s, had a memorable introduction to Mahoney's close ties with the White House. Confronted with the task of getting appropriations from Congress for a national network of health centers, he asked a friend, "How do you raise money for health care?" "It's very simple," she responded, "there's a woman in Washington named Florence Mahoney who's raised funds with Mary Lasker for all the federal health programs. The way you raise money is talk to Florence Mahoney." English promptly called her up and said he would like to accept a previously proffered invitation to dinner. "Why?" she asked. "I am now involved in health care for the poor," he said, "and I'm told that to get more money from Congress, I've got to convince you it's important."

"Nobody's ever called me like *that* before!" she laughed, adding, "How about Sunday night?" English "appeared at her table," whose guests included Senators Walter "Fritz" Mondale and George McGovern, HEW Secretary John Gardner, and presidential domestic counsel Harry McPherson.

"I was at the end of one table, she at the other," English recalled. "I was sensible enough to be silent while the dinner conversation went on. Florence finally said, 'I brought you here tonight because Dr. English has some ideas about improving health care for the poor in the United States, and rather than I tell you about it, I thought you should hear him.' I started talking and that began a friendship with John Gardner that ended bureaucratic squabbling between HEW and OEO and began unprecedented cooperation between them. We soon had $100 million for neighborhood health centers. It started around Florence's dinner table."

But a continuing appropriation to keep the programs running subsequently was held up. Again English found himself invited to dinner at Mahoney's. When he arrived, he was visibly downcast. "What happened to *you* today?" Mahoney asked. English demurred but she pressed him. "It must have been something awful — you look terrible." "It's my problem," he said, "I don't want to bother you with it." To which Mahoney said, "You're not going to get dinner until you tell me the problem." When he told her, she exclaimed, "Oh is *that* all you're worried about? I think we should get this cleared up before dinner."

She went to the telephone, and English heard her saying, "We have this young doctor here, he has all these good programs — it's just what your husband is wanting to do; it may be the most important health program in the administration, but it could go down the tubes." English realized with astonishment that she was talking to Lady Bird Johnson. When she hung up, Mahoney told him that Mrs. Johnson had promised, "Don't worry about it, we'll take care of it." When he reached his office the next morning, he had a call from the president's press secretary, Liz Carpenter, who said, "Joe, I don't know how you pulled this off, but your program has just become one of the five great pieces of legislation in the Johnson administration. I thought I should tell you, and Mrs. Johnson is about to make a tour of the five great achievements — including the Kennedy space program and the redwood forest — and we've decided to add the Denver neighborhood health center as another example. We want you to come on the First Lady's plane and brief Mrs. Johnson before she visits Denver." She added, "Does this have anything to do with the continuing appropriations?"

"I could tell you lots of things like that about Florence," English mused in retrospect, "who, by the way, a lot of people in Washington didn't know!"[37]

Mahoney also was close to John Macy, chairman of the Civil Service Commission (1961–68), who handled all personnel appointments during the Johnson administration. When Johnson faced choosing a new surgeon general in 1965 (after the resignation of Luther Terry), she had Macy "alone to dinner so we could discuss everything. There are so many applicants for surgeon general that it makes you ill," she wrote Lasker of what she considered a number of unsuitable candidates. "I explained the facts to Macy and am not worried." Sidney Farber "thought it would be a good idea to make Shannon SG and get him out of NIH," she added. Since they had not been consulted for their ideas on the HEW Secretary, she "was glad we are making this move" to influence the choice for surgeon general. Their first choice, Dr. Robert Aldrich from the University of Washington, was not selected although new HEW Secretary John Gardner considered him a good candidate. But he "was not *about* to let Jim Shannon go" as head of NIH, Gardner said years later, considering him a fine administrator and savvy politician who could give the secretary "seasoned advice."[38]

Basic versus applied research — struggle for control

The secretary would need good advice. Another long-standing debate was energized by the scrutiny of NIH in the 1960s — whether *basic* or *applied* research should be given priority by the government.

Basic research, the term used for studies of fundamental mechanisms of biology and other sciences, permits scientists to probe such things as the inner-workings of genes and origins of diseases without preconceived notions of the usefulness of such knowledge. *Applied* research puts to use discoveries and knowledge that benefit human health. Shannon defended giving priority to basic research. Forcing discoveries to be applied before they were thoroughly proven, he believed, was wasteful not only of money but scientific manpower and time and narrowed opportunities for the kinds of innovation that was often produced by basic research in unexpected and rewarding ways. "The development of diagnostic, therapeutic, and preventive capability [i.e., applied research] will continue to be dependent upon empirical approaches, serendipity, and the brilliance of too few gifted individuals" who undertook basic research, he stated publicly in a lecture in 1966.[39]

Shannon, and the scientific community who backed him, now appeared to laymen to be thwarting efforts to get medical advances to people who were suffering and to be opposing the position held particularly by Lasker. She turned to the White House after it was occupied by her friends Lyndon and Lady Bird Johnson, pressing the president to back her stance in favor of more applied research, arguing that scientists should start applying their findings from clinical tests when they were only 60 percent confident of positive results rather than 100 percent.[40]

Mahoney, while not as emphatic as Lasker in pressing for applied over basic research, wanted to see results *and* support of innovative research. Her self-education and years on NIH advisory councils had taught her to understand the importance both of fundamental research and the need to prod bureaucrats to move with greater dispatch than some wished.

She also recognized the political fact that research that focused on curing diseases resulted in funding. "It was the only way we ever got money for anything," she said. "It would be ideal if you could collect all the money that was needed for basic research, but since it was utterly impossible to be able to do that, you had to categorize it, or you never would get any money at all."

In that respect, Mahoney was like Fogarty and Hill, who shared a respect for basic work but made it clear that Congress' legislative intent was to progress as quickly as possible toward cures and breakthroughs. The coalition was experiencing what White House health-aide Douglass Cater termed "creative tension."[41]

While Lasker turned to the White House, Mahoney brought scientists, legislators, and policymakers together to talk. Both women were harder at work than ever, as were their professional allies, cajoling Congress for a variety of things they thought warranted immediate action by NIH.

One example of Mahoney's and Lasker's desire to see therapeutic results from research was in the development of chemical agents against cancer (chemotherapy). Lasker and Farber, both members of the National Cancer Advisory Council in 1963, urged the institute to begin widespread testing of the agents. They asked the council to invite industrial laboratories (as opposed to not-for-profit university or research institutions) to submit proposals to NIH in the form of contracts rather than grants. Congress had reinforced their position by earmarking considerable sums of money for the program. But NIH directors demurred, saying advisory councils did not have statutory authority to review contracts, only grants. In addition, although chemotherapy by the early 1960s suggested advances in cancer treatment, NIH opposed such approaches until better management of contracts was in place. That seemed ridiculous to the likes of Lasker and Farber.[42]

Another issue was the development of drugs to treat mental diseases, something that Mahoney particularly backed. Based on problems with the cancer chemotherapy program, however, the National Institute of Mental Health director believed that a large clinical-testing program was premature, as he had told Mahoney and Gorman, arousing the ire of the Committee against Mental Illness, which publicly accused the NIMH director of blocking the program.[43]

On still another front, Michael DeBakey's efforts to get NIH support for development of an artificial heart were blocked in 1966 because Shannon believed that, too, was premature, likening such haste to the Salk polio vaccine, which had been hurried into use despite the fact that an improved version was imminent.[44]

Mahoney and Lasker went to their Capitol Hill allies, and in the 1964 funding bill the Senate Appropriations Committee directed the cancer council to review contracts as well as grant applications. But Shannon went to his secretary, Gardner, who asked the congressmen not to press the matter until he could fully analyze its impact. They agreed, and Gardner appointed a committee to review the issue. Again the so-called health triumvirate was not a part of the committee, which ended by siding with Shannon, who had threatened to resign if the contract matter were not resolved in his favor. Not only did Shannon feel vindicated, but his position, with the backing of his boss in the executive branch, was strengthened against the Mahoney-Lasker coalition.[45]

Lasker, increasingly frustrated at Shannon's stone-walling her initiatives, again went to the top, urging President Johnson, the heart-attack victim, to call NIH to task. "'Give me a memo . . . ,' he said, and I appeared with it on June 15, 1966," Lasker recalled. "He used it at once," summoning Shannon and his directors to a meeting on June 27 along with the surgeon general and Secretary Gardner "to ask them what they were doing to save lives," as Lasker put it.[46]

Johnson called it a "strategy council in the war against disease," quoting extensively from the Lasker memo. Was "too much energy being spent on basic research and not enough on translating laboratory findings into tangible benefits for the American people?" he asked, posing a series of questions that had been composed by Gorman and Lasker. For two hours, Johnson reiterated that he wanted "results" from research and pointed to statistics showing that the United States had surprisingly poor overall health compared to other developed nations (it ranked eighteenth in life expectancy for men, eleventh for women). "I think the time has now come to zero in on the targets by trying to get this knowledge fully applied," he said. He concluded by telling the NIH leaders to reexamine the institutes' priorities with that objective in mind. He personally would follow up with a "checklist" — "like when you take a car in to get . . . the tires filled and the radiator checked and all those things . . . we will see what specific efforts they are going to make to reduce deaths among the leading killers . . . . In my judgement, *research* is good, but results are *better* . . . . We must make sure that no life-giving discovery is locked up in the laboratory."[47]

The scientific community was stunned. Well aware of Lasker's influence and agenda, researchers took the president's action as anti-basic science. What did the president know about such things anyway, they wondered? He had likened himself to an auto mechanic rather than a scientist and clearly was taking advice from lay people, not experts. "This is not an issue which should be decided on the basis of who happens to have the president's ear," wrote one critic. But Lasker felt that Johnson's action "reoriented the institute directors a little. Not Shannon, however," who she felt fought the president's message "with double-talk." One of her "great hopes" was that he would retire and not take "another job to make more confusion for us." His opposition stemmed from being "afraid of clinical research," she told an interviewer for an oral history in 1967.[48]

To counter Johnson's move, university researchers coalesced as never before and went to Congress to protest. Gardner had to calm them, explaining the president's rationale while assuring scientists that HEW had not changed policy away from supporting basic research.[49]

The scientific outcry was so vigorous that the president, through in-house advisers like Gardner and Philip Lee, heard the scientists' side of the argument. Medical cures could not be produced without tedious and time-consuming underpinnings, just as the nuclear bomb, developed by the Manhattan Project, could not have been produced without an understanding of basic physics and mathematics, he was told. The president, aides argued, had harmed himself by allying too vocally with one camp, and they concocted a brilliant public-relations countermove.

On a warm summer day in July 1967, Johnson boarded a presidential helicopter on the White House lawn, accompanied by a phalanx of reporters and photographers, and flew over the Capitol city to the Bethesda campus. Aboard the helicopter, Lee and other staff bent the president's ear about "why it was so important not to reduce NIH expenditures, what the payoffs were" of a solid research program.[50]

After a tour, Johnson told the assembled researchers in carefully crafted words, "The government supports this creative exploration because we believe that all knowledge is precious, because we know that all progress would halt without it." He rebutted what he called the "hot-shots" who "think we have reached what you might call a stalemate because we have not found all the answers . . . since we last ran our check," a backhanded slap at the Lasker camp. The president concluded by proudly calling the whole operation "the world's greatest research enterprise" — in short, he reiterated twice, it was "a billion-dollar success story." [51]

"We need a one-liner," Douglass Cater had said en route when Johnson asked him to cut his talk down a bit, but the president ended by ad libbing at length. "Billion-dollar success story" was the only quote reported in news accounts that evening, Lee recalled, noting how much more there was to tell. The president "not only was warmly received by the people out there but obviously reacted very favorably and very warmly to the whole business, and just kept on talking," he remembered.[52]

Scientists privately called the president's conciliatory act "the Pedernales solution," a reference to the river that ran through his Texas ranch where he took people to persuade or reconcile with them. NIH nevertheless "calmed down," as Lee recalled.[53]

Mahoney was delighted. "I keep hearing how great you were at NIH Friday," she wrote Johnson immediately after the visit. "Just spoke to one doctor who said he had never been close to you before and that you were so handsome and that your pictures do not do you justice." To which the president responded, "Your warm letter brightened my Saturday working day. Your reports on Secretary Gardner and Dr. Lee are very encouraging. I am grateful for your good opinions — and for all your good and tireless works."[54]

Mahoney at first had been astounded at the choice of Gardner to head

HEW. Presidential assistant Jack Valenti promised to arrange a dinner "so we could meet," she wrote Lasker soon after Gardner's appointment in the summer of 1965. "Says he is very nice. I don't know what he knows about health but he knows about education, and perhaps he will just leave the health part to [assistant secretary] Wilbur [Cohen]. Anyway, that seems to be the way it is and I was very much upset when I first heard it, having a Republican and no one with health interests" named to such an important health post. Neither Senator Hill nor Mahoney's group had been consulted about the appointment, which she thought surprising. The dinner took place a week after Gardner was sworn in. "The Valentis were going to have me meet him at their house but they have no cook so we are coming here. Have got the Hills coming," too, she reported to Lasker a few weeks later.[55]

Gardner, however, turned out to be a positive force for the health cause. "You have made such a good politician out of Mr. Gardner that we are always plotting who can help him," she would write Johnson two years later.[56]

Of Mahoney Gardner said, "She would introduce me to people, speak well of them, do what she could to build my good impression of them" in a low-key way. "Florence was so sensitive and skillful in her relations with people that I don't remember any pressures," rather, "lots of conversation, give and take, meeting people she wanted me to meet, that kind of thing. People who press too hard burn the ground around them — and that's the mistake that Florence never made. She just made very sure that I knew the people she regarded as good people. I think my very good relations with Lister Hill were unquestionably traceable to Florence." He counted Mahoney among a number of "great mentors" who guided him "through the mine fields" of Washington. Like Wilbur Cohen, Mahoney found "the way through in that kind of gentle, infinitely purposeful, but not confrontational, quiet way. That put her in a better position, really; at least, it certainly did with me."

He was struck by her ability to listen, to be interested in others' points of view. "Everyone wants to be interesting — but the vitalizing thing is to be *interested*," he often said in motivational speeches. "Every time I use that, I think of Florence. Those qualities are impressive in a person with the strong sense of purpose that she has." That "pulled her" and kept her "in contact with life."[57]

Fortunately for Mahoney's causes, Gardner also admitted to having "a fundamental bias in favor of the NIH," finding that, contrary to many government-run research efforts that he had observed, NIH's were "really quite good." He was "very conscious of the fact," however, that it was "on an upward curve that couldn't go on forever" and warned the NIH hierarchy accordingly.

It was clear that the times called for changes in federal priorities. People wanted to experience the fruits of their tax-supported endeavors, a campaign to which Mahoney and Lasker lent their backing.

Bringing research to the people

The battle lines between applied and basic research were drawn in another health-policy arena in the 1960s: the creation of federally funded Regional Medical Centers to make advances in research more accessible to the general public.

During the first years of the Kennedy administration, the Mahoney-Lasker team had begun to press for the creation of clinical centers throughout the country where promising new leads in heart, cancer, and stroke research could be tried on people. (Mahoney in time would suggest applying the concept to child-health research.) It also was another way to directly improve the health of the nation's citizens.

Gorman had persuaded the Democratic Party in its 1960 platform to call for a White House study of heart disease and cancer, which the Kennedy administration agreed to. Coincidentally, on the same day (April 21, 1961) that the president received news of an anti-Fidel Castro invasion into Cuba, he also got the health study. Unremarkable for its lack of ideas, Kennedy refused to make it public, and it was sarcastically labeled the "Bay of Pigs Report," reflecting the debacle in the Cuban harbor where the U.S.-backed invaders were captured. The concept appeared to die an early death, to the relief of Surgeon General Luther Terry and Jim Shannon.

Regrouping, Mahoney, Lasker, and Gorman decided that a proper commission — patterned after Truman's on the nation's health needs — would be a better approach to putting the idea forward. President Kennedy, although lukewarm to the idea, was considering naming a Commission on Heart, Cancer and Stroke — the last added as a consideration for his father, who recently had suffered one — when he was killed.[58]

By 1963 both House and Senate appropriations reports for several years had urged NIH to develop such centers, but Shannon had stubbornly resisted doing so, increasingly opposed, as were many scientists, to categorizing research by diseases. He even had cut his budget, under a directive from HEW Secretary Abraham Ribicoff, for the clinical-research program.

That infuriated Mike Gorman. He boldly went so far as to tell the House Appropriations Committee, in testimony as an "interested individual," that Shannon, who favored a "multi-categorical approach — which presumably covers everything from the one-day cold to the seven-year itch — has chosen to misunderstand" the clinical centers idea "for reasons of his own .... He did not," Gorman snorted, "take one dollar from his precious multi-categorical, amorphous, metabolic, or whatever, program centers."[59]

The idea of a nationwide network of centers where research could be combined with training and patient care was attractive to Lyndon Johnson, who knew about heart disease from personal experience. What Mahoney, Lasker, and Gorman envisioned made sense to Johnson, who shared the ideal that people everywhere should have access to the latest treatments.

The president, only a month after being elected, on February 10, 1964, announced the establishment of the Commission on Heart Disease, Cancer and Stroke, with DeBakey as chairman and Mahoney as one of about twenty-five members. "The President is very much pleased to have your assistance," Johnson's deputy special counsel wrote Mahoney, saying the objective was to "chart a course whereby our full capability in the health sciences can be brought to bear most rapidly and effectively on these three major causes of death and disability." Other members included Johnson's heart physician, Dr. J. Willis Hurst of Emory University, Mrs. Harry Truman, Dr. Howard Rusk, and others who shared the same objective. As Gorman put it, tongue-in-cheek, "We had a quorum."[60]

"Health is something that we treasure in this house," Johnson told commission members assembled in the Rose Garden. He exhorted them, in extemporaneous remarks, to "stay awake at night, roll over, go get a glass of water and come back and think some more on how to get the results that we know are within our reach . . . . We must conquer" these diseases, he went on, impassioned. "I am firmly convinced that the accumulated brains and determination of this commission, and of the scientific community of the world, will, before the end of this decade, come forward with some answers and cures that we need so very much. When this occurs — not 'if,' but 'when,' — . . . we will face a new challenge . . . what to do within our economy to adjust ourselves to a life span and a work span for the average man or woman of 100 years." Mahoney was photographed standing next to the president on what would turn out to be a historic occasion.

One historian wrote that it was "the major health event of 1964." Commissioners "went to work with a surge of excitement, moved by the need to go beyond the mere support of medical research to some new strategy that would really make a difference . . . . They saw theirs as the chance of a lifetime to influence policy at the highest level, and they were in a hurry to give the president something to use in his next State of the Union address, something practical, 'something other than poetic expressions,'" as one member put it.

By the end of the year, the commission had made its recommendations — promising "miracles" that might not occur, another member observed, to which DeBakey responded, "Miracles have been around the corner for a long time." The final report, heavily weighted in favor of applied science, retained the expectation of "miracles," given a massive expansion of research and manpower to mobilize a nationwide network of treatment centers. It was widely publicized — the prestigious *New England*

Journal of Medicine said it portrayed "an idealistic state of future well-being" — and Congress acted quickly on a bill that the president cited as a high priority. Within a year the Regional Medical Centers program — "a bunch of little Mayos," the president called them — was authorized.[61]

The concept was not without its critics, who on one hand thought it smacked of "socialism" and on another that it targeted diseases affecting only the elderly, from which people generally died anyway. Shouldn't more focus be on cures that benefited the young, they asked?[62]

The program as enacted would be watered down somewhat from the commission's original intent. The AMA opposed the measure as infringing on its fee-for-service system with salaried, government doctors. "There is much opposition against the centers," Mahoney recorded after dinner with Lasker, DeBakey, Farber, and Bo Jones, adding "We need all help" possible.[63]

She went to work, backing the White House Conference on Health, which would push the program forward, and recommending a number of experts who could help. "The goal of the government should be one level of health for all the people and that should be top quality," she wrote Douglass Cater April 22, 1965. "Have talked to Cater about names for a W. H. conference and about having a commission appointed by the President to study the population problem, and gave him names to be on it, and in touch often with [Wilbur] Cohen for a few names for the cancer council," she recorded in her journal. (Many of the participants in the health conference, held November 3 and 4, 1965, were suggested by Mahoney.)[64]

She organized a number of strategy sessions with key Members of Congress, including a new one, James Mackay from Georgia, whom she had helped get appointed to the Interstate and Foreign Commerce Committee. "I am certain it is all settled now and . . . Mackay could swing another vote and with his own" get the bill out of committee. "The best thing to do is educate Mackay right in the beginning. Have sent the Pres.[examples of] his letters home [to constituents] and will get . . . the Pres. to take notice," she wrote Lasker in August.[65]

The pro-centers forces gathered in Washington to push the bill when it became obvious that it was in trouble. "Sidney [Farber] is here for testimony tomorrow in the House for heart, cancer and stroke centers," Mahoney recorded in her journal. "The administration's testimony did not go well last week so it has to be saved by Sidney and Mike [DeBakey]."[66]

Johnson himself had to reiterate his commitment to the bill at the swearing-in of his new HEW Secretary Gardner on August 18, 1965, and to meet personally with AMA leaders, instructing Under-secretary Wilbur Cohen to work out the objections the doctors had to the bill in order to get it through Congress.[67]

"I hope you and Mary Lasker are leaving no hours unattended by work on all the medical bills we have before Congress," Johnson wrote Mahoney in September. "There is so much needed work to be done in this area and you and Mary are the pioneers who can be hugely helpful." Amendments were drafted that appeased the AMA, and Congress passed the measure for the president's signature in October.[68]

Mahoney and Lasker, at the bill signing in the East Room, sat just behind Mrs. Johnson, Gardner, and Senator Hill. Ironically, Johnson himself was about to enter the hospital for gall-bladder surgery. Lady Bird wrote in her diary that he "was having a whirlwind of a day . . . as though to show the world how tough, how indestructible he was."[69]

Mahoney sent him two books while he was recuperating. "I shall love reading Valley Forge aloud if he'll be still," Lady Bird said in thanking her, "or just to *me*, if he doesn't!" The president wrote Mahoney, "I appreciated your good letter about the White House Conference on Health. It is comforting to me to learn your appraisal of my new health team. I expect great things of them."[70]

The Regional Medical Center program, however, never developed as initially envisioned by its proponents because Medicare and Medicaid insurance coverage largely fulfilled the objective of making medical care available to the aged and low-income populations.

Population control and children

Mahoney took advantage of having friends in the White House during the 1960s to also further her interest in population control. She "had continuous input" to family-planning policymaking in HEW and the Agency for International Development (AID), according to Dr. Philip Lee. Her travels and association with Margaret Sanger had given her credibility: "She knew a *lot* about that subject," said Lee.[71]

Mahoney in 1962 had prevailed upon AID to reverse a decision cancelling the appointment of Dr. Russel Lee as an international consultant. Among other matters, he was to study population problems. "He called me and told me they had decided against his trip," said Mahoney. "I was *so* mad because it had all been arranged with AID." Soon after that she found herself sitting next to AID Administrator Fowler Hamilton at the home of *Washington Post* publisher Katherine Graham. "I talked to him all during dinner about how awful I thought it was that they had cancelled Russel Lee's trip. Finally Fowler said to me, 'If you'll be quiet about'" Lee's advocating population control — "'we don't want it intimated'" that he is pushing that through AID — "'I'll see what I can do.'" True to his word, Fowler called Lee back, "and off he went!"

"Florence really put the heat on him," Philip Lee joked, and with "several other people worked very hard" to get his father's "mission around the world" reinstated.[72]

It was during the Johnson administration that the U.S. government issued its first policy statement on population control. It was a "very tricky issue in those days," as David Bell, Fowler's successor, put it. It took another forthright woman advocate, Dr. Leona Baumgartner, then assistant administrator at AID, to articulate the way for a change in the government's position. On her return from a conference in New Delhi, Bell related, Baumgartner told him, "'I think I have figured out how U.S. policy can be presented so that we can help on the population issue. First we say that we will support only *voluntary* family-planning activities, and then only if they have a *method of choice*.' That meant that the Catholics, who had a method of choice" — abstaining, as Mahoney had noted in her communiqué to Pope John XXIII — "would be included." Politically it was doable, Bell realized. When a leading Catholic congressman with whom he discussed the idea said he would not object, "that was the turning point for U.S. population policy," Bell said.[73]

To avoid the words "birth control," AID called its department the "Office of Population Reference and Research," a reflection, Lee recalled, of how controversial the subject was. After joining HEW he was asked by Secretary Gardner to draft a family-planning policy like the one he had helped draft at AID. At HEW the words "family planning" were chosen over "birth control," again to assuage opponents. "President Johnson was the one who moved this and gave us the overall umbrella" in a "breakthrough" State of the Union Message in January 1965, recalled Lee. "It was the first time a president had ever given population control that kind of recognition," opening the way for government assistance, he said of Johnson's boldness.

Lee credited Mahoney with helping influence the president. "Her conversations had an effect. She didn't lose a beat" when the presidency changed following Kennedy's death, and she "constantly helped us," thanks to her easy access to the Johnsons. "Few people had more influence on that subject than Florence — more so than Margaret Sanger," he believed.[74]

The HEW statement — which "we worked and worked on," according to Lee — specifically made clear that it was not a "pro-abortion policy" so that Catholic hierarchy at least would be silent on the government's position. But at the White House Conference on Health, with which Mahoney was closely associated — "the first time a federal conference included a discussion of family planning," Lee noted — one speaker uttered the forbidden word, "abortion," causing consternation from Catholic leaders, who felt the White House had "reneged on our agreement." "People were very sensitive in the fall of 1965, ten months after the president's State of the Union Message, about this issue, and particularly about a government conference on the subject," as Lee remembered. Family-planning clinics for needy women nevertheless were set up throughout the country, funded with federal Office of Equal Opportunity (OEO) money as part of the government's anti-poverty program.[75]

One of Mahoney's major concerns for some time had been the lack of research activity on contraception. She found that Secretary Gardner shared that concern and wanted to encourage such research. With an infusion of earmarked money (about $1 million, Lee remembered), "people immediately started doing research on it." Prior to 1963, when the birth-control "pill" was first produced, there had been very little research in the field. "That was another area where Florence was very active," Lee said.

A related subject that commanded her attention in Johnson's "Great Society" era was helping children at an early age. A visit with Lady Bird Johnson on one occasion gave Mahoney the opportunity to explain a radical new approach being tried in Russia that she had heard about from a social psychologist and fellow NICHD Advisory Council member, Dr. Urie Bronfenbrenner. "He'd been to Russia off and on and came back and explained what they were doing with tiny children. They took them away from their parents and put them into beautiful houses with everything for them, even nurses. They could go home on weekends, but they had this place where they took these new babies, who were brought up properly. I kept thinking about how many babies were brought up in this country" without basic care and educational benefits.[76]

"I had plenty of trouble on *that* one," she recollected. "I had a lot of trouble getting things done on that council. So I had a dinner and asked all the best columnists to come so they could talk to Dr. Bronfenbrenner, but they actually drank too much before they got a chance to listen to him, so they didn't learn much from that. But then I asked Lady Bird if I could bring him over to see her and suggested that she invite all the wives of cabinet people. So she did, and she got so much out of it that I think that was the beginning of 'Head Start.'"[77]

"On Friday, March 6th at 4, a friend of Florence Mahoney's, Dr. Urie Bronfenbrenner, is going to show Mrs. Johnson his slides of the Russian education system," an invitation from the White House stated in 1964. The "Head Start" program that soon evolved — providing federal assistance for education and social services for poor preschool-aged children — became one of Johnson's most successful and long-enduring antipoverty programs. Mrs. Johnson became directly involved with "Head Start" from the outset and was its honorary chairman. She hosted a tea in the Red Room of the White House in February 1965 to help promote the idea.[78]

Vietnam War

By the middle of Johnson's term, the war in Vietnam was beginning to overshadow domestic issues. "The town is now divided into two groups," Mahoney wrote in early January 1966, "the hawks and the doves, and you can sense a reluctance on the part of people to have them together in small gatherings. Very subtle, but there."[79]

As the war escalated, Mahoney sent President Johnson encouraging words. "I like for you to have bright spots *when ever* possible," she wrote him in September 1967. "My son Michael said he hoped that you knew how many people shared Jack Valenti's sentiments and thoughts about sleeping better. Michael thinks Jack will get credit in history for having said it, too." Her reference was to Valenti's saying, in the face of growing public opposition to the war and anger with Johnson's policy, that he "slept better at night knowing that Lyndon Johnson is in the White House."[80]

The war prompted Mahoney to send the president information about a pet idea that she had been pushing for some years: "The reference to drafting females is an interesting one and one that I have talked about for some time because of the nursing shortage," she said of an editorial in *Modern Medicine* magazine, "sent to me by a doctor when I was on the committee to study how to help the shortage." One idea that she got HEW to consider was Dr. Paul Sanger's suggestion in 1968 to develop nursing courses for vocational training in high schools. Another advocate of taking students directly from high school into medical training was Dr. Grey Dimond, who set up an accelerated study program at the University of Missouri in Kansas City. Joseph Califano [special assistant to President Johnson] felt it had "merit" and urged the president to consider putting it into legislation. "I found the suggestions for pre-medical and continuing education to be of particular interest and I am having them carefully staffed out," Califano told Mahoney in March 1968. "In addition, as you know, we have already launched the effort to encourage nurse and home-healthcare training in high school. With thanks . . . "[81]

Mahoney's efforts gained acceptance and would have far-reaching effects for the future of nurse training. "We will be pushing the idea of nursing education for high school girls as part of the Volunteer Program announced by the President in the Health Message," Califano told her a few weeks later. "This will be done in several ways including the development of nursing curricula in vocational high schools and the development of vocational high schools oriented toward health occupations. In addition, our legislative program includes a request for authorization to strengthen the links between universities, junior colleges and other nursing schools to take full advantage of their training capacity. We will also encourage the States to introduce nurse training into their high school curricula. With thanks again for all your help . . . "[82]

The war, Mahoney soon found, was having a large impact on long-range health care matters. Soon after enactment of the Regional Medical Centers bill, Johnson put forth across-the-board budget cuts that surprised and aroused the health community. The pesky conflict in Southeast Asia was placing huge demands on federal coffers, forcing cuts in domestic spending. No one was more surprised than friends of the health cause. Howard Rusk, who had been sent to Vietnam by Johnson as a special envoy, wrote in the *New York Times* January 2, 1966, that it was "inconceivable" the pro-health Johnson "would give the indiscriminate axe treatment" to the "crusade."[83]

NIH particularly looked like a fattened calf that could be slimmed down and, like other agencies, suffered presidential restrictions on what it could spend. Congress nevertheless raised its funding in 1967. Its actions afforded another opportunity for critics to come forward, resulting in at least one instance of bad publicity for the cause. "The National Institutes of Health, one of the the few agencies on which Capitol Hill regularly showers more money than it requests, may get $4 million it did not seek this year for a heart drug study it did not recommend," the *Washington Post* blared on its front page September 3, 1967. The article went on to describe how Senator Hill had added $4 million to test a drug shown in British studies to lower cholesterol, a boon to people with heart disease. Congress' action was unusual because it rarely gave specific research instructions to NIH without its prior agreement.[84]

Behind Hill's action was Lasker's hand. She had become familiar with work on hormones to control cholesterol by a female professor at the University of California, Doctor Jessie Marmorston, whom Lasker also had recruited to treat Margaret Sanger. Convinced by the researcher's testimony, and DeBakey's favorable comments, Hill had ordered the money added to the Heart Institute's appropriation. It turned out, how-ever, that the institute already was testing the drug. Hill lost that round (the $4 million was deleted), and for the fourth time in twenty years, Congress in 1968 actually lowered NIH's budget.[85]

But even more momentous changes were in the wind.

Death and retirement

To Mahoney's dismay, and Washington's shock, on the day that Con-gress convened in January 1967, John Fogarty suffered a massive heart attack and died in his office. He had served for sixteen years as chairman of the House appropriations subcommmittee on HEW.

Fogarty was succeeded by a former Shakespearean actor, Daniel J. Flood of Pennsylvania. In addition to his dramatic flair, manifested in a long, curling handlebar moustache and red-lined cape, Flood had ex-perienced a brush with cancer. If he at first lacked Fogarty's expertise and interest, he soon developed both and became a major supporter of the NIH.[86]

Fogarty's death was followed by further shocks as the year progressed. Senator Hill announced that he would retire at the end of his 1968 term, in the midst of the unpopular Vietnam War and civil-rights unrest, lacking the spirit for a tough reelection fight and because his wife's health was deteriorating. The news "absolutely stunned" Mary Lasker. Although Mahoney understood Hill's motives, she recognized that things would never be the same for them in Congress. Hill, who had served for forty-five years, would be remembered as a "statesman for health" and hon-ored by having a new Center for Biomedical Communications (part of the National Library of Medicine) named for him on the NIH campus.[87]

Mahoney had maintained her tight relationship with Hill. "Have some very good ideas for you, re: education," she wrote in a note at the end of 1964. "You could do a National Institute for Education from kindergarden through high school for research in learning — on NIH grounds. All new methods could be tried for a national program: how to teach teachers and how to get children to learn the most, etc. [It] would help all programs and 'Great Society.' We have national schools for [the] army — why not a 'Hill bill' for one as a pilot school for all schools, even try out visual aids, etc.?" It was something that she had conceived while a member of the child-health advisory council, which, she was pleased to tell him, had approved a training grant for the University of Alabama. She also suggested names for a director of the institute and for members of the council.[88]

Shannon soon followed Hill and announced that he, too, would retire in 1968. NIH Deputy Director John F. Sherman remembered that Shannon and Wilbur Cohen had come to loggerheads over some issue and Cohen had issued an ultimatum, hinting that "it was about time" Shannon considered retiring. NIH and its budget no longer were sacred and safe from budget cutters. A "political dynasty," as HEW historian Rufus Miles called it, was truly ended, one that had been "without precedent and may never be matched again" for NIH and health policy in America.[89]

Critics

Despite their triumphs — though occasionally mitigated — during the Johnson years, Mahoney and her group were not immune from public criticism. Their successes in part prompted grumbling from those who thought they were amateurs meddling where they had no expertise. Lasker was the lightening rod that attracted particular attention because of her adamant stances on getting the earliest possible pay-off from tax-supported research.

The criticism reached a high point at the end of 1967, when *Atlantic Monthly* Washington-correspondent Elizabeth Brenner Drew wrote a tough analysis that the magazine featured on its December cover with the provocative title, "The Health Syndicate: Washington's Noble Conspirators."

Few had dared speak openly against the advocacy in which Mahoney was deeply involved, but Drew quoted unhappy scientists such as Shannon who described the negative effects that poorly designed, prematurely accelerated research might produce, such as deaths from experimental artificial hearts that were not thoroughly tested. The "extraordinary growth of the federal role in medical research," Drew wrote, was due to a "unique historical phenomenon" that had produced "some distortions and questionable departures in federal health policy." She focused on Lasker as the fulcrum behind a network of private citizens with "unparalleled" influence that one federal official called a "noble conspiracy" and on Gorman, "a high class kind of subversion." "We're not second-story burglars," he was quoted as saying, "we go right in the front door." Drew raised pointed questions about such power, which Johnson-aide Douglass Cater had admitted (at a Lasker Awards luncheon) "set a new fashion in lobbyists. The moving and shaking done by such womenfolk affects everybody, including the most obdurate politicians. Be glad for them, for our children's children will reap the benefits." Drew, however, wondered if such methods — translating "personal experience . . . into national health policy" — led to "a good deal of flukiness."[90]

Still, Mahoney's group had backers in Hill and Fogarty, both of whom liked to see results from their largesse in appropriations. "There is nothing more important than getting the findings . . . out to the patient's bedside," Drew quoted Hill as saying.

For all the criticism, however, it was hard to ignore the many changes for the better that had occurred because of the "syndicate's" persistence over a quarter century, and by association Mahoney received praise for what she and Lasker had been doing. Their instincts were correct, another government official told Drew; no one could disagree with the merits of building up the national research effort to the point that it had reached by the late 1960s, nor with the idea that its results should be made as widely available to every citizen as soon as possible. It was not the women's fault, Drew conceded, that the "U. S. Public Health Service, a quasi-military corps based on an 18th century concept, has been so lacking in courage and imagination, so deferential, in dealing with everything from disease prevention to pollution control."[91]

Lasker and Gorman in particular felt betrayed by Drew and her article, which predicted that "the voice of the health syndicate will be diminished." After all, Drew pointed out, Fogarty was dead, Lister Hill about to retire "in political trouble," and "Mary Lasker and Florence Mahoney are no longer young women." (They were sixty-six and sixty-eight, respectively.) "The health syndicate," Drew conceded nevertheless, while "probably unparalleled," was "certainly an important one. There may never be anything like it again."[92]

Even with those kudos, Lasker called it "a vicious article." It "tried to describe our activities over the last few years in a really unfriendly and scurrilous manner," she told an interviewer soon afterward. She had spoken only briefly with Drew on the telephone, and Gorman, in agreeing to talk to the reporter, had "thought she was sympathetic and was giving her background material," unaware that he was being quoted verbatim. "It was really a very unsympathetic piece, written, as Philip Wylie said, 'by a fool,'" Lasker felt. "All the criticism and snide attitude that [the heart, cancer and stroke centers program] was a mistaken policy is really vitiated by the fact that she didn't know her figures, as most readers wouldn't know either" — ie., the fact that "cancer and heart are the major causes of death from the age of one to ten and twenty to forty as well as from forty on."

Reflecting her contentious attitude on NIH Advisory Councils, Lasker attributed much of the article's negatives about her to a "power-drunk" director of the Cancer Institute, Doctor Kenneth Endicott, "who resented the fact" that she had urged the cancer council to approve $70 million in contract funds which he opposed. She believed that Endicott was retaliating against her because he "hated women and anybody like me who wanted to have anything done in a more orderly fashion. So what was critical [in the article] I can tell was either said by him or one of his henchmen. But the overall article is really contemptible, because it's unsynthesized, phony and poorly informed, but damaging."[93]

"Mrs. Lasker is admired," Drew had written, "Mrs. Mahoney is liked. Mrs. Lasker has been considered an able woman who has done good things but is too covetous of power, too insistent on her pursuits, too confident of her own expertise in the minutiae of medicine. Mrs. Mahoney is seen as gentler and warmer, and since she has never made the same claims, she has been easier to take."[94]

The article created a minor sensation, sparking one analysis in the national magazine *Newsweek,* which noted that a Lasker awardee that year was sixty-seven-year-old Claude Pepper, "one of the chief advocates of the categorical approach to medical research" that Drew was criticizing. A physician reader was so angry that he wrote *Newsweek*'s editor, "It appears that your medical writer misconstrued the intent of the Lasker-Mahoney combine in reviewing the unjust *Atlantic* article" to which he had written a rebuttal, "correcting the injustice done to the whole-hearted women who devote so much of their time and money to help the nation now and not in some nebulous time."[95]

The *Atlantic* printed a long letter to the editor from Gorman, refuting, point by point, what he called Drew's "inaccuracies." He had been misquoted as saying that Lasker "made" Fogarty by teaching him "everything he knew." "Mrs. Lasker taught him everything that *she* knew," Gorman said. "No one taught John Fogarty his magnificent parliamentary skills, his sense of timing, his great dedication, and so forth." The group, he retorted, was not as narrowly focused as Drew implied. "Since the mid-1940s, we have been deeply concerned with the shortage of doctors and other key medical personnel in this country," as well as with mental-health needs and training. Furthermore, "the whole point of the Regional Medical Program in the fields of heart disease, cancer and stroke, which [Drew] accuses us of rushing through the Congress with unseemly speed," was to improve access for the population at large to quality treatment at university centers . . . . We hope that the regional centers eventually will move into other disease areas," he added.[96]

Other letters attacked Drew for giving "an inaccurate and misleading account" of the centers' legislation and objectives, and for her charge that the "prevention and postponement of death among the aged may not be the most important priority in medicine." To the contrary, one physician wrote, "Science, for the first time in human history, has reached the stage where the prevention of aging is no longer an impossible dream."[97]

Mahoney and her stalwarts were not daunted by Drew or other doubters, but set about revitalizing their coalition and becoming acquainted with their new congressional and NIH leaders: Flood, Warren Magnuson of Washington, who took over the Senate Appropriations subcommittee, and Dr. Robert Q. Marston, the new director of NIH. That same year (1967) Mike Gorman got Senate Majority Leader Mike Mansfield to host a luncheon for his colleagues to hear DeBakey and other cardiologists describe the latest developments in heart research. Gorman joked that his role was to make sure the food was edible and "the tables were bussed properly."[98]

They would need all the help they could get because Congressman Fountain again was on the attack. This time he accused NIH of favoring a small number of medical schools in grantmaking, and, worse, he challenged the quality of research that it supported. Those factors, ironically, may have been a result of President Johnson's pressure to push for more applied research than NIH had supported previously. One grant in particular came in for criticism — a five-year commitment to the Sloan-Kettering Cancer Institute in New York. [99]

The diplomatic and thoughtful Secretary Gardner again was called in to fight NIH's battles. The agency defended itself against the accusations. But it needed all the friends it could muster.

That same year, the National Institute of Mental Health was removed from NIH and made a separate bureau within HEW. That was something that Mahoney and her fellow advocates had pressed for, believing that mental-health programs would fare better if outside NIH. The agency also had developed into more of a service than a research program.

But greater challenges were to come.

End of an era

As the war worsened and Johnson's expected reelection loomed in 1968, Mahoney and her friends rallied behind him. "In the last two days I've had calls from Mary Lasker, Mike DeBakey and Florence Mahoney," a memo to the president stated March 29. "Each one volunteered a willingness to support you in any way that we may wish. Dr. DeBakey said he would be glad to contribute money to a newspaper ad whenever it seems best."[100]

Unbeknownst to them, however, a major surprise was in the offing. President Johnson stunned the world by announcing a few days later, on March 31, 1968, that he would "not seek . . . [nor] accept, the nomination of my party for another term as your President." Still, he had nine more months to push his programs.[101]

The next week Mahoney was invited to the White House for a small dinner for departing cabinet members — "very small and interesting. Have kept notes." They were revealing of the First Family:

Pat Nugent [Luci Johnson's husband] left at 7 p.m. for Viet Nam. Little Lyndon, 9 mos. old, walking and so good. Conversation at dinner re: Larry O'Brien leaving and asked to see the President yesterday. Had cried and said how he hated leaving . . . . The President said [Secretary of State Dean] Rusk in pain and quite ill — stomach — and that he [was] the greatest Roman of all . . . . The President [went] to see the baby in crib after dinner . . . . President talked about [his] Library and how he wanted to train boys in political science [with] fellowships. Said it would be bigger and better than Hoover's or Roosevelt's, Eisenhower's or Truman's or Kennedy's . . . wouldn't ask anyone for money . . . . Showed Mary and me the new pictures in bed room . . . [reminisced that it had been] 31 years last p.m. since he had won his first squeaky election . . . [talked about] Chuck [Robb, his other son-in-law, a Marine officer] being already in combat . . . [and about] turning direction of Hanoi, soul searching.[102]

"I still remember seeing the president telling Pat Nugent goodbye at the elevator upstairs," Mahoney recalled of the moving scene. "He [Johnson] looked so *sad*. He was just sick. He was very fond of those girls, a wonderful father."

Mahoney would visit the White House several more times as Johnson's tenure wound down, including the swearing-in of Wilbur Cohen as HEW Secretary on May 16, 1968 — "the President and Wilbur both made amusing speeches" — and with Lasker, DeBakey, Rusk, Farber, and Mike Gorman to meet with the president on July 15.[103]

A year later, after Johnson had retired to his ranch in Texas, he wrote Mahoney, who was still sending him clippings, "It is beautiful here. Flowers are blooming everywhere, the countryside is a lush green and the air is laden with Spring. The evening drive to watch the deer is a pleasure I look forward to every day. It is respite for the soul just to drink in nature's generous offerings." It would be one of her last communications from him.[104]

When he again suffered heart problems in the spring of 1972, Lady Bird Johnson told Mahoney, "The high spot of these long hospital days comes when I walk into Lyndon's room with a big handful of dear letters like yours. They do more to cheer him than anything else imaginable," adding in her own hand, "After the flurry of extra heart beats on Monday, Lyndon has once more reached a stable situation and we're beginning the long, slow return to activity with a good deal of cheer and *all* determination."[105]

Unfortunately Johnson, who had worked so hard to expand such research, was unable to benefit from subsequent discoveries in the treatment of heart disease and died of it the next year at age sixty-five. His daughter Luci wrote Mahoney after his death, "Your friendship through the years has always been a source of happiness for our entire family. Your recollection of those special magical moments we were privleged to share with Daddy will ease the pain of facing tomorrow without him."[106]

Mahoney disagreed with critics who accused Johnson of responding to laymen rather than knowledgeable experts in his health policymaking. She believed that he had a genuine commitment and personal interest in fostering biomedical research and solutions without damaging the integrity of basic science, which he continued to support along with efforts to bring new findings to the bedsides of afflicted people. Nobody wanted those more than the afflicted Johnson. His idealism — that all people should enjoy the quality care that he had — and his hopeful expectations for improved treatments injected the research cause with an energy that it had not enjoyed from any previous president. He embodied the views of the Mahoney-Lasker team, which had told him, when presenting him a Lasker Award in the Cabinet Room on April 7, 1966, for "leading this God-inspired crusade against needless disability and death": "We glory in your impatience with things as they are."[107]

A Republican administration moved into Washington in 1969 and its leader, Richard Nixon, the White House. His team quickly instituted rigorous military-industrial management practices and ruthless budget cuts, particularly in those agencies like NIH that had grown fat during a decade of Democratic regimes.[108]

With its champions gone, Congress failed to raise the NIH budget in 1969, and the next year actually reduced it. The first Nixon budget request for NIH, for fiscal year 1970, was $35 million below the previous year's appropriation; for FY 1971, it was $20 million below the previous year's appropriation. The Nixon administration also put preference on breakthroughs showing promise for application as opposed to basic research. Now people at NIH had reason to worry about political interference.[109]

If some proclaimed that the "golden years" of NIH had ended, that was a red flag to Mahoney, Lasker, and their allies. But they would have to adapt to new political policies. They had no friends in the White House and had to court new members of Congress. Although, as Drew had said, they were "no longer young women," their activities did not reflect slowing down. Lasker renewed efforts backing a national health-insurance plan. Mahoney continued her form of lobbying and advocacy through personal friendships and social gatherings at her home, particularly with newcomers to Washington.

Among new and vocal allies were university scientists and administrators, who became less timid about speaking out before Congress in defense of their work to counter the enemy, now more than ever, the Budget Bureau.

Both women felt a political sting, however, when their terms on NIH advisory councils expired in 1970, and they were not reappointed. It was the first time in eighteen years that Lasker had not been on a council. Mahoney had served intermittently for more than twenty years. "Some thought the medical research lobby was through," wrote Strickland of that move.[110]

"One of the really extraordinary lobbying jobs of our lifetime"

The research effort had continued to thrive through the 1960s despite periodic lack of political support in the White House, friendly and unfriendly reviews by various committees, hostile investigations by a not-always-understanding congressional committee (Fountain's), unfavorable press at times, and a constantly vigilant Budget Bureau. The quality of NIH research, however, was rarely questioned again after Fountain's concerns were rebutted. It was a testament to the merits of the agency's oversight, and to ever-curious and persistent scientists, that it continued to produce positive results that would make life better for all humankind. The United States by 1970 led the world in science, especially biomedical sciences, thanks in a significant degree to Mahoney's and Lasker's and their colleagues' enduring belief in the merits of what they espoused.[111]

Mahoney and Lasker, in John Gardner's perception, "did one of the really extraordinary lobbying jobs of our lifetime. Compared to the enormous power circles that characterize Washington, they didn't have many battalions," he laughed, "but they got something done. It's a story for any history of our time in Washington. They were two absolutely dedicated people."[112]

Few disagreed with NIH claims, articulated by the president of the Association of American Medical Colleges in 1970, that over a twenty-year period, its work had "revolutionized the range of diagnostic, therapeutic and preventive capabilities; advanced prognostic expectancies in many disease areas; [and] opened penetrating insights into nature and processes of life." Once widespread infectious diseases by then were virtually eradicated in the United States.

DeBakey boasted that for heart disease "more progress has occurred in the past fifteen years than in all previously recorded history, owing almost exclusively to laboratory research." The heart-lung machine, a perfect example of that progress, was being "used daily in operating rooms around the country to support blood circulation while surgeons repair diseased hearts or segments of the circulatory system in patients who previously would have been doomed to death."

New anti-cancer technologies were curing one in three cancer cases. Even the controversial chemotherapy program was now given marks for causing remission in twenty-one different types of cancer, as were drug treatments for mental illness. There were breakthroughs in curing or treating hypertension, German measles, and Parkinson's disease, some sup-ported by federal agencies other than NIH.

Most of the advances in biomedicine were the direct result of the taxpayer-supported federal program at NIH, however, which in turn had stimulated research in the private sector. More scientists were being educated, more physicians graduated than ever before in the United States, thanks to federal underwriting of medical education, a correlating benefit of the enterprise in which Mahoney had figured so prominently.[113]

Wilbur Cohen, in an oral history of his years at HEW, declared, "There were . . . four women who I think were more influential with Johnson than almost any other people . . . . Mrs. Johnson, first and foremost, secondly, Mrs. Mary Lasker, third, Mrs. Arthur [Mathilde] Krim [a close friend of the Johnsons], and fourth, Mrs. Florence Mahoney. If you really want to find out how things got done in the Johnson administration, you've got to find out from those four women, because . . . when I couldn't get something done, I worked through those four women. I was more successful in working through [them] than I was with the White House staff. That's an interesting observation, isn't it?"[114]

Cohen learned an interesting lesson about how the women operated. When he complained to Krim that Johnson was becoming irritated by all the pressure he was receiving from the women, she replied, "Don't let it bother you. The president likes to be pressured by us. That's something that he knows and understands. While he objects to it verbally, if you didn't do it to him, he wouldn't know how to deal with it. So let's just go ahead and put the pressure on him." It was an astute observation, Cohen realized, and one that Mahoney also understood. "He honestly wanted these women's views," said Cohen, "so he would alternate between fussing at them and at the same time inviting their pressure." If he did not hear from them for a time, Cohen felt that Johnson probably would call them up and ask what they thought about some issue.[115]

He went on to describe Mahoney as "one of the women who, as far as I know, had direct access to President Johnson on the telephone, easily, conveniently and quickly." She, like the other three, had Johnson's attention, because "He was the kind of man who would be perfectly willing to repeatedly listen to the views of certain people whose contact and friendship had been built up over his lifetime, and who he had fixed in his mind did not have any ulterior purpose [or interest] in embarrassing him . . . . The four women . . . had this common element — that President Johnson could talk with them, get their comments with the ultimate feeling that [they] were loyal, friendly and trustworthy."[116]

Mahoney would not have the same relationship with the man who succeeded Johnson to the presidency. But she now had her own agenda, which transcended partisan politics.

7

It's about Being Healthy
While You're Here

———————————◆———————————

T HE DECADE OF THE 1970S would be momentous in the history of
Mahoney's accomplishments, a decade in which she and Lasker led
personal campaigns in different directions. The "medical research enterprise" of which they were considered a vital part "was still largely intact,"
historian Strickland wrote after the election of Richard Nixon, and although it "might have lost some of its force," it had developed "a life and
momentum of its own." That enterprise, however, was about to be tested
as never before, and Mahoney, then in her seventies, would branch off
on her own, taking the initiative in a single-handed effort that would
succeed only because of her conviction and persistence.[1]

The lobby's first challenge was the fact that Nixon was not as generous
to NIH as previous administrations had been. Nixon and his staff were
out for budget cuts — his first budget director, Casper Weinberger, was
dubbed "Cap the Knife" — and Nixon wielded the veto with dispatch,
especially on an issue that would be dear to Mahoney's heart.[2]

Scientists and their advocates like Mahoney and Lasker would have to
become better at explaining what they were doing. The scientific com-

228

munity, principally academic medical-center researchers who benefitted from NIH's largesse, represented by the Association of American
Medical Colleges (AAMC), during this period grew into a sophisticated
and vocal constituency that could aid the women in their pitches.
Mahoney's many friends at universities in those years would come
forward to testify or visit their legislative delegations and government
policymakers in person, often at her urging.[3]

"She would say to a member of Congress, 'There's a doctor I want you
to meet,' and the next day he would be invited to cocktails or dinner or
whatever," Strickland observed of her putting such people together in
those crucial years. She used such gatherings sparingly and purposefully,
however. "She didn't overload" her politically savvy dinner parties with
scientists, remembered Assistant HEW Secretary for Health Dr. Charles
Edwards, a frequent guest. "She used science when she needed science."[4]

"Trying to land a man on the moon without knowing Newton's laws of gravity"

Lasker on her part launched what would be her most daring — and controversial — campaign. It was one that Mahoney would not share, either
in belief or actions.

Partly influenced by others and partly by her own convictions, Lasker
honed in on the most feared disease, cancer. What was needed, she and
her backers believed, was a full-scale "war," and in December 1969, a
Citizens' Committee for the Conquest of Cancer (whose address was the
same as the Lasker Foundation's) placed a full-page ad in the *New York
Times* remonstrating, "President Nixon, you can cure cancer." Lasker
joked that while the ad cost her $22,000, it resulted in 6,000 to 8,000
letters to the White House.[5]

One of their arguments was that decisions at NIH had to go through
"six layers of HEW bureaucracy" from laboratory to human tests. Why
not eliminate those layers by taking the cancer research program entirely
out of NIH and HEW?

It all sounded good to the unknowing public, even to many in
Congress.

Early in 1970, with oncologist Farber prominently at her side, Lasker prevailed on Senate Labor and Public Welfare Committee Chairman Ralph Yarborough to employ her oft-used and seemingly nonpartisan "white-paper" tactic: He appointed a Committee of Consultants on Cancer (thirteen scientists and thirteen lay persons) to review current cancer research and recommend ways to "achieve cures" for its "major forms by 1976 — the 200th anniversary of the founding of this great Republic," calling "the conquest of cancer . . . a highly visible national goal." It was in part an effort to boost Yarborough's reelection. A few months later, with little discussion or contemplation, Congress, in a nonbinding resolution, expressed what was thought to be a harmless "sense" that a "national crusade" against cancer was needed.

The "consultants," however, had a war plan. Chosen from a list specifically drawn up by Lasker and her colleagues, they included allies from old battles — Elmer Bobst, a personal friend of Nixon's; Emerson Foote, the former advertizing executive; Anna Rosenberg Hoffman; Dr. Mathilde Krim. Sidney Farber was vice chairman and a former law student of Yarborough's, Benno C. Schmidt, a wealthy investment executive and Republican, was named chairman.[6]

Now, rather than a friend to NIH, Lasker would become its chief antagonist. Mike Gorman and Luke Quinn were the lobbyists for what would become Lasker's toughest fight.

"None of us could understand her rationale," said Dr. John F. Sherman, then NIH deputy director. Edwards, who had joined the Nixon administration as head of the Food and Drug Administration in 1969 and subsequently became HEW's assistant secretary for health, believed that Lasker was "manipulated by lots of people" in the cancer endeavor — unlike Mahoney, he noted, whom "no one manipulated," and who took no part in the cancer endeavor.[7]

With such a make-up, the consultants committee, not surprisingly, in November 1970 recommended an assault on cancer directed by an independent National Cancer Authority responsible only to the president.[8]

Yarborough, though, suffered a primary defeat and was retired that same year. Massachusetts Democrat Edward Kennedy became chairman of the Senate's authorizing health subcommittee in 1971 and took over the cancer fight, introducing, with Republican colleague Jacob Javits of New York, the Conquest of Cancer Act, reflecting the panel's recommendations. President Nixon, not to be outdone by a potential future presidential rival (Kennedy), tried to one-up Congress by suddenly adding $100 million to the 1971 NIH budget specifically "to find a cure for cancer." He echoed the consultants allusion to its being comparable to a "Manhattan Project" or "moon shot," the successful government efforts to develop the atomic bomb and land a man on the moon.[9]

The bill in effect moved the Cancer Institute out of the NIH and gave it special standing with funding to be appropriated "as may be necessary" — an unprecedented arrangement. NIH leaders and scientists throughout the country were appalled.

Their reason, as NIH Director Marston put it, was that separating one research effort from others was foolhardy because biomedical work benefitted from interaction among researchers. That was how serendipitous discoveries occurred. Besides, as cancer experts themselves stated, the basic knowledge for such a "moon shot" did not yet exist. The origin and causes of cancer still were elusive, despite years of hard work to find out what caused the disease and the most effective antidotes to cure it. "An all-out effort at this time," stated one eminent cancer researcher, "would be like trying to land a man on the moon without knowing Newton's laws of gravity."[10]

Opponents of the bill argued that expecting cures from a targeted "war on cancer" was a fallacy at that point. Many avenues still were being explored — anti-viral vaccines, antagonistic chemicals, genetic possibilities. More dangerously, separation from NIH threatened to shift emphasis away from basic research, which produced the kind of information conducive to finding cancer breakthroughs. Changing federal bureaucracies would not change the state of research, would do harm to scientific practice and expend funds that could not be efficiently used. The whole idea was anti-science, they felt.

One member of the Senate health subcommittee — Democrat Gaylord Nelson of Wisconsin, whose father had been a country doctor

— in preparation for the first hearings on the bill in March 1971, had done some digging. He had talked to a number of scientists and medical experts who laid out strong reasons to oppose what appeared on the surface to be a good idea.[11]

Nelson, who with his wife Carrie Lee was a good friend of Mahoney's, learned privately that Nixon's HEW Secretary Elliott Richardson was not sold on the bill either. Neither was the president's science advisor, Dr. Edward David, Jr., who favored leaving NCI within NIH's administrative purview. In fact, the administration did not actually anticipate changing the organizational status quo. Nobody disagreed that the research effort should go forward.[12]

Nelson, during the hearings, surprised Richardson by bluntly asking his views and evinced from him a confession that a separate cancer agency was not a good idea.[13]

The Lasker forces were furious. They countered with a major media coup — this time, without any of Mahoney's help. Lasker contacted her friend "Ann Landers," a.k.a. Eppie Lederer. She ran a personal plea in her column April 20, 1971, that began, "If you are looking for a laugh today, you had better skip Ann Landers." She asked readers to write their senators and demand the separate cancer agency.[14]

"We're going to blow you out of the water with an Ann Landers' column," Gorman had boasted to Phil Lee in advance of its appearance, and "they did," Lee admitted. Within days, congressional offices began receiving huge mail bags stuffed with postcards and letters, the public's emotional response to Landers' column.

Opponents of the concept still had only the one voice on their side in the Senate. But Nelson was fully convinced of the wrongness of the approach advocated by Lasker and company. He retorted on the telephone to Lederer, whom he had known when both were building a fledgling Democratic Party in Wisconsin, "Eppie, it may be politically smart but scientifically it's the stupidest g--d--m thing you could possibly do." To threats that she and Lasker might not back him in future reelection campaigns, he shrugged.[15]

The scientific community began to take heart from Nelson's courage and forthrightness. Backed by NIH leaders who secretly worked with Nelson's staff, they began to mobilize their own constituency to counter Lasker's and bring reason to the debate, writing and calling on their congressmen in unprecedented numbers. Nobelists and leading scientists came out of their laboratories to meet with senators and their aides. No senator, however, wanted to appear pro-cancer, and the bill moved forward as if unstoppable.

Nelson warned his colleagues that separating cancer from other research activities portended the disintegration of the world's finest biomedical enterprise. Heart disease lobbyists, after all, were waiting in the wings to follow suit as were other disease-oriented interests. Three distinguished scientists on the original consultants panel, encouraged by Nelson's outspokenness, publicly dissociated from it and supported his position. NIH leaders privately backed him to the hilt. Philip Lee, by then chancellor of the University of California Medical School, read into the hearing record the now-retired Shannon's testimony opposing the idea of a separate cancer effort as "dangerously destructive," warning against the possibility that "uncritical zealots, experts in advertising, and rapacious 'empire builders'" — an attack on the Lasker forces — would dominate the program. Nearly eighty university medical-school chairmen and their deans, organized by the AAMC, joined the outcry in favor of keeping the research effort within NIH, and thirteen leading scientists (including five Nobelists) signed a letter to the New York Times saying the Senate bill was not "a rational approach to the conquest of cancer because it narrows the scientific focus."[16]

Their outcry was beginning to be heard, but only slightly. The Senate bill was redrafted, giving the cancer program direct budget lines to the president (bypassing HEW and Budget Bureau clearance) and the president authority to appoint its director, in effect eliminating control by the institutes over cancer research. That still augured disaster for the future of NIH, Nelson and his scientist allies believed.

When the bill came before the full Senate in July, Nelson boldly voted "no." The count was 79 to 1. Afterward, several senators, meeting him in an elevator, admitted that he was right in opposing the bill, that they had not had the courage to face angry constituents by voting in a reasoned way rather than bowing to emotional pressure. Nelson's was the loudest vote cast in recent Senate history, Assistant HEW Secretary for Health Affairs Dr. Merlin K. DuVal remarked afterward, one "that was to echo down the years and be heard again," according to historian Natalie Spingarn. Editorials nationwide praised his wisdom and courage "on a highly emotional issue," one calling him "the only person in the U.S. Senate with guts enough to risk a charge of having voted in favor of a horrible disease."[17]

The House then took up the matter. Nelson was the leadoff witness before Representative Paul Rogers' health subcommittee and set the tone for a more balanced bill. "If the Congress adopts the ... Senate bill, it is the first giant step in the dismantling of the National Institutes of Health," Nelson stated. "Next will follow the National Heart and Lung Institute with a political case for independent status equally as compelling .... I emphasize the word *political* as contrasted with *scientific* because no scientific case whatsoever has been made for separatism. In fact, the scientific case is overwhelmingly against it. What we are dealing with ... is a mischievous political compromise of a very important scientific matter.... The enormous irony," he concluded, "of proposing a moon-shot-type agency for cancer is that the breakthroughs to date have occurred *because of the capabilities* of the National Institutes of Health and its National Cancer Institute, *not in spite of them*."[18]

Again the Lasker camp responded with publicity, placing full-page ads in committee members' districts, funded by the American Cancer Society and the Citizens' Committee for the Conquest of Cancer, chastising representatives for thwarting the "war" effort. The plan backfired, though, angering congressmen, who raised questions about the society's tax-exempt status when it was clearly lobbying. Nelson's initially lone stance now had adherents in the House. The final compromise bill resulted in a largely symbolic change in how the cancer budget would be handled at the federal level. The scientists had preserved the integrity of their institution, but at some political price: Both the NIH and Cancer Institute directors henceforth would be appointed, not by the HEW secretary and NIH director, respectively, but by the president.[19]

The great cancer debate thus put a large political foot in NIH's door. Scientists who received grants or contracts from the other institutes worried that their funding levels would be reduced while cancer's grew. Other disease interest groups took note. It would be hard in the future for Congress to keep them in balanced perspective when their advocates marched on Capitol Hill demanding a cancer-like "war" on behalf of diabetes, arthritis, AIDS, and other afflictions. Ironically, the very fears expressed to Senator Pepper's committee in 1944 were resurfacing among the scientific community; one scientific spokesman warned, "Much of the freedom of science is now being legislated away and we are approaching the Russian system of directed research."[20]

Nixon's heavy hand was felt in 1972, when, under the new law, he dismissed Marston as NIH director, a move widely considered a political decision to replace an appointee of the previous Democratic administration.[21]

Grumbling rose in the mid-1970s that NIH's advisory councils were threatened with politicization, something Mahoney had experienced in the Eisenhower days when Senator Hill's recommendation of her had been turned down. During the Nixon administration even Congress balked when it was rumored that politicians were "clearing" council members based on party affiliation.[22]

Sadly, several of the players in the cancer debate, notably Luke Quinn and Sidney Farber, would die of the disease not long afterward.

Defection

Mahoney conspicuously parted ways from Lasker on the cancer issue. "Mary didn't understand why Florence was taking time away from cancer," as Gorman saw it. But she considered Lasker's approach wrong and ill-conceived. "I think that was another thing that endeared Florence to me," commented John Sherman.

"Florence was very skeptical about that," Strickland remembered, probably because "she kept in touch with scientists as well as legislators. One reason people liked and respected her was that she was willing to listen to other views. She was more reasonable, would listen to the other side. She was deeply interested in research and science, whereas Mary was interested in results, how you got there. She wanted to push the consistently slow scientists. The cancer issue gave momentum to a diversion of interests between Mary and Florence."[23]

"I didn't see any point in taking it out of NIH," Mahoney reflected of her position. "I thought it was a dumb thing to do, bad publicity — and unnecessary, in the first place. We had spent all that time getting NIH organized — why do this? There was plenty of money for cancer research at that point. And nobody wanted it done, but Mary was very determined about anything she set her mind on."[24]

Gorman, the long-time proponent of "categorical" research, later confessed that he, too, thought that pulling cancer out of NIH "was stupid . . . . I talked to Mary and told her there was no logic in taking it out. The fundamental thing was that we had been trying to add more to the NIH for twenty years, and here she was trying to get a major program taken out." As a result of his promoting a "deal" to establish a three-person presidentially appointed cancer panel, Gorman said, "Mary's hard line about taking the war on cancer out of NIH was finally shelved."[25]

Mahoney, meanwhile, was involved in a campaign of her own.

An institute on aging

"I'm working now for a bill that would create another institute for the National Institutes of Health," she told a reporter in 1974. "This one would serve as a center for research into aging. I am convinced that if we get one, within a few years — with drugs and knowledge — we would prevent or slow down the disease of aging."[26]

This time she was on her own. Lasker did not participate in the aging crusade although she was mildly encouraging from the sidelines. "She was delighted that it was going on, she wasn't against it, she just didn't do any work on it. Mary was of the opinion that once you solved cancer and heart disease, you solved aging. I thought that was ridiculous," Mahoney said.

She had become aware that the Institute of Geriatrics in Bucharest, Romania, was studying chemicals aimed at the prevention and treatment of aging. Russian leaders, including Nikita Khrushchev, were going to Bucharest for rejuvenation treatments, and the Soviet Union set up its own research institute of gerontology to study chemicals such as Gerovital and Procaine, which purported to slow the aging process.

Mahoney, increasingly frustrated that no similar research was going on in the United States, wrote the Romanian woman, Anna Aslan, who was the treatment's principal proponent and obtained the serum, according to Charles Edwards, then FDA administrator, and his wife Sue. Mahoney introduced them to the Romanian when she visited the United States. "Florence took that religiously and asked me to try it, saying, 'I want your reaction to it,'" recalled Sue Edwards. For the head of the FDA, it "presented a dilemma" because the substance was not approved for use in the United States. "How she got it, I have no idea!" Edwards remarked with bemusement years later. Mrs. Edwards, reflecting on Mahoney's long and healthy life, thought that there might have been something to the treatment.[27]

Dr. Grey Dimond, in a memoir published in 1991, commented on Mahoney's occasional attraction to unorthodox remedies: "Flo did not encumber herself with trying to understand the basic science involved. This was not her special skill. She did work hard at knowing the people in the research labs and knowing what they needed. Her accuracy in separating real science from charletan science was not precise; she occasionally backed a rejuvenation expert who had mastered promotion and mystique." The serum treatments later were proven to be not effective in slowing aging or lengthening life. "In retrospect, it was probably a terrific placebo rather than an actual chemical effect," according to a leading gerontologist.[28]

As a member of the NICHD Advisory Council (1963–67), Mahoney had noticed that gerontological issues got short shrift. Its emphasis was primarily on child health, reproduction, and fertility, a reflection of the discipline of its director, Dr. Robert Aldrich, a pediatrician, and of President Kennedy's intent in directing its establishment by executive order.[29]

"Every time a grant came up about aging, it was turned down," Mahoney said in published interviews. "Everyone said aging came naturally.

I never believed the effects of old age were irreversible." Perhaps drugs, like those being studied in eastern Europe, could counter the fact that "30 percent of the brain's cells die with old age," could "keep people from a certain kind of aging, or the lack of memory. We know nothing about diet," she told a writer, "all we know are vitamin requirements. We talk about vitamin E but nobody has done anything about it. Maybe by special treatment of diet and drugs, we might keep people out of nursing homes and if we can keep people at home, and their minds are all right, they'll be better off and so will the country," to say nothing of the reduction in cost for care in institutions where little was being done for seniors. [30]

"I kept telling them not to discourage those grants, or they would have to have another institute," she said. People laughed at her at the time.

NICHD had set up a Gerontology Research Center in 1968, but it was inadequately funded and staffed. Adding that aspect to NICHD's responsibilities came in response to a recommendation of a 1961 White House Conference on Aging.[31]

Another White House Conference on Aging in 1971 had taken cognizance of the NIH's inattention to the subject and recommended the establishment of a separate institute, validating Mahoney's arguments. The American Gerontological Society also began to push for it, "which is not to take away from Florence's role," a member said.[32]

Over the years Mahoney had visited a number of facilities where the aged were cared for or treated and had worked to increase funding for Veterans Administration (VA) aging programs. "Going this next Friday to Boston to see the aging center there with the Vet. Hosp. and Boston Univ.," she had written Lasker in the 1960s. "The Vets. now have 8 centers so let's hope they do well." In another letter in 1965, she reported, "Am doing all right with Mr. Driver, [administrator] of the Vets and our aging program, and he has already put it into the budget for '66 and it has passed that part of the hurdle. Now I have to talk to the BOB [Bureau of the Budget] man . . . . What a relief not to have to work with what we had to in the past." Referring to conflicts between medical and military personnel in the agency, she said, "The doctors could not even communicate with the General except through echelons and my having Dr. Myers [head of the VA aging program?] and Driver for lunch got that cleared up."[33]

She learned a great deal from her travels to such medical centers where researchers were uncovering new information. One researcher's work on antioxidants in particular caught her attention. As Phil Lee put it some thirty years later, "The guy was absolutely right, but nobody was paying any attention to this stuff in those days." As with many scientists with promising leads who were not getting attention, Mahoney introduced the man to people like Lee at her house.[34]

A number of people shared Mahoney's interest in promoting better aging research, treatments, and lifestyles. Russel Lee, she had noted to John Macy in 1965, had built an assisted-living complex "which is similar to a hotel with private apartments, for people past 65. He can explain how it can be done all over the United States through private enterprise and may be one of the important answers to housing for the elderly, besides giving many people work. I should have him submit the whole plan to you because it is a good one."[35]

Another person who had an abiding interest in the subject of research and aging was Paul Glenn, an investment broker who "became interested in biochemistry at Princeton and now knows all the research going on in the United States in the biological field and is interested in the aging research program," Mahoney told Macy. Glenn in 1965 had called on Mahoney to learn "how you believe a non-scientist can make an effective contribution in gerontology." Mahoney credited Glenn as "the only person who helped me with the institute in the beginning."[36]

She was then trying to interest President Johnson in backing more research on aging. "I think from a tactical standpoint," she told Glenn at the time, "the only thing to do for the present is to move ahead as fast as we can under the present institute structure as it is so complicated to get a bill through . . . . What we need most is to mobilize the field, create interest in it, get more training and more grants and more research in the field. Concentrating our efforts in this direction will be more beneficial in the long run than trying to change the structural setup now. I'm sure you agree that the most important part is to get research in the field."

Mahoney subsequently, according to Glenn, "provided the inspiration for" a Foundation for Medical Research that he created in 1965 and served on its board of directors.[37]

But the idea of another institute was not thought of favorably by NIH leaders or others in government, including Edwards. "They all tried to keep me from doing it," Mahoney recalled. Nor had a significant lobby constituency yet developed to prod Congress on behalf of senior issues. Government officials argued that another institute was expensive and work already was underway within the existing structure; others maintained that the caliber of aging research was not at the level that warranted its own institute, "had turned up little of real value," as one commentator wrote.[38]

"The whole concept of an aging institute had its followers and detractors," Edwards recalled. "You can argue whether we needed such an institute because most things related to aging were disease-specific, i.e., heart. It wasn't without controversy. Although I had nothing but the highest regard for Florence, and understood and in a way admired her position, I wasn't enthusiastic for it. And there was a lot of resistance at the White House to it — particularly at a time when the HEW budget was going up, up, up. Some thought it didn't make sense."

But "Florence plugged away for that and worked on everybody who could do something on it," Gorman recorded of her persistence. "I worked with her on it a little but there weren't many allies for it at first. Everyone would say that there were already enough institutes, and then the Association of American Medical Colleges, which had a wonderfully consistent record of being supportive of every other institute established, was very vocal against it .... By that time Lister [Hill] had left office, and I didn't know whom to get to support it, but Florence worked unrelentingly to get support for it."[39]

She first approached the logical person to carry a bill — Chairman Yarborough. "I had given him some valuable books — he loved old books. But he got interested in something else and didn't pay attention to my bill idea."

Mahoney then fixed on a Senate "freshman," Democrat Thomas Eagleton of Missouri, who chaired a newly created subcommittee on aging. "I talked to him at dinner one night — there were about six for dinner." He jumped at the chance to carry the bill. After it was introduced, Yarborough called Mahoney and "gave me hell because I had given it to Eagleton." Congressman Paul Rogers, chairman of the Subcommittee on Health and the Environment, agreed to sponsor the bill in the House.[40]

"Early in my Senate career," Eagleton recalled of his involvement, "Florence came to me and said, 'Tom, our country needs a National Institute on Aging. We have Heart, Cancer, Eye Institutes (and many others), but it is old age, in its generic sense, that ultimately takes all of us.' I took this on as a most worthy legislative endeavor."[41]

"I am glad to know that Paul Rogers and Senator Eagleton will introduce your bill for a new Institute on Aging Research," Lister Hill wrote Mahoney in November 1972. "Knowing you as I do and how influential you are, I am sure you will get the bill passed."[42]

But the bill and Mahoney's efforts would not travel an easy road to their destination. What now seemed like an obvious solution to her was not so to most policymakers. "People would say to me, 'Nobody wants to live *that* long.' But I said this is not about living longer — it's about being healthy while you're here."[43]

The bill was designed around that theme. It's aim, Eagleton's legislative counsel James Murphy said, "Was to explore problems of the 'healthy old' in order to keep them healthier — to differentiate between the frail elderly, who need institutional care, and others who need other kinds of support. But it was mainly to promote research, find out why people age differently, what their health problems are." To critics who charged that the state of research did not justify a separate institute, its proponents said it would be the "carrot" that stimulated new research.[44]

"We had a pretty elaborate set of hearings," Murphy remembered, which Mahoney always attended. Four gerontological professional organizations backed the bill. The Nixon administration continued to oppose it, in part because other disease-based interest groups were pressing for their own separate institutes, such as one dealing with diabetes.

John Sherman presented the official departmental position in testimony, but when Senator Edward Kennedy asked him what NIH would do if Congress went ahead and enacted the institute anyway, Sherman replied, "We would try to make it the best possible institute we can." John Zapp, the HEW legislative liaison representing the Nixon administration, whom Sherman described as his "chaperone," "looked at me when I said that as if he would throttle me!"

Senior-citizen lobby organizations were noticeably quiet on the issue, concerned that funding for grants they received for service programs like "Meals on Wheels" might be siphoned off by a new institute. But "they couldn't really *oppose* it," Murphy pointed out. A separate, non-legislative Senate Special Committee on Aging also held hearings in members' states, which helped "stir people up in favor of the institute."

Significantly, the bill provided for research not only on biomedicine but also on social, economic, behavioral, and mental-health matters. That would turn out to be far-sighted. "That was one of the things the Gerontological Society insisted on," said Murphy, "that it not be strictly a lab-bench or clinical institute but that it cover more broadly the problems of aging." There also was emphasis on encouraging geriatric education in medical schools.

Mahoney's hand was evident in the large number of Republicans who began to support it, "who had no reason to be on the bill except that she must have contacted them," said Murphy. "She would call me regularly to tell me that she was talking to this guy or that guy and had gotten a favorable response. No doubt about it, she was very busy keeping the thing going, keeping the momentum up. She really mobilized forces."

When the bill came before the House in July 1972, Congressman Tim Lee "Doc" Carter, Republican of Tennessee, summed up the views of many of his colleagues, who wanted to know why women generally lived longer than men: "I have never been quite satisfied that men do not live as long as they should," he said on the floor. "It has always been strange to me that a good man is soon called to his reward, but it seems a rascal will live forever, and I want to find the reason."[45]

"I share the gentleman's concern in that regard," said Rogers. "May I say too . . . [that] this committee has gone into the question [of aging research] with witnesses and with great concern." Then he added some poignant words about Mahoney:

> I particularly want to mention one person who has been a constant promoter of research on aging and who has urged that Congress take this action — Mrs. Florence Mahoney, who has done a magnificent job of bringing the need for this institute to the attention of this committee and the Congress.

The bill, Rogers emphasized, would make sure that "traditional programs of the National Institutes of Health" continued. "We are not basically putting a lot of new authority here. We are simply setting up a focus for research to be done on aging."

The ranking Republican committee member, Ancher Nelson, noted that "the role of older people in American life has changed dramatically in recent decades," that the number of people sixty-five years or older — twenty million at the time — had increased more than six times since 1900, compared to a less-than-threefold increase in the population of those younger than sixty-five. One in ten Americans by 1972 was a "senior citizen."

"Our knowledge about the health impairment of age is embarrassingly small," Democrat Michael Harrington of Massachusetts stated. "Our efforts to confront the health aspects of this crisis have been piecemeal and haphazard. The problems of the aged have had to compete for funds and attention with the whole spectrum of other concerns in various agencies and departments." The bill brought "under one roof the resources and personnel to concentrate" on "the physical and mental capabilities" of the aged.

The institute would "fill a long-recognized but long-unmet need to greatly expand biological and behavioral research into the aging process," said Eagleton when the bill was presented for a vote to the Senate in October. "Basic research in the process of aging is widely recognized in the scientific community as an idea whose time has come." Current

knowledge offered opportunities for "major breakthroughs" in understanding degenerative diseases, he said. A compelling argument for
more work in the area lay in future demographics and health costs:
within thirty years, more than forty-five million people would be older
than sixty-five and consume two-thirds of national healthcare expenditures while only one-tenth of 1 percent went for aging research.

Shortly before the Senate vote was taken, Eagleton, too, praised
Mahoney's efforts:

> I cannot let this opportunity pass without paying tribute to a very
> distinguished lady, Mrs. Florence Mahoney of Washington, D.C.,
> whose intelligence, determination and concern for the creation of a
> National Institute on Aging contributed in very large measure to the
> enactment of this legislation. Indeed, were it not contrary to the ac-
> cepted practice, I would suggest that the new institute might appro-
> priately be known as the Florence Mahoney Institute on Aging —
> her role has been of that great a significance. I am grateful to Mrs.
> Mahoney for the encouragement that she has given and the support
> she has mobilized on behalf of the establishment of this institute.
> While I do not presume to intrude on the prerogatives of the Secre-
> tary of Health, Education and Welfare, I strongly commend Mrs.
> Mahoney to him with the hope that he may find her to be a suitable
> nominee for a position on the advisory council of the new
> institute.[46]

With no opposition, the bill was approved without a roll-call vote.

However, a major obstacle loomed. President Nixon would not sign
the bill, subjecting it to a "pocket veto."

The legislative process had to begin all over again in 1973. "Both the
House and Senate have reintroduced the bill," Mahoney told Lasker in
March from a "very scientific" conference that she was attending on the
biochemistry of aging, "and are having hearings middle of this month,
briefly. Yesterday Rogers interrogated [HEW] Secretary Weinberger all
day. He said he had a good head for figures." Reporting on the Nixon

administration's failure to appoint a new NIH director, she said, "The news from people who work at HEW and NIH is that morale is low and all is chaotic. Sounds familiar."[47]

Congress reenacted the institute bill, but Nixon, by then consumed with scandals, again refused to sign it, knowing that if he vetoed it, there were more than enough votes to override him.

"She worked, she called everybody," said Phil Lee of Mahoney's building insurance to override a veto. "Please don't give up on the Institute for Aging!" Lasker wrote her of the setback.[48]

Congress took up the bill a third time in the spring of 1974.

"Bravo! Mrs. Mahoney," an author friend wrote her in early May. "When I attended the hearings of Mr. Rogers' subcommittee, I thought for sure the administration's point of view would prevail. Of course, I realize that there is another hurdle, but I think you'll make it. At any rate, congratulations on your skillful management of the situation. And the climate at NIH is just right for this institute — 'people-related' research in behavioral areas . . . and so on."[49]

Mahoney's persistence finally paid off. On May 31, 1974, the bill was signed into law by Nixon. (Two months and nine days later, he would resign under threat of impeachment.) It was the eleventh National Institute of Health, and Mahoney duly was named to its advisory council.[50]

"Congratulations on . . . your initial insight," a professor of behavioral studies wrote her. "I have long considered this a most urgent investigation for 'the human condition' and I suspect the 'yield' on knowing about pathology and life itself and how to maximize individual and societal opportunities will be greater in this research area than most people dream . . . . In no other area has our culture been so negligent and so lacking in compassion and knowledge. You deserve a great deal of credit."[51]

"I never worked so hard for anything in my life," Mahoney later recorded. "It took five years, and the president, NIH and HEW all were against it." She felt well-rewarded for her tenaciousness twenty years on. "I didn't feel so old then, but I have good reason for working for it now," she joked in her ninety-ninth year. "I wasn't thinking about that then," although at the time she had been in her early seventies. She had not been motivated by fear of sickness either, having been blessed, unlike Lasker, by good health throughout her life. "So it had *nothing* to do with that."[52]

Once the Aging Institute was enacted, Mahoney became deeply involved in finding a director, knowing that whoever undertook the job would be critical to the success of the new institute. "We are now working hard to get it organized," she wrote one of its supporters, former Arkansas Congressman David Pryor, who was running for governor. Pryor had a special interest in the subject, having disguised himself as an aide in a nursing home and exposed abuses that he witnessed. "My file on you and nursing homes is rather substantial and coming in very handy," Mahoney told him.[53]

"As you know, the President finally signed the bill for the Institute for Aging and now to get the right people to make it work," she told former Senator Hill. "People are always longing for the good old days when you did all the work."[54]

Mahoney, though, had fixed on her own candidate for institute director. She had been "very impressed" by a just-published book, *Why Survive? Being Old in America*, by Robert N. Butler. "I called him and told him I wanted to see him. He asked if I would come and have lunch with him." She forgot the appointment, however. "But I was not so dumb as to remind her of that!" Butler laughed. "Then she invited me to her house for coffee and we talked."

Mahoney immediately was convinced that he was the man for the job and went to work in her quintessential way, knowing that it would be another uphill battle. Butler, after all, was not a renowned academic or biomedical scientist; he was a behavioral psychiatrist specializing in gerontology but with little administrative experience. Starting right at the top, Mahoney went to see the director of NIH, Dr. Donald Fredrickson, and presented Butler's credentials.

"This man is available, you can get him to do aging," she urged. "But we don't even have a director," Fredrickson demurred. Never mind, Mahoney pressed. "You can get *this* man as a director. He's very good."[55]

She then made sure that the search committee listed Butler among several others recommended for the post. But NIH officials "were looking around for a gerontologist," Phil Lee remembered. "And here's Bob, a psychiatrist." Mahoney nevertheless was undaunted and kept pushing from the sidelines.

Months of deliberation ensued, according to Sherman, who headed the search committee. Gradually even diehard, biologically-research-oriented administrators began to come around to Mahoney's way of thinking. A year after its enactment, Butler, to the amazement of many, was picked as "director designate" of the institute.

"That was a remarkable departure," Sherman noted, "and a fortunate one," he added of the unprecedented choice.

Butler would be the first behavioral scientist to head an institute. Coincidentally, as if to validate the decision, "the very first day that I was on the job officially was the day the Pulitzer Prize was announced." He had won it for his book.[56]

"She was your number-one advocate," Fredrickson confided to Butler years later. "Talk about having someone on your team! My own personal opinion is that I never would have gotten the job without Florence Mahoney," Butler readily admitted. It changed "my whole life. You don't get an opportunity like that very often to build something from scratch."

Nor would the institute have existed without Mahoney. "We in the academic community could have screamed bloody murder for a long time, but it took Florence and her dining room to put it together, to get people like Eagleton, Paul Rogers, and others on board. I think it probably never would have happened without her. She got two key sponsors, and despite opposition from every side, 'Florence the Indomitable' pulled it off!" Butler laughed.

Her motives, he believed, were pure: "Here was an opportunity to improve people's lives. I think she was interested in helping people live long and vigorous lives. The idea of being locked up in nursing homes would have been horrible to her. Anything to reduce that would have appealed to her. And she understood that there was an important opportunity for research, including the basic sciences."[57]

Mahoney also made sure that Butler met the relevant committee members and staff who would fund and forge the new institute, such as health appropriations subcommittee aide Nicholas Cavarocchi. "I remember her bringing him around to meet us," Cavarocchi said. "Then she hosted a couple of dinners for staff at her house with Butler, so a rapport began to develop between us. She did a number of those over a year or so when he was first there. She made sure these folks got to know him and what he was doing — so there was a comfort level between us." Mahoney also talked to Chairman Dan Flood and other committee members "to make sure there was funding for the institute," according to Cavarocchi. It initially was given money even before an official budget request was made.[58]

In 1976 Mahoney would write Lasker, "In retrospect, more has been accomplished than seemed possible. It took forever to get Dr. Butler really there as Director of the Institute. Thank goodness it is he, though, for he is wonderful. By great good fortune, he got the Pulitzer award for the non-fiction book of the year and that made the Institute have visability (although) the *N. Y. Times* first story called it the Institute of Dying until some bright *Times* editor got the message. There is *now* a change in attitude re: the whole problem with even doctors and medical schools thinking about it — or *are being told to.*"[59]

By 1981 she could tell Lasker, "At the Plenary sessions of the AAMC last week, there was talk of the medical schools' changing their curriculum to include more teaching in the field of geriatric medicine. [AAMC president] John Cooper has appointed a group to assist the medical schools and asked me to help . . . . The veterans are serious now re: their aging research and programs."[60]

The institute's broad mandate afforded Butler a rich palate. Eagleton aide James Murphy had written the legislation's intent — its "whereas" clause — on his dining room table one night, "and ever after that, Bob Butler used it as his mandate."[61]

"The beauty of the Research on Aging Act," Butler later would say, "was that it was very broad-based. I thought it justified taking the wider view." Institute priorities, as a result, emphasized promoting physical independence by fostering research on a wide range of subjects from nutrition and the adverse effects of prescription drugs to the basic biology of aging, economic aspects like the impact of retirement, and mental factors like bereavement, which was found to affect the immune system. "We didn't know all that then" Butler noted of such findings. "Aging is cross-connected with everything."[62]

At the outset, as Mahoney had observed, there was little funding for such research. "I personally counted only twelve grants in 1975, at an average cost of about $60,000, totaling some $700,000, on dementia and aging of the brain," Butler remembered of the token activity. "That is partly why I decided that we really had to do what the other institutes had done to survive — they had 'disease missions.' The ordinary person didn't think you could *do* anything about aging. I thought we needed a terrible disease to publicize, and picked Alzheimer's," a form of senile dementia. Butler realized that a debilitating disease with which many people could identify was the key to attracting money from Congress for his institute — the "health politics of anguish," he termed it, on which interest-group constituencies were built.[63]

"Public relations people said, 'You have to change the name'" for a national awareness campaign. Butler refused.

Mahoney, too, thought that should be done — "no one could even pronounce the name." "When they first started talking about Alzheimer's," she said of her involvement, "I saw an Alzheimer's brain dissected. One day this doctor who was the leader in Alzheimer's research called me and asked if he could come and see me. He thought we should start a foundation or something. 'Yes, I said, but you can't *call* it that. Call it *organic brain disease* or something, otherwise it will scare people.' But he said, 'This is what it *is*,' and talked me into the fact that it should be called Alzheimer's. So we started a small foundation just to get people interested."

With Mahoney's and Butler's help, the American Alzheimer's Disease Association was founded in 1976. The name soon became familiar to all Americans, and federal funding for Alzheimer's research grew from $3 million in 1976 to $396 million by 1999. Still, the disease (the fourth leading cause of death and one of the three common reasons for nursing-home admissions in the 1990s) continued to elude researchers and to be one of medicine's greatest challenges.[64]

"The key issue," even Edwards later conceded, "is not whether the institute was right or wrong. We've got it, and as time has gone on, it's probably a good idea. Now it's taken on a life of its own. That isn't to say that [aging research] might not have gone forward in a different direction, within each institute. But the key issue is that it wouldn't ever have happened without Florence Mahoney." And, unlike the concept of separating a discipline from the mainstream as the cancer bill might have done — "which was wrong then and wrong today," Edwards believed — "the Aging Institute is not wrong. You can argue whether it should have happened, but there is nothing wrong with it; it's part and parcel of our national health effort."[65]

"Aging well"

When NIA celebrated its fifth year in 1980, Mahoney, Rogers, and Eagleton were given awards for their roles in starting it. Mahoney by then was widely known for her association with aging causes. Pepper, chairman of a Select Committee on Aging and a senior citizen himself, still turned to her for advice and help. "Besides discussing any legislative issues in which you are interested," he wrote in an invitation to lunch in 1984, "I would like to tell you about an exciting project in gerontology at Florida State University . . . . I believe it will be important to you."[66]

Mahoney would be honored many times in succeeding years for her farsightedness and persistence, which were validated by numerous scientific advances. In 1987 the NIA, honoring her "lifetime commitment to medical research and its benefits to people worldwide," established an annual Florence Mahoney Lecture on Aging. The first lecturer was eminent health historian, philosopher, and author Dr. Lewis Thomas.[67]

By the beginning of the twenty-first century, the Aging Institute's budget had risen from $19 million (in 1976) to nearly $615 million. Its central theme remained "aging well," as its director Dr. Richard J. Hodes told Congress in 1999, "critical" because the population of older Americans continued to expand rapidly: people over sixty-five comprised the fastest-growing demographic group in America, numbering 34.7 million in 2000, and U. S. Census Bureau projections for 2050 were that one in every eight people would be seventy-five or older.

There was good news, though: America's older population was becoming healthier and more fit. Rates of disability in older persons had declined since 1982, and the ability to function had improved most notably in people over eighty.

"A revolution in aging research" was unfolding, Hodes testified. The "rapid pace of discovery" was fueling "important opportunities . . . to delay or to prevent . . . conditions that were once thought to be a normal part of aging." Such advances held "the promise of adding years to life as our nation ages," he told the congressmen.[68]

Alzheimer's disease, however, still affected some four million Americans by the end of the millennium and continued to be a priority for the institute. Beginning in 1999, drugs were being tested in humans for their ability to delay or prevent the onset of the disease. Research on its underlying pathology was producing hopeful leads about effects on the brain. Another exciting advance was the discovery that adult brain cells reproduce, offering the possibility that memory loss might be reversed.

"We used to say, 'too bad, you're old, nothing can be done'"

While such advances in gerontology could only hearten Mahoney, she kept up her aging advocacy long after the institute's founding. "Give me one breakthrough that extends human life and I'll get you all the money you want from Congress," a seniors' publication in 1991 quoted her as telling researchers.[69]

Not only were many impressive breakthroughs occurring but, as other causes of death were conquered and old age became its major perpetrator, geriatrics gradually became a medical specialty, something that Mahoney and Butler had pushed. At the time of the institute's establishment in the mid-1970s, only 2 of the nation's 125 medical schools required students to take courses in geriatrics or gerontology. Doctors had to go to other countries to study the discipline. By the 1990s a number of specialty programs had been set up, such as the Geriatrics and Adult Development Department at New York's Mount Sinai School of Medicine, one of the first, established by Butler in 1982 when he left the institute.[70]

"We used to say, 'too bad, you're old, nothing can be done,'" Butler's successor, Dr. T. Franklin Williams, commented. "Now, we know that much *can* be done," and age is "no longer a barrier to restoration" procedures like joint replacements and coronary bypasses.[71]

"Many wonderful pieces of the puzzle have already been put together," Mahoney reflected about the advances achieved since she had started her campaign. Her view that "it's about being healthy while you're here" was vindicated by the work that not only was extending but actually enhancing the quality of life for the elderly. "I know a lot of people who have never been as happy as after age 65," she said at the age of 91. Life expectancy by 1999 was 79.4 for women, 73.6 for men, and centenarians — as Mahoney would be — were the fastest-growing age group (they numbered more than 70,000 in the United States).[72]

She herself had been reluctant throughout her life to tell people her age, long a source of speculation even among her closest friends, because, as Grey Dimond wrote in a memoir, "she maintained a youthful demeanor, a grace in movement, and a full head of hair with a youthful sheen." The mystery was "good evidence that her campaign against aging had merit." "Ladies just don't disclose their age," Mahoney once remarked to John Sherman's wife. She ignored queries that might date her and did the same for others' ages, assuming "the most blank, uncomprehending expression if an untrained guest" asked how old a certain senator was. "Age is not even . . . in Flo's vocabulary but [as] a disease to be eliminated," Dimond said admiringly.[73]

"An older person needs a dream as well as a memory"

Mahoney was a premier example of what another active senior citizen promoted, public servant Arthur Fleming, who said on his ninetieth birthday that his formula for a long full life was to "Stay involved.

Reminiscing is great, provided it's linked to the future. Someone once said, 'An older person needs a dream as well as a memory.'"[74]

Mahoney did just that, keeping busy on a variety of fronts like presidential elections in her later years. Her notes on the 1972 race reflected Democrats' bitter infighting (Hubert Humphrey, George McGovern, and Maine Senator Edmund Muskie were vying for the nomination) as they tried to field a candidate who could remove Nixon from the White House. Clark Clifford told Mahoney in May that he thought "both McGovern and Muskie could defeat Nixon," although many people in those "seemingly unstable" times unfortunately considered "emotional outbreaks" like Muskie's speech in New Hampshire, with "his voice breaking" to rebut a newspaper's allegations about his wife, "a weakness" in men.

In a June memo following dinner at her house, Mahoney recorded an account of "how really angry some of the men were re: delegate selections for the convention — actually screaming, etc." John Gardner told her that if "HHH got the nomination, it would not be worth a nickel" and that McGovern's "mind was working well and he had a dignified burning anger. Spoke to Eleanor McG [his wife], she said Geo. [was] too good and honorable probably to be Pres. They had liked Carter of Ga., said his ideas for budget [were good] and he had done much for [the] state with re-distribution of moneys." Gardner also told her that an effort would be made to "to get [Ted] Kennedy to be compromise [candidate] or pull together, he [being] acceptable both to the young and blue-collar workers and the Blacks, etc."[75]

George McGovern, for whom Mahoney had hosted a large fund-raising event, was the eventual candidate but lost to Nixon in a landslide in 1972.

Democrats regained the White House in 1976, following Nixon's Watergate debacle, with the election of Jimmy Carter. "The first time I ever heard Carter talk, I *knew* that he was going to be president," Mahoney recalled. "He had wonderful rapport with people. I paid $5 to hear him speak. He never looked at *other* people while he was talking to you, he listened to what everybody said."

She considered Carter "extremely intelligent," "a brave personality," and helped promote good publicity for him and his wife. On March 1, 1976, she "spoke to Daniel [Mahoney, her son] re: Carter and Mrs. Carter and story in paper." The next month, she "spoke to Clifton [Daniel] re: story re: Rosalynn and editorial lunch for Governor C[arter]. Jim Bellows [managing editor of the *Washington Star*] said good story on Mrs. Carter and his sister in Sunday paper coming up. Clifton wants copy of story from Palm Beach paper . . . . Clifton said [there would be an] editorial lunch in NY on St. Pat's day, 17th."[76]

Mahoney brought the head of the federal anti-poverty program's health services, Dr. Joe T. English, to the attention of Carter and his wife during the campaign. "The man with the little liver pills?" English asked Mahoney when she first mentioned Carter, whom she was convinced would be elected. Mahoney suggested that English talk to Rosalynn Carter, then Georgia's First Lady, who volunteered at a neighborhood health center and was to be a keynote speaker at an OEO convention in Atlanta. When English said that he was referred by Florence Mahoney, Mrs. Carter took note, telling English that when her husband was president, she wanted to place special emphasis on expanding mental-health programs nationally. "If I hadn't been cued by Florence, I would have thought that Mrs. Carter needed psychiatric help!" English joked of her confidence in the election's outcome. Forty-eight hours after Carter's inauguration, however, English got "a call from the White House," asking him to meet with the president and Mrs. Carter to discuss their plans. "Florence was behind the scenes in all of this," English acknowledged.[77]

Carter, at Rosalynn's instigation, established the Presidential Committee on Mental Health, and Mahoney, again in presidential favor, was appointed to its aging task force and traveled to hearings aboard Mrs. Carter's plane. Mahoney also served on the citizens' advisory council to the Association of American Medical Colleges during that period.[78]

"I have never known so much to be done and so little time," Mahoney wrote Lasker just before Christmas in 1976. "Fortunately some of our endeavors go well. Delighted re: [Joseph] Califano [as HEW secretary] and interesting that Ted Sorensen is taking CIA." "I went to the unveiling of [James] Shannon's bust," she said of Lasker's long-time antagonist. "Lots of old faces and quite touching. Shannon looks well and young. I seemed to be the only person [there who was] outside [of NIH]."[79]

Mahoney maintained her brand of continuing education, telling Lasker (then recovering from a bout of shingles), "The National Academy of Sciences conference on Care of the Elderly was good (enclose program), also excellent Institute of Medicine seminar on the Health Sciences and Burden of Illness. Your award winners this year were very exciting and you must have been very pleased," she added. "Cheers and congratulations, also for the new 'Fact Book' — missed aging, though, and now [there are] good statistics on various diseases, i.e., Alzheimer's and the dementias. We will have a meeting after Jan. 1 and you must advise *avec* ideas. The Gordon Conference on biology of aging always good. Butler is sensational and with superb ideas. The conference on genetics at Jackson Lab this fall also good with lots of new investigators in the field."

An expense voucher for 1977 showed that she traveled to meetings nationwide during eight months out of the year — conferences on long-term care, medical-school training, aging research, a Veterans Administration symposium on aging, and a "health enhancement meeting." She maintained a similar travel schedule in 1978 — then seventy-nine years old.[80]

As with previous Democrats in the White House, Mahoney had a good relationship with the Carters. "Jimmy and I appreciate all that you have done for us and will always deeply value your friendship and support," Rosalynn wrote her in 1981 after leaving the White House. A few months later she said, "I want to take this opportunity to tell you once more how much I appreciate the generous assistance you provided to me during the past few years. I am very grateful."[81]

Among Mahoney's other interests in those years was funding for the Lister Hill Center for Biomedical Communications at NIH. "Steve Strickland and I are lobbying madly for appropriations," she wrote Hill.

"We have spoken to all those dear young men in the right places and are optimistic. If we get $10 million this year, the building can be started and they can finish it next year."[82]

Mike Gorman in 1978 enlisted Mahoney's help for a bill to benefit "that group of patients whom I refer to as the 'socially disabled.' They are at least several million in number .... Congressman Michael Harrington introduced a bill several years ago to provide a very large sum of money for long-term care of terminally or permanently disabled persons of all types for whom no further medical intervention was indicated .... I suggest that you check his office and get a copy of the bill. Awfully good to talk to you," he added. "We must get together some time and talk about old times in Idaho, particularly the day I fell off the horse."[83]

Mahoney did not involve herself in an effort to create a separate arthritis institute ten years after the cancer fight. Lasker again was identified as a "key figure in the extraordinary success of the proposal," as was Pepper, whom Lasker had convinced to sponsor the bill. "I think there is no problem with proliferation of institutes as long as there is proliferation of disease," she retorted to opponents of the idea. She was considered either "the *grande dame* of the NIH" or its "*enfant terrible*," a *Science* magazine commentator wrote. Gorman, too, was "plugging away" for the institute, lining up "prominent people who were arthritics" to endorse it. "We were going to get [actress] Rosalyn Russell but unfortunately that dear woman died before we had the chance."[84]

The arthritis institute was another example, the *Science* writer stated, "of masterful lobbying by a powerful combination of supporters." NIH again opposed the categorical move as making "little administrative, fiscal or scientific sense."

"Where does it stop?" NIH director James B. Wyngaarden asked, as diabetes research advocates clamored for equal status. A National Institute of Arthritis and Musculoskeletal and Skin Diseases nevertheless was established in May 1986, separate from the newly constituted Institute of Diabetes and Digestive and Kidney Diseases.[85]

With Republican Ronald Reagan's election in 1980, health budgets once again were threatened. (The White House would remain in GOP hands for the next twelve years with Reagan's successor George Bush.) The same charges of politicization made about Nixon's administration would recur in Reagan's. In 1982 several scientists complained that presidential appointments to the National Cancer Advisory Board replaced distinguished scientists with political favorites.[86]

While Mahoney focused more specifically on aging issues in those years, Lasker continued to be a proponent for NIH. "I think the House did very well by the NIH funds," she wrote Mahoney in 1986, "but I still fear we can be vetoed. What do you think?"[87]

When Bill Clinton and Senator Al Gore Jr., were running for the presidency and vice-presidency in 1992, Mahoney wrote Gore in September, "It is such a joy to hear you on television. It is wonderful that the campaign is going so well. It seems too good to be true. I know how pleased your mother and father are with you."

She enclosed an article regarding Dr. Bernadine Healy, a cardiologist who had served as Reagan's science advisor and was the first woman to head NIH. Her appointment had come after a two-year hiatus (1989–91) during the Bush administration when no director was named. Despite Healy's political association, Mahoney liked what she was doing although she was controversial among scientists and morale at NIH was low during her directorship. "Please keep her in mind," Mahoney nevertheless urged Gore. "That position was never political until Mr. Reagan [meaning Nixon?] made it so and she is the first person, for years, who has come up with any new ideas for the future of NIH."[88]

After Clinton's election in 1992, Mahoney told a friend, "I never thought I would live long enough to see another Democrat in the White House." "At least it's much more interesting now in Washington than last year," she wrote David Pryor. "It's such a joy to have a new president. He certainly has a lot of energy and there is so much to do."[89]

As she approached her centenary year, Mahoney observed the national scene more from the sidelines than from the center of influence, but with no less respect from those who recognized her remarkable accomplishments.

8

An Early Visionary

———————◆———————

*C*ONTEMPLATING HER OWN MEMOIRS, in a letter to Lasker written sometime in the 1960s, Mahoney had said, "I am fascinated now at times when I hear things about NIH that have *not much* to do with the facts, but it's too much trouble to try and educate [people]. I hope you will put all of your notes together in a book for you like Margaret Sanger" as part of "making 20th-century history. I have all my files but will never have time to organize them."[1]

She spent years trying to do just that, not so much because she wanted *her* story told but because she wanted the story of the NIH told.

Michael Mahoney likened his mother to the explorers Lewis and Clark, who doggedly proceeded on their long trek across the continent, despite great obstacles. So did Mahoney through her full life although the daily pace in her seventies occasionally seemed daunting, as she wrote to Lasker in June 1976 to thank her for remembering her seventy-seventh birthday.

258

My favorite title has always been "Stop the world, I want to get off." I haven't recovered from the '48, '52, '56, '60 and '72 election years yet and now they throw the Bicentennial on this one. I try 6 hrs. sleep and various other short cuts trying to get just part of the things done that seem necessary. Always so much I want to discuss with you and the time is always 1 or 2 AM . . . .

First I want to thank you for the basket of white azaleas that came on Apr. 20th. I was at a meeting at USC and didn't even remember the date. You were dear to remember but now we forget to remember.

To briefly tell you what I have been up to — was in Ariz. end of Dec. and part of Jan. Was a consultant to the Nat. Comm. on Arthritis, etc., and they had hearings in Ariz. and at an Indian reservation. Then to the Gordon Conference on biological research in Santa Barbara and some meetings in Seattle, so back and forth with Aging Council meetings here, plus working with our friends on the Hill, plus everyone coming and going, and going out too much.

Have all of our friends writing material for Carter [during the presidential campaign] . . . [2]

Mahoney would keep busy well into her ninth decade. She read national newspapers daily as well as science journals, kept up with political changes, and delighted in every new medical discovery reported by the media.

"People who don't read papers must be out of their mind!" she said in mock derision.

She continued to clip articles and forward them to people who shared her interests and communicated her ideas to Members of Congress, many of whom still contacted her. One with whom she maintained a friendship over the years was Democratic Congressman Andrew Jacobs of Indiana. "If I wanted to be introduced to somebody on the Hill, he would do it," even if not involved in the issue on which she was working, Mahoney said of their relationship.

"Your taste, dear lady, is refreshingly honest and without unnecessary complication. I guess that makes you Lincolnesque," he mused in a note to her.[3]

A physician new to Congress in 1971, Dr. William R. Roy of Kansas, told Mahoney, "There are very significant roles for all of us to play if we are to meet our national responsibilities regarding the health of our people, especially our older people. My role is, of course, a new one; yours is only a continuation of the great service that you have rendered during the years. Thank you for your attention to me." He looked forward to a "productive and very pleasant continuing relationship" but unfortunately his congressional career ended in 1975.[4]

Mahoney maintained contacts with old and new friends in and out of public office. "Thanks for the articles," Thomas Eagleton wrote her in 1992 after retiring from the Senate, "I still love to read," he joked. "Many thanks for Dr. Healy's speech and *The New Yorker* column about Canada's health system," Senator Lloyd Bentsen of Texas wrote the same year. House Democratic Whip Chester G. Atkins of Massachusetts thanked her for "kind words of encouragement and support regarding my Op-Ed piece on international family planning. I am pleased to know that you share my concerns about reproductive freedom and over-population." New York Senator Daniel Patrick Moynihan in 1994 was grateful for Mahoney's backing in his fourth successful Senate race, in which, he wrote her, "there was peril aplenty." (He won by more than 600,000 votes, "the highest margin of victory among the 35 Democrats who ran for the Senate" that year, he boasted.)[5]

National health insurance was foremost on her mind in correspondence with John Dingell, chairman of the House Energy and Commerce Committee in 1992. He appreciated her "very kind comments about my father and his good work on behalf" of Truman's bill. "Many of the old and hollow arguments about national health insurance are steadily but slowly being demolished as the sheer madness that is today's health care system proves the need for a universal system," he wrote.

"I still can't understand why so many people are against the government's being a payee [meaning payor?] instead of having so many different insurance companies," she responded. "I'm certain the AMA is using all the influence it can to defeat it!"

She also urged Dingell to use his influence to keep Bernadine Healy as director of NIH. "If you and Dr. Healy could put your ideas together, you could accomplish anything....[I]f we win in November [the presidential election], she can be kept on to accomplish new directions. You are both so important and such good leaders — together anything could happen." (Healy, however, was replaced in 1993 by Dr. Harold E. Varmus, a Nobel Prize winner for findings on cancer-causing genes.)[6]

"An early visionary"

In 1996 the National Institutes of Health Alumni Association surprised Mahoney with a Public Service Award for "her life-long dedication to improvements in the mental and physical health of all humans" and "her effectiveness in marshaling public opinion to the importance of sound research."

It was notable that the three previous awardees had been a chairman of the House Appropriations Committee and two distinguished NIH scientists. "We believe strongly that you belong in this unusual company," awards chairman John Sherman told Mahoney.

"Mrs. Mahoney was an early visionary in the realization that advances in the diagnosis, treatment, cure and prevention of physical and mental illness would be greatly dependent on new methods," the award stated. "In an unusually perceptive fashion, she also recognized that research was the ultimate key."

"As a firm believer in the power of the federal government to achieve well-selected national objectives," it continued, "she strove in highly effective fashion to convince the country's political leadership to provide the NIH with the legislative and financial resources . . . to improve health for its citizens. Her crowning but far from sole achievement was her largely single-handed effort that culminated in the passage of legislation establishing the National Institute on Aging."

She was commended for "her dogged persistence and her shrewd and well-prepared arguments on behalf of better health through support of medical research which eventually overcame opposition from a variety of sectors."[7]

The award ceremony fittingly took place in the Mary Woodward Lasker Center on the NIH campus, a tribute to Mahoney's partner over many years and endeavors. NIH acknowledged that although Mahoney was "publicly less well known than Lasker," her talents "melded well with the attributes of her associate, making them a formidable team." Mahoney "was a person of her own mind, however, differing with Lasker on occasion and pursuing her own convictions," the citation noted.[8]

End of a team

Lasker had attended the center's dedication in September 1984, despite suffering several strokes in the 1980s that slowed her down. Then pushing for a separate arthritis institute, she still was widely regarded as a leading advocate for health. "For nearly half a century, Lasker has been the fairy godmother for U.S. medical research," a *Business Week* article stated, calling her "among the most powerful lobbyists on Capitol Hill," known for "tough-as-nails prodding" and reliance on celebrities to tout her messages before Congress. Her emphasis then also included AIDS (she had gotten actress Elizabeth Taylor to testify for more funds to combat the growing epidemic) and endocrine diseases such as osteoporosis, diabetes, and growth disorders. "You can solve any problem if you have money, people and equipment," she was quoted as saying.[9]

Mahoney and Lasker, however, no longer traveled together or saw one another often. "It isn't quite the same," Mahoney said of their lives as octogenarians, "you don't see each other as much as if you were doing things together."

The third member of their original team, Mike Gorman, died of septicemia on April 1, 1989, at the age of seventy-five. He had retired the previous year, having worked for Lasker and the causes that she and Mahoney espoused for forty years.[10]

Lasker succumbed to heart failure in February 1994 at the age of ninety-three. Jonas Salk called her "a matchmaker between science and society." Senator Edward Kennedy referred to her "integrity . . . authenticity and commitment." In addition to her medical advocacy and urban philanthropy in New York City, she was praised for helping make possible masses of colorful flowers that graced Washington, D.C., and its environs as part of Lady Bird Johnson's beautification program. At the time of her death, fifty-one Lasker awardees had received Nobel Prizes.[11]

Mahoney could no longer keep her age a secret when she reached a milestone 100th birthday in 1999. To honor her, an American flag was flown over the Capitol on April 20, the Aging Institute conducted a special symposium as part of the lecture series in her name, and the *Washington Post* ran a feature story about her.

"Flo — and other people who have strong interests — do seem to live long and enjoy it more," Robert Butler said of Mahoney as a role model for seniors. She and her allies, as Alliance for Aging Research director Daniel Perry put it, had helped bring about "a new era for the federal government in health research."[12]

Past and future — more to be done

Indeed, Mahoney and her friends had done their job extraordinarily well, but many of the same battles they had fought would continue — as did Mahoney's brand of soft outrage over work still to be done.

She could take comfort in the fact that life expectancy for Americans had increased steadily over the last fifty years, rising from 68.2 years in 1950 to 73.7 in 1980 and 76.7 in 1998 (the United States, however, still ranked behind other industrialized countries, tied for nineteenth among men and seventeenth among women in 1995). Mortality rates for two of the three most deadly afflictions — heart diseases and strokes (cerebrovascular diseases) — had fallen 58 and 71 percent respectively from 1950 to 1998. The death rate for cancer (malignant neoplasms), after rising steadily for forty years, began to drop in the 1990s to slightly below the 1950 level (from 125.4 per 100,000 in 1950 to 123.6 per 100,000 in 1998). While improvements resulted from many factors, including social and environmental changes, research discoveries had enormous influence.[13]

Mahoney also could only have been heartened by headlines at the end of the twentieth century that announced such good news as "New weapons in battle against flu" (which killed up to 40,000 Americans a year), "Why we're healthier today," "Miraculous medicine," "Dramatic leap in life span from small advances." A vaccine had been found that showed promise of preventing Alzheimer's, another had been developed to combat Lyme disease. Advances were promising for the future of organ transplants, engineered proteins to rebuild bones, and "stem-cell" remedies for a variety of disorders, including stroke, epilepsy, and Alzheimer's and Parkinson's diseases. "Some of the most startling discoveries predicted for the next century are based on 20th century strides in molecular biology, microsurgery, drug therapy and genetic engineering," one science writer reported, a validation of Mahoney's advocacy.[14]

Still, the World Health Organization in 1999 warned that infectious viruses and bacteria were killing thirteen million people (AIDS continued to be virulent), and a disastrous international epidemic loomed because of bacterial resistance to antibiotics, a result of human overuse. Editorials called for "more money for research, education and infection control" to ward off such eventualities. "Science marches on, but so do human folly and complacency. We haven't licked disease yet," the San Francisco Examiner cautioned.[15]

Mahoney's view precisely.

Neither had another of her lifelong concerns been achieved as a new millennium approached — population control. There would be more than six billion people on earth by the beginning of the year 2000. Although birth control had become widely accepted, it was still not practiced or was controversial in many parts of the world, as was abortion. Some women, like a valedictorian at Mills College, had resolved not to bear children, calling the future a "cruel hoax" that promised an overpopulated world of starving people. Indeed, in the twenty-first century, three of ten children were likely to be born into extreme poverty — more than ever before and more than ever likely to die from malnutrition and preventable diseases.[16]

Right-to-life movements retained enough clout to try to thwart the use of human embryo and fetus "stem cells" for valuable research that might uncover clues to heart disease and diabetes, even reverse the effects of aging.[17]

More than forty-three million Americans still were without health insurance. Mahoney, observing the national crisis that she had worked to correct beginning in the 1940s, predicted that "managed care would lead to national health insurance" as people grew increasingly frustrated with an impersonal system over which they had little control.

Advocacy by disease, which still governed American policymaking, despite its successes remained controversial. "Whoever has the loudest voice gets the money," a spokesman for the American Diabetes Association candidly admitted on a television news program in 1998.[18]

"One of these days, we'll have a left-eye institute, then a right-eye institute, and then we'll start on the ears," health appropriations chairman Dan Flood had once humorously deplored at a hearing. "Little does he know," committee aide Nick Cavarocchi laughed in hindsight, "that we now have a Deafness Institute!"[19]

"We've all learned from AIDS activists that sometimes you need to toot your own horn and shake the tree a little bit," the president of the American Society of Clinical Oncology told cancer-research advocates at a rally in Washington in 1998. Theirs were the same arguments heard during the cancer debate of the early 1970s: "Clinton vows to increase efforts to fight cancer, promises better access to clinical trials, focus on research, prevention .... Clinton, whose mother died of cancer [as had Vice President Al Gore's sister], said he was ordering wider access to 'cutting-edge clinical trials' in hopes of spurring breakthroughs in cancer cures."[20]

The debate thus continued — sometimes fiercely — over the merits of basic-versus-applied research. Nobel Prize-winning cancer researcher Harold Varmus in 1993 had been one of three medical-school professors to warn in a *Science* magazine article that the previous decade had "witnessed an accelerating erosion of the infrastructure for fundamental research in the United States. If that erosion is not reversed soon, the pace of discovery will necessarily decline, with widespread consequences for industry, health care and education."[21]

It was basic research, after all, they noted, that had fostered progress "far beyond anything anticipated a generation ago. The benefits . . . include . . . a revolution in preventive medicine, novel approaches to the diagnosis and treatment of cancer, heart attacks, infections, inherited diseases and other ailments." Knowledge of gene behavior, a prime example of serendipitous research discoveries, had greatly accelerated promising treatments for AIDS.[22]

Reiterating Mahoney's and Lasker's oft-made argument, the researchers believed that, contrary to increasing overall costs, "biomedical research typically generates simpler and less-costly devices," such as vaccines that saved billions in treatment. Still, they felt, as Mahoney and Lasker had fifty years before, that American research programs were "threatened by inadequate funding . . . flawed governmental oversight of science, confusion about the goals of federally-supported research, and deficiencies in science education." The nearly $10 billion annual appropriation that NIH then was receiving was "too small," the scientists complained. It represented less than two percent of the federal budget allocated to study diseases, and fewer than fifteen to twenty-five percent of approved NIH grants were being funded compared to thirty percent in the previous two decades.[23]

Varmus soon would be in a position to act on his complaints: He was named Director of NIH shortly after the damning article appeared and deftly set to work educating Congress to his point of view. Although continually pressed by vocal advocacy groups to favor high-profile diseases such as AIDS, breast cancer, and prostate cancer, Congress now embraced the concept of underwriting basic research, even though it did not always produce instant cures and applicable results. As a result, according to a New Yorker profile of Varmus in 1999, "the secrets of biology, principally in the area of genetics, are being revealed at an unprecedented rate," something that could only bring enormous satisfaction to the lay student of science, Florence Mahoney.[24]

In a coincidence that must have struck her as deja vu, Varmus was being compared to World War II's Dr. Vannevar Bush for championing government-supported science. Varmus, in turn, was practicing lessons that Mahoney and Lasker had pioneered — putting public advocates on NIH advisory panels.[25]

Credit due

Mahoney's humility in not seeking accolades for her work endeared her to many followers, but the lack of public credit for her remarkable contributions to national health policy caught their attention as they reflected on those who had been major influences on NIH for more than half a century. Phil Lee cited James Shannon, Lister Hill, House health appropriations subommittee chairman William Natcher — "and Florence Mahoney," who "never asked for credit" for what she accomplished. Charles Edwards agreed: "She was one of the two or three most effective people in terms of promoting health policy that we've had in this country in the last fifty years. And she did it her own way. What you saw was what you got. She put on no airs. And she did it by herself."[26]

Former NIH Director Donald Frederickson expressed a similar sentiment: "'Florence Mahoney really hasn't received the credit she is due for what she did for NIH,'" he told Butler at a meeting in 1998, "which is quite a statement," Butler noted.[27]

She had a genuine "lifelong interest in these things," historian Stephen Strickland reflected. "From an early point — even taking time out to raise two boys and to be a mentor to young people — she honed and moved her personal interests into the sphere of public policy, and learned how to make things happen."

"We liked to call her the 'poor man's Mary Lasker,'" John Sherman remembered, "since she seldom got credit for things because she preferred to work behind the scenes." Mahoney had an "interesting and challenging way of doing what she wanted to do: She had patience, but that was almost an oxymoron because she wasn't patient in terms of what she wanted — in pursuit of it, she was determined." She also "was dedicated to the public good in a selfless manner," he felt, "which is rare these days when people pushing public-policy agendas tend to do so for crass reasons and personal glorification. Florence was the opposite."[28]

"She just wanted to get things done," Cavarocchi observed of the fact that Mahoney "was always *out* of the spot light, Mary was always *in* it. 'I'm just happy that I made those contributions,' she would say. 'I don't need any more than that.'"[29]

"Lister Hill, John Fogarty and Mary Lasker get proper credit for their influence on legislation and budgeting for health in the United States," Grey Dimond wrote in his memoir, "but an unseen spinner of the finest web of them all was Flo Mahoney." If her skills "were at their highest when a Democratic president was in the White House," her ability to "reach into friends in the Senate and House" during GOP administrations "was a delight to observe." She and her accomplishments also seemed to be timeless. She worked her "magic" on a "stage that remained active for more than fifty years . . . . Her efforts spanned so many administrations and so many players . . . that it is, in reality, past, present and future time."[30]

There was evidence of her bipartisan skills during the Nixon Republican administration. "We were having a terrible time" with the health budget, Health Services and Mental Health Administrator English recalled, but "Florence didn't give up. She invited [domestic policy chief] John Erlichman to dinner, and it had a positive impact."[31]

As Boisfeuillet Jones put it, "Florence was involved in practically everything that had a social significance." Looking over the 1960 Committee of Consultants report to Senator Hill, Jones could "see Florence's hand in practically *all* of it. I think she has done more for the health of the American people than anybody I know, but she was always in the background."[32]

To Senator Eagleton, Mahoney was "a superbly polished 'Molly Brown' — she's unsinkable," one of the "most talented individuals in terms of influencing health care legislation — never 'pushy'" but "always persuasive . . . always persistent."[33]

She had an "uncanny way of persuading you to do things, even if you didn't agree with her," said Butler.[34]

A particularly striking aspect of her life, as Mrs. Charles (Sue) Edwards pointed out, was that Mahoney "was operating in a man's world *long* before many women were"—and "was truly effective," Dr. Edwards added. "Men didn't control Florence — she controlled them, by her presence," he said. "When she walked into a room — she was not tall — she was special. You just *looked* at her," both recalled. Part of her attraction was not only her simple, elegant appearance but the fact that "she was a very sensitive, caring person who knew how to treat everybody as an equal," men and women alike. "She wasn't trying to impress anyone," Sue Edwards learned from experience. Wives and children received the same attention from Mahoney as important husbands.

"She really liked women; she honestly enjoyed conversations with them and wasn't putting it on. She always cared about our children, knew their names, cared terribly about her sons and their children, and talked about her grandchildren's future. She is an amazingly interesting woman, in her intellect."[35]

Mahoney's sense of humor became a trademark that enhanced her capabilities throughout her career. She liked telling stories with amusing punch lines, especially if they put self-importance in its place. One that she heard during the Vietnam War lightened an otherwise dark time, as she wrote a friend: "Seems a young teacher, who was trying very hard, kept a young girl after school who had come wearing a sweat shirt with the words across the front, 'Make love, not war.' The teacher told her he thought that not very dignified and she said, 'That was just like the older generation, they thought that to make love meant a lay.' The teacher . . . told it to Fred Friendly [the television journalist], who told it to Walter Lippmann, who said, 'What is a lay?' And Friendly told that to his daughter, who said, 'Who is Walter Lippman?'"[36]

"I can remember anything like that — funny things," Mahoney said of herself, "but I can't remember a joke. I've never remembered a joke in my life. But a funny line just fascinates me."

Mahoney also became well known for helping young people. Not a few, like Bruce Babbitt and Bob Butler, attributed their future success, in many different fields, to her encouragement and aid. She made special efforts to place them in jobs where they could move forward and demonstrate their abilities.

"One of her special skills was to spot young, coming talent," Dimond recorded. "She always had a stable of new, bright potential stars. She enjoyed bringing them along, showing them off, opening doors for them."[37]

"Apropos the young man I spoke to you about," she wrote a White House aide to President Johnson, "he was just graduated from Georgetown University . . . and has been interested in oceanography for some time. He tried to get into the Environment[al] Science Services Administration but did not have enough science credits. Thanks for any help or advice you can give, for he is uniquely qualified in certain areas." The aide promptly forwarded Mahoney's query to another White House staff person for attention.[38]

Her beneficiaries were not limited to aspiring public servants or politicians — they included artists and writers. The walls of her homes were covered with paintings by people whom she patronized, a veritable gallery that displayed art to other potential buyers.[39]

"A non-paid lobbyist in the health field for many, many years"

Mahoney's career might best be characterized as one of "advocacy." She referred to herself in a letter to President Bill Clinton as "a non-paid lobbyist in the health field for many, many years." That summed it up.[40]

Of the impact she had, the millions of people who benefitted from her years of advocacy, Florence Mahoney was modest: "You don't think about it every day. And then there's always something else that you try to do, another idea" to promote. "I can always think of some ideas that should be followed but nobody seems to follow them up as I think they should."

She conceded that her efforts had resulted in research in the United States that "changed the whole world."

She also realized that she had had many memorable experiences: "Oh, very!"

Mahoney counted no one thing as her proudest achievement. "They all blend together. I never really thought very much of [the relative importance of] anything I was doing. It was just there to be done, and you did it."

NIH at the millennium

By the year 2000, the National Institutes of Health had become indisputably the world's leading research entity across the spectrum of biomedicine. Research supported by U.S. taxpayers constantly improved medical techniques and knowledge that contributed to longer, better, and healthier lives from cradle to grave.

It had grown to twenty-five research institutes, the National Library of Medicine (where Mahoney's papers were archived), and the Clinical Center, where some 10,000 patients underwent trials on new treatment methods each year. NIH employed 13,000 scientists on a 322-acre site. Its budget was nearly $16 billion and likely to continue rising.[41]

A description of its mission at the end of the century echoed Mahoney's and Lasker's objectives when they had set out on their campaign some sixty years earlier. Carefully balancing basic with applied research, NIH portrayed its goals as "science in pursuit of *fundamental* knowledge about the nature and behavior of living systems, and the *application* of that knowledge to extend healthy life and reduce the burdens of illness and disability" [emphasis added]. To those ends, the NIH was pledged to "enhance the nation's economic well-being and ensure a continued high return on the public investment in research, and exemplify and promote the highest level of scientific integrity, public accountability and social responsibility in the conduct of science."[42]

Mahoney justifiably could be proud.

Notes

◆

– CHAPTER 1 –

1. Birth certificate, Florence Amelia Sheets, Delaware County Department of Health, Muncie, Indiana; "Synoptical Family History, Giving Sketches of the Glendoyn-Glendenning-Clendenin-Clendening, etc., Family, Historical and Inferential," copy from "Archives and History Collection, West Virginia," Florence S. Mahoney Personal Papers, hereafter cited as FM Personal Papers; "Clendenins in Mason County, West Virginia," History of Mason County, West Virginia, 1987, 69470, copy in FM Personal Papers.

2. Robert S. and Helen M. Lynd, *Middletown: A Study in American Culture* (New York: Harcourt, Brace and Company, 1929), 6–9, 25, 37, 93, 100–02, 111.

Muncie was the setting for the Lynds' classic sociological study, published in 1929, of a midwestern city evolving from the industrial revolution in the early 1900s. They portrayed a small urban community over a period of 35 years, beginning in 1890, which includes Mahoney's years there, 1899–1917. Muncie's population in 1920 included 2 percent who were foreign-born and 6 percent who were African-American; four out of five salary earners were male; within the state, one woman in six made a living on her own.

3. Muncie High School yearbook, 1917 class information.

4. Frank Smith, *Robert G. Ingersoll, A Life* (Buffalo, N.Y.: Prometheus Books, 1990), 7–14.

Ingersoll, credited with stimulating a free-thought movement in the United States, was reputed to have addressed more Americans than anyone during the last two decades of the 19th century. He popularized many ideas that previously had not had wide currency.

5. *Ibid.*, 8.

6. Russian ballerina Anna Pavlova (1881–1931) was considered the greatest of her time.

Dr. Dudley Allen Sargent (1849–1924) founded in the 1880s the Sargent Normal School of Physical Training as part of Harvard University curriculum. His educational approach emphasized the importance of physical activity as a factor in the prevention of disease and the improvement of health. Modern rehabilitative medicine and physical therapy owe much to Sargent's pioneering work and theories. George K. Makechnie, *Optimal Health: The Quest, A History of Boston University's Sargent College of Allied Health Professions* (Boston: Boston University, 1979), v, 16, 22–23, 38–39,46–47, 52–53.

7. "Demonstration of Physical Work is Great Success," undated, unidentified newspaper article, courtesy J. Michael Mahoney.

8. Carolyn Saunders, "Folklore, Roaring '20s," *Sask Report Newsmagazine*, December, 1988, 54; "United police raid alleged opium dens here Saturday night," undated, unidentified newspaper article, 1926; Leith Knight, "1920 prohibition stories tell drinkers of euphoria," Moose Jaw *Times-Herald*, July 31, 1987; Milton Cust, "Author says city roared in 1920s," *Times-Herald*, July 11, 1975; Susan Tinker, "Moose Jaw in 20s 'nice quiet place to live,'" *Times-Herald*, August 7, 1985.

9. George Dixon, "Mrs. Mahoney," *Washington Post and Times Herald*, 25 March, 1956.

10. *International Encyclopedia of Dance* (Oxford University Press, 1998), s.v. "Luigi Albertini . . ."

The Institute for Crippled and Disabled was located at 400 First Avenue near Bellevue Hospital, with which the institute was connected.

11. WIOD radio program, "Let's Look It Up," 28 February, 1953, Florida Collection, Miami Public Library.

Hereafter Florence Sheets will be referred to as Mahoney except to distinguish between her and her husband.

12. "Mr. Miami Beach," *American Experience*, PBS Television, 1998.

13. Fisher built the "Dixie Highway" from Indiana to the foot of Collins Bridge to make it easy for midwesterners to travel to the sunny vacationland. He also developed Montauk Point on Long Island.

14. WIOD radio program.

15. Captain Joe Maggio, "Miami: In the Wake of the *Santiago*," *Sea History* 85 (Summer, 1998), 16–17, citing 1924 photographs, courtesy Historical Association of Southern Florida, Jean Taylor Collection.

16. "In Miami's realm of social activities," *Miami Daily News*, Wednesday, 13 October, 1926; photo caption, "Mildred Sheets and Mrs. Dan J Mahoney (Florence Sheets)," *Miami Daily News*, 17 October, 1926.

17. "Daniel Mahoney, Miami publisher," obituary, *New York Times*, 2 April, 1963.

Cox served in the 61st and 62nd Congresses from Ohio's 3rd district (1909–13) and as governor for three terms (1913–15, 1917–19, 1919–21). He was a prominent supporter of President Woodrow Wilson and the League of Nations. In 1920 he lost soundly to Warren G. Harding, who did not support U. S. participation in the League. Cox was credited with forging a coalition of urban-industrial Northerners and Southerners to redirect the national Democratic Party in the 1920s and 1930s and considered running for U. S. Senate in 1930. He was active in a movement to stop the 1932 presidential candidacy of his former running mate, Franklin D. Roosevelt. Cox nevertheless campaigned for Roosevelt but refused offers to serve in his administration (as ambassador to Germany and chairman of the Federal Reserve Board). Cox did serve as delegate to the World Monetary and Economic Conference in London in 1939 and generally supported Roosevelt's New Deal policies, which he publicly stated were saving capitalism through government intervention.

Cox died of heart failure at age 87 on 15 July, 1957, at "Trailsend," his Dayton home for more than 40 years, leaving an estate valued at $10 million to son James, daughters Anne and Barbara, and wife Margaretta Blair Cox. Daniel Mahoney was a trustee of a fund controlling stocks of the Dayton, Miami, and Springfield newspapers. James E. Cebula, *James M. Cox, Journalist and Politician*, (New York & London: Garland Publishing, Inc., 1985), 133–36, 138.

18. Cebula, 127, 128, 138–39, 168 n3 citing Daniel J. Mahoney to Cox, 18 April, 1923.

Two years after its purchase, Cox commissioned an elaborate and colorful building with a 279-foot "Freedom Tower" to house the re-named *Miami Daily News*, the city's first skyscraper dominating the sky line along Biscayne Bay.

19. Biographical sketch, James M. Cox manuscript collection, Wright State University, Dayton, Ohio, hereafter cited as Cox Papers; Cebula,132; James M. Cox, *Journey through My Years* (New York: Simon and Shuster, 1946), 394–95.

20. FM interview with Stephen Strickland, no date, FM Personal Papers, hereafter cited as Strickland interview.

21. Cebula, l28–29, 168 n6, citing Cox to Daniel J. Mahoney, 22 November, 1924; "Tributes tell loss a city feels," *Miami Daily News*, 2 April, 1963.

22. Helen Muir, *Miami, U. S. A.* (Miami: The Pickering Press, 1953), 187–88.

23. John Crittenden, *Hialeah Park: A Racing Legend* (Miami: The Pickering Press, 1989), 49.

24. *Ibid.*, 53–55.

25. *Ibid.*, 56; Muir, 188–191; William Tucker, "Mahoney gave Dade colorful

leadership," obituary, *Miami Daily News,* 2 April, 1963; Lawrence Thompson, "Publisher, UM leader Daniel Mahoney dies," *Miami Herald,* 2 April, 1963.

The *New York Times,* in its obituary of Mahoney (2 April, 1963), stated that "His direction of newspaper reports on Miami's gambling establishments was credited with the formation of congressional investigations [led by Senator Estes Kefauver] and the eventual dissolution of the gambling syndicates."

It was during the heyday of gangster violence that the Cox-owned *Daily News* won its first Pulitzer "for the most disinterested and meritorious public service rendered by an American newspaper in 1938." Its nine-month series of articles led to a recall election the following year that rid city government of what the *Daily News* derisively called "the termites," commissioners whom it accused of "boring from within," insidiously undermining representative government by "terrorism." Dan Mahoney, then general manager, as well as the newspaper were named as defendants in a $1.6 million libel suit by one person targeted in the series. *Editor and Publisher,* December 1938, 4.

26. Tucker, "Mahoney gave . . .,"; "Daniel Mahoney," obituary, *New York Times,* 2 April, 1963.

27. WIOD radio program; Thomas J. Wood, "Dade County: Unbossed, Erratically Led," "City Bosses and Political Machines," *The Annals of American Political and Social Science,* American Academy of Political and Social Science, May 1964, 69.

Mahoney served on many civic organization boards, including chairman of the University of Miami trustees for 10 years (until his death in 1963), where a women's residence hall was named in his honor.

28. The Union Pacific railroad purchased 4,300 acres near the declining mining village of Ketchum and built the Sun Valley resort to attract passenger-train traffic to the West.

29. FM notes, FM Personal Papers.

30. Tucker, "Mahoney gave . . ."; Michael Mahoney, "Report from Africa," 17 columns written for the Cox newspapers, Papers of Harry S. Truman, Post-Presidential files, Harry S. Truman Library, hereafter cited as Truman Papers.

Florence Mahoney in 1999 had six grandchildren and 12 great-grandchildren.

31. FM notes, FM Personal Papers.

32. Strickland interview; FM to Mary Lasker, Saturday P.M., 1950, Mary Lasker Papers, Rare Book and Manuscript Collection, Columbia University, hereafter cited as M. Lasker Papers.

Daniel J. Mahoney died 1 April, 1963, at age 75 on the operating table at a New York hospital from the effects of an anesthesia explosion while undergoing surgery for the removal of part of a lung. His obituary and a report of the cause of his death were carried in the *New York Times.* Tucker, "Mahoney gave . . ."; "Surgery death laid to gas explosion," *New York Times,* 3 April, 1963.

— CHAPTER 2 —

1. Strickland interview; Cebula, 139.

2. Cebula, 137, citing Cox, *Journey through my Years.*

3. Strickland interview.

4. Cox to Mrs. Albert D. (Mary) Lasker, 26 September, 1946, Cox Papers.

5. Cox to Dan Mahoney, 30 July, 1945; Cox to "Mrs. Doc Mahoney,"13 August, 1945, both in Cox Papers.

6. Cox to Mrs. D. J. Mahoney, 28 July, 1947, Cox Papers.

7. Cox to Mrs. "Doc" Mahoney, 31 August, 1945, Cox Papers.

8. Cox to Mrs. D. J, Mahoney, 20 August, 1945, 7 August, 1946, 12 August, 1946, Cox Papers.

9. Cox to Mrs. D. J. Mahoney, 31 October, 1945, and 31 August, 1945, Cox Papers.

10. Cox to "My dear Doc," 6 February, 1948, Cox Papers.

11. FM column excerpts, no dates, FM Personal Papers.

12. Florence Mahoney, unsigned column, "About People," *Miami Daily News*, 27 January, 1946.

Cox had informed her of Albert Einstein's comments in a letter, 31 October, 1945, Cox Papers.

13. FM column excerpts, no dates, FM Personal Papers.

14. "About People," *Miami Daily News*, 16 January, 1949, 15 March, 1953.

15. "About People," *Miami Daily News*, 4 January and 15 March, 1953.

16. "About People," *Miami Daily News*, 17 May, 1953.

17. "About People," *Miami Daily News*, 8 February and 15 March, 1953.

18. Philip Wylie, *Generation of Vipers* (Normal, Illinois: Dalkey Archive Press, Illinois State University, 1970, copyright 1942), ix–xii.

Generation of Vipers depicted American society as hypocritical, crazed and at the same time inhibited sexually, driven by advertising to buy useless objects, and badly governed, a society in which women were condemned to ineffectual, dilettantish lives and men to making money. The book had wide appeal: from the 4,000 copies initially published in January 1943 by Farrar and Rinehart, it had gone into more than 20 printings, with sales exceeding 180,000 copies by 1955, when Wylie revised the book and wrote an introduction to the new edition. Wylie was ahead of his time in both sociological views and as a conservationist. In 1951 he wrote in *Life* magazine that Miami was a "polluted paradise" and Biscayne Bay an "open sewer," which led the city to begin a massive cleanup campaign. An ardent outdoorsman and fisherman,Wylie also led the fight for establishment of the Everglades National Park. Martin Arnold, "Philip Wylie, author, dies; noted for 'Mom' attack, prolific iconoclast," *New York Times*, 26 October, 1971.

19. Strickland interview.

20. Wylie, xiv–xv, 194, 195, note.

Wylie in *Vipers* created the word "momism" to describe what he considered uniquely American domination by women of their sons, causing tyranny over their intellect and wills.

21. Strickland interview.

Rusk was in charge of setting up convalescent training centers in several locations, including one in Coral Gables, Florida. He subsequently became an associate editor at the *New York Times*, for which he wrote a weekly column, and in 1948 established the Rusk Rehabilitation Institute in New York. He was the recipient of several Lasker Awards (for significant contributions in health fields), "a whole shelf full," as his daughter Martha (Mrs. Preston) Sutphen put it. Sutphen interview with author, 3 May, 1999.

Mahoney during the war met people by helping them, relating: "Every hotel practically was taken over in Miami Beach for people to live in because the air force and army people were [stationed] there. So I went around and tried to find places for wives and people to live."

22. FM, "Memos Plans 1947, Programs for 1947," FM Personal Papers.

23. "Dr. Brock Chisholm, former W. H. O. head, dies," Associated Press, *New York Times*, 5 February, 1971.

George Brock Chisholm (1896–1971) served as an infantryman in the Canadian Army in World War I, enlisting in 1915 at the age of 18. He received his medical degree from the University of Toronto in 1924 and became Toronto's first practicing psychiatrist. In World War II, he headed the Canadian army's medical services. Immediately after the war he raised the specter of the potential dangers of germ warfare, which he argued gave small nations or groups equal destructive capacity to those with extensive hardware resources or the atomic bomb. Chisholm served as Canada's deputy minister of health and welfare after the war, became executive secretary of an interim committee of the World Health Organization (WHO) in 1946, and was elected director general in 1948. He retired in 1953 and died at age 74 in 1971.

24. Mahoney wrote about the Churchills frequently in her column during their 1946 visit. "About People," *Miami Daily News*, 20 January, 3 February, and 3 March, 1946.

25. "Dr. Brock Chisholm . . ."

26. Mike Gorman, "Oklahoma Attacks Its Snake Pits," *The Reader's Digest*, September 1948, 145, "condensed from his forthcoming book," *Oklahoma Attacks Its Snake Pits* (University of Oklahoma Press, 1948).

The title referred to Mary Jane Ward's novel, *The Snakepit*, published by Random House and condensed in the May 1946 *Reader's Digest*.

Another exposé at the time was *The Shame of the States* by journalist Albert Deutsch, describing visits to twelve institutions, which Mahoney also read and referred to in a letter to Mary Lasker.

27. Mike Gorman, interview with Stephen P. Strickland,1987, Mike Gorman Papers, 1946–89, MS C 462, History of Medicine Division, National Library of Medicine, hereafter cited as Gorman Papers.

28. Elizabeth B. Drew, "The Health Syndicate: Washington's Noble Conspirators," *Atlantic Monthly* (December 1967), 76; Stephen Strickland, interview with author, 24 September, 1998; John Foord Sherman, NIH deputy director (1968–74), interview, 5 February, 1998.

29. Strickland interview, Gorman Papers.

Gorman in 1949 was chosen one of the nation's 10 outstanding young men by the United States Chamber of Commerce for his crusading efforts in the field of mental health. Mike Gorman, *Every Other Bed* (Cleveland and New York: The World Publishing Company, 1956), "About the Author," and "Mike Gorman," *Current Biography*, [1956], 20, Gorman Papers.

30. Strickland interview, Gorman Papers.

31. *Ibid.*

Gorman's first article in the *Miami Daily News* appeared on 28 March, 1949 under the headline "How we treat our mentally sick in Dade County." It was prefaced with an editor's note introducing Gorman's background, saying that "he visited the Miami Retreat yesterday . . . to compare it with hospitals he has visited in 21 states."

32. *Ibid.*

33. "Jack" Kennedy to FM, [1944], FM Personal Papers.

Barbara Cox Anthony, a daughter of James Cox, was the "Mrs. Ripley" referred to in Kennedy's letter.

34. "Jack" Kennedy to FM, 5 September, 1944, FM Personal Papers.

35. *Ibid.*

Karl Augustus Menninger (1893–1990) with his father Charles Frederick (1862–1953) founded the Menninger Clinic in 1920 and were joined by Karl's brother William Claire (1899–1966) in 1926. The clinic was conceived as a place to gather many specialists in one center. The Menninger Foundation was created in 1941 to foster research, training, and public education in psychiatry. The Menningers also were instrumental in founding the Winter Veterans' Administration Hospital in Topeka at the close of World War II, for many years the largest psychiatric training program in the world. Karl Menninger's books *The Human Mind* (1930), *Love Against Hate* (1942), and *Man Against Himself* (1938) would have been the books that FM referred to Kennedy in 1944.

36. Claude Denson Pepper (1900–1989), Democratic Senator (1936–51) and Representative (1963–89) from Florida, was considered a populist liberal and advocate of social reform and international cooperation with the Soviet Union, for which he was accused of being pro-Communism. In later years as a member of the House of Representatives and chairman of the Special Committee on Aging, Pepper was influential in causes benefitting the aged. Muir, 179.

37. Claude D. Pepper with Hays Gorey, *Pepper: Eyewitness to a Century* (New York: Harcourt, Brace, Jovanovich, Publishers, 1987), 110.

38. Margaret Truman, *Harry S. Truman* (New York: William Morrow & Company, Inc., 1973) 323–24, 437–38, 443.

Vice President Truman was sworn in as president 12 April, 1945, on the death of President Franklin Roosevelt, and again 20 January, 1946, his first inauguration.

39. M. Truman, 396, 399.

Truman continued to visit Key West after leaving the presidency in 1952.

40. "About People," *Miami Daily News*, 3 February, 1946.

41. M. Truman, caption to photo number 23; "About People," *Miami Daily News*, 27 November, 1949.

Clark M. Clifford (1906–98) served as counsel to President Truman from June 1946 until he resigned in 1950 and established a law firm in Washington. Clifford would serve Presidents Kennedy, Johnson, and Carter in special roles related to defense, foreign intelligence, and diplomacy and was Secretary of Defense, 1968–69.

Mathew J. "Matt" Connelly was a government investigator whom Truman hired for a Senate committee that he chaired in 1941 to investigate waste and mismanagement of the nation's wartime defense program. Connelly served as speech writer and appointments secretary in the 1948 presidential campaign.

– CHAPTER 3 –

1. John Gunther, *Taken at the Flood: The Story of Albert D. Lasker* (New York: Harper & Brothers, 1960), 180–81; Florence Mahoney, "About People," *Miami Daily News*, 10 March, 1946.

2. Gunther, 1–3, 33, 294; "A. D. Lasker dies; philanthropist, 72," *New York Times*, 31 May, 1952.

Lasker served several presidents of both parties in important posts: He was assistant to the secretary of agriculture (1917) in President Wilson's administration and chairman of the United States Shipping Board (1921–23) in Harding's administration. In 1940 Lasker was a delegate to the Republican National Convention that nominated Wendell Wilkie for president and served as Wilkie's floor manager for Illinois. He also was a trustee of the University of Chicago (1937–1942).

3. Gunther, 5, 36–40, 63, 72–74, n7, 167, 195; "A. D. Lasker dies . . ."; Gary Cohen, "Epitaphs," "A tobacco fortune for a cancer cure," *U. S. News & World Report*, 29 February, 1994.

Lasker married Flora Warner in 1902; she died in 1936, leaving three children, Mary (Mrs. Leigh Block), Edward, and Frances (Mrs. Sidney F. Brody).

Lasker determined to make it acceptable for women to smoke in public after a restaurant manager asked his wife Flora to refrain from doing do. He put together a creative marketing strategy and hired actresses, opera singers, and other well-known women to endorse *Lucky Strikes,* and sales within one year shot up 312 percent. Lasker also was the first to use coupons to entice buyers to untried products and to exploit radio serial "soap operas" and entertainers for advertising.

4. Gunther, 112–13; "A. D. Lasker . . ."

5. Gunther, 113–114.

6. *Ibid.,* 113–14, 177–78.

7. *Ibid.,* 224–25, 235.

Lasker's feelings of frustration and desire to cure his and his wife's ailments prompted him in 1928 to give the medical faculty of the University of Chicago $1 million to study aging, geriatrics, and degenerative diseases (he was a trustee of the university, 1937–42). Asked why he picked those for his generosity, he said that he wanted to live to a very ripe old age. He grew discouraged, however, when that effort did not appear to lead to progress in curing diseases. Gunther, 13–14; Stephen P. Strickland, *Politics, Science, and Dread Disease* (Cambridge, Massachusetts: Harvard University, 1972), 34.

8. Gunther, 236–38; Eric Page, "Mary W. Lasker, philanthropist for medical research, dies at 93," *New York Times,* 23 February, 1994; "Moving Force in Medical Research," *Medical World News,* 20 November, 1964, 86; Claudia Levy, "Philanthropist Mary Lasker Dies at 93," *Washington Post,* 23 February, 1994.

Mary's parents were Frank Elwin Woodward and Sara Johnson. Mrs. Woodward gained recognition for leading an anti-pollution crusade, the Outdoor Cleanliness Association, to force utilities to curb smoke emissions in New York City. Both parents died of stroke, Mary's long-time maid of cancer. Strickland, *Politics,* 33.

9. Gunther, 236–38; Page, "Mary W. Lasker"; "Moving Force . . ."

10. Gunther, 239.

Mary Lasker sold much of her and Albert's art collection later in her life because she "wanted to be able to give away the money" realized from the sales. The Albert Lasker collection was exhibited twice after his death in 1952 (in Dallas, 1953, and San Francisco, 1954) for the benefit of the American Cancer Society. Individual works also were loaned periodically to major museums, including the Louvre and the Metropolitan Museum of Art, New York City. Gunther, 314.

11. *Ibid.,* 239, 260, 268.

12. *Ibid.,* 269–72, 287; "A. D. Lasker . . ."

13. Gunther, 238, 240–41; "Medicine, Fanning the Fire," *Time,* 30 August, 1948.

14. Gunther, 319, 321, 325; Drew, 76; "A. D. Lasker . . ."

The motto over the door to the Albert and Mary Lasker Foundation office in the Chrysler Building, New York, was a quote from Belgian poet and philosopher Maurice Maeterlinck (1862–1949): "*At every crossing on the road that leads to the future, each progressive spirit is opposed by a thousand men appointed to guard the past,*" a credo that Mary Lasker quoted and believed. Gunther, 299.

15. Gunther, 326; Gloria Donaldson, "Lasker Foundation's president holds numerous medical honors," Honolulu *Star-Bulletin*, 8 March, 1955.

The Lasker Foundation also supported beautification projects in New York and the arts.

Among Lasker Foundation awardees over the years who would figure in Mahoney's story were: Dr. Howard Rusk (three awards), Dr. Brock Chisholm (two), Margaret Sanger, Dr. Paul Dudley White, Senator Lister Hill (two), Rep. John E. Fogarty, Rep. Melvin Laird, Rep. Claude Pepper, Karl and William Menninger, Dr. Leona Baumgartner, Dr. Jonas Salk, Dr. Sidney Farber, Dr. Michael E. DeBakey, Ann Landers (Eppie Lederer), Mike Gorman, and President Lyndon B. Johnson.

16. Gunther, 323.

17. *Ibid.*, 321–23.

18. *Ibid.*, 321–22; Elmer Holmes Bobst, *Bobst, The Autobiography of a Pharmaceutical Pioneer* (New York: David McKay Company, 1969), 224–27, 29.

Bobst later became board chairman of Warner-Lambert Pharmaceutical Company.

19. Strickland, *Politics*, 36.

20. Bobst, 256; Gunther, 323.

21. Gunther, 324–25.

22. *Ibid*, 288-89, Bobst, 229, 256.

Anna Rosenberg Hoffman (1902–1983) was a personal representative in Europe for Presidents Roosevelt and Truman, reporting on problems of returning G.I.s. When named an assistant secretary of defense in charge of manpower in 1950, she assumed the highest post ever held by a woman in the national military establishment.

23. Gunther, 298; "A. D. Lasker . . ."; Page, "Mary W. Lasker," citing *New York Times* column by Meyer Berger, 1953.

24. Gunther, 299, 316; *Margaret Sanger,* The Margaret Sanger Project, television documentary, 1999; Ellen Chesler, *Woman of Valor, Margaret Sanger and the Birth Control Movement in America* (New York: Simon & Schuster, 1992), 388–89, 394.

Albert, according to Gunther's biography, claimed to have suggested changing the name of Sanger's organization to Planned Parenthood Federation because he thought the term "birth control" created negative images for people. Sanger, however, reportedly hated the new name, adopted in 1942, and objected to the organization's being restructured and run by men, for a time disassociating with it. Mary Lasker also considered the male head of Planned Parenthood overly cautious and lacking in crusading spirit.

The Laskers were the largest individual supporters of birth-control programs in the United States in the 1930s and early 1940s, according to Sanger biographer Ellen Chesler, who wrote that it was their funding of her organization's "Negro

Project" in the South that convinced Eleanor Roosevelt to get involved in the birth-control movement.

25. FM to Albert and Mary Lasker, July 1942, M. Lasker Papers.

26. M. Lasker to FM, 31 July, 1942, M. Lasker Papers.

27. M. Lasker to FM, 11 June, 1943, M. Lasker Papers.

28. Bruce Babbitt, interview with author, 15 January, 1999.

29. Cox to A. Lasker, 25 September, 1939, Cox Papers.

30. A. Lasker to Cox, 28 September, 1945, Cox Papers.

31. *Ibid.*

32. Cox to A. Lasker, 18 December, 1951, Cox Papers; Gunther, 262 n2, citing *Chicago Daily News*, 12 October, 1943.

33. A. Lasker, telegram to Cox, 21 December, 1951, Cox Papers.

34. Gunther, 312 n298, 338–39, 343, 345–46; Strickland, *Politics*, 299, n3.

Lasker, according to a tax appraisal of his $11.6 million estate, bequeathed $5.6 million to the Albert and Mary Lasker Foundation, Inc., and an equal amount to Mary Lasker. "$11,574,455 Lasker net," *New York Times*, 11 March, 1955.

35. Strickland, *Politics*, 45–46, 137; Drew, 77; Gorman, *Current Biography*.

The committee's first lobbyist was Lynn Adams. Lasker's sister, Alice Fordyce, was secretary.

– CHAPTER 4 –

1. FM note, undated, FM Personal Papers; Paul Starr, *The Social Transformation of American Medicine* (New York: BasicBooks, 1982), 340.

2. Starr, 340–41; Strickland, *Politics*, 15–31; "Hearings, Wartime Health and Education Subcommittee of the Committee on Education and Labor, U. S. Senate, 78th Congress, Pursuant to Senate Resolution 74 authorizing an investigation of the educational and physical fitness of the civilian population as related to national defense," Part 7, 14–16 December, 1944, Sen. Claude Pepper, chairman, 2285, citing Exhibit 6, "The Future of American Science," by Kirtley F. Mather, Harry Grundfest, Melber Phillips, United Office and Professional Workers of American, Congress of Industrial Organizations (CIO), 1944, hereafter cited as Pepper hearings. See also "One giant step out," editorial, *New England Journal of Medicine*, 5 September, 1968, 546; Charles V. Kidd, "The NIH Phenomenon," book review of Strickland's *Politics*, *Science*, 19 January, 1973, 270; and "James A. Shannon dies, scientist, NIH Director," *Washington Post*, 23 May, 1994.

3. Strickland, *Politics*, 15–31.

The OSRD and its Committee on Medical Research were disbanded in 1947.

Similar post-war plans for strengthening and developing science that were being considered in Great Britain and France influenced policymakers and scientists in the United States as well as scientific planning in the Soviet Union. Pepper hearings, 2287.

Truman headed a committee responsible for planning the peacetime economy, beginning in 1943–44, when he was being rumored as a potential vice-presidential candidate in Roosevelt's forthcoming campaign. The Truman committee's report on reconversion pointed up opportunities for using resources and facilities developed during the war. M. Truman, 164.

4. Strickland, *Politics*, 38.

A few far-sighted government officials, including Surgeon General Dr. Thomas Parran and NIH Director Rolla E. Dyer, in 1944 proposed attaching the OSRD's Committee for Medical Research (CMR) programs to the existing Institute of Health. In the debate over what kind of government entity should take over the wartime OSRD activities, a CMR advisory panel influenced by medical-school representatives adamantly opposed federal control of medical research, preferring a separate, autonomous foundation over the PHS. Director of OSRD Vannevar Bush and several members of Congress realized, however, that Congress would never allow federal funding of research without its and federal agency oversight. For accounts of the transition of government-administered biomedical research programs from war- to peacetime, see: Richard Mandel, *A Half Century of Peer Review, 1946–1996*, Division of Research Grants, National Institutes of Health, Bethesda, Maryland, 1996, 11–13 and *passim*; and Donald Swain, "The Rise of a Research Empire: NIH, 1930 to 1950," *Science*, 14 December, 1962, 1235.

5. Strickland, *Politics*, 44; Pepper hearings, 2200–01.

6. Strickland, *Politics*, 38, citing Richard H. Shyrock, *American Medical Research* (New York: The Commonwealth Fund, 1947), 104.

7. *Ibid.*, 37, citing Daniel S. Greenberg, *The Politics of Pure Science* (New York: The New American Library, 1967), 134.

8. Gunther, 316–18.

9. *Ibid.*, 318; Strickland, *Politics,*40, citing Dr. Vannevar Bush, *Science: The Endless Frontier* (Washington: U. S. Office of Scientific Research and Development, 1945). See letter in Pepper hearings, Part 7, 2285–86, Exhibit 6, "The Future of American Science," quoting President Roosevelt to Dr. Vannevar Bush, 20 November, 1944.

10. Swain, 1235.

Although the PHS had authority to make grants to nongovernmental entities, the Bureau of the Budget refused to allow the payments from the federal purse. It took the Pepper hearings to spring the coffers loose and prod the budget agency to release extramural research grant money.

11. Strickland interview, quoting FM:

"Senator Pepper was in a very important spot in the Senate . . . and he was a friend of Mahoney's. So we decided to go and talk to him about holding hearings. He was running for reelection and he wanted the support of the papers, so we went to see him. He had a great deal of influence. He said he'd be delighted to hold hearings. These were the first health [research]–related hearings ever held at the time. I came from Miami to Washington for the hearings."

12. Gunther, 318–19; Strickland, *Politics*, 19.

13. Drew, 76; Pepper, 111.

In his autobiography Pepper said, "I read some statistics that caused me grave concern. They made me wonder about the health of the American population . . . . . [O]ur selective service system had discovered that young Americans were not in very good shape . . . Nearly 2.5 million [29.5 per cent of potential draftees] had been rejected for military service because they were educationally, mentally, physically or morally deficient; another 300,000 had been turned down because were illiterate. This was the situation in the richest country on earth, rich enough to do something about it . . . I was able to win a small appropriation and to borrow federal personnel to launch a study of this depressing phenomenon, which I felt reflected poorly on our society."

14. Strickland, *Politics*, 34; Drew, 76; Gunther, 330–331.

Albert Lasker wrote Pepper in 1944: "The government collects and spends, in the course of time, billions in social insurance, veterans' aid to men stricken with post-war disabilities, and those who cannot take their place as producers in society (on account of illness or disability). A comparatively few millions spent [for medical research] annually over a period of a decade might make the need for such vast social security and veteran expenditures largely unnecessary."

15. Strickland, *Politics*, 38.

16. "Memoranda book, personal," undated, FM Personal Papers, hereafter cited as "Memoranda."

17. FM to ML, "Saturday P.M.," 1944, M. Lasker Papers.

18. Swain, 1233; Gunther, 319, 331; Starr, 340; Strickland, *Politics*, 25–27, quoting PHS memoranda, 1926–29.

The National Institute of Health was created by the Ransdell Act of 1930, which reorganized and expanded the Hygienic Laboratory, reflecting a shift in research policy from infectious to chronic diseases and an expansion of federally funded medical research. The National Cancer Act of 1937 established the Cancer Institute within the NIH and for the first time authorized grants to nongovernment researchers as well as a program of training fellowships to institutions like universities. In 1938 the total PHS research budget was $2.8 million compared to $26.3 million for research in the Department of Agriculture.

19. Pepper hearings, 10 July, 1944, 1613.

20. *Ibid.*, 14 December, 1944, 2177.

21. *Ibid.*, 2186, 2196, 2198, 2200.

22. *Ibid.*, 15 December, 1944, 2218–19, 2233, 2238.

According to testimony, private industry in 1941 had spent some $270 million on biomedical research principally aimed at producing profitable commercial products while foundations were thought to be giving less than $5 million for medical research.

23. *Ibid.*, 2201–02; Starr, 341.

24. Pepper hearings, 15 December, 1944, 2245.

25. *Ibid.*, 2228, quoting Dr. E. V. Cowdry, professor of anatomy, Washington University School of Medicine, and director of research, Barnard Free Skin and Cancer Hospital, St. Louis, Missouri; and 2239, quoting Henry S. Simms, Ph.D., Columbia University College of Physicians and Surgeons.

26. *Ibid.*, 2229–31, quoting Lawrence S. Kubie, M. D., College of Physicians and Surgeons, Columbia University, who testified: "With a minimum nationwide need for 20,000 psychiatrists, we have barely 3,000; yet our training facilities cannot turn out more than 150 to 200 a year, barely enough to cover the annual retirement from old age." Kubie further testified: "The result is, of course, that each such incapacitated person represents not only a tremendous economic problem to himself and dependents but to the entire community. He doesn't die. He is still there. He has to be taken care of," at a cost of $40,000 if in a veterans' facility. If "$25,000 invested in research [or in training a psychiatrist] succeeds in keeping one man from becoming a chronic patient, that would represent a saving of $15,000 to the government [or] community."

27. *Ibid.*, 2238, 2241, 2244, citing figures "Compiled by Mrs. Albert D. Lasker"; and 2220, 2224, quoting Cowdry.

A side issue was raised by the spokesman for science workers — the need to make medical-school entrance requirements "free from the various discriminations due to race, sex, creed or color." "We have a very obvious sex discrimination in medicine," he testified. "Very few women in this country are given the opportunity to enter into medical research and into the practice of medicine. Some schools bar women entirely from studying medicine. Other schools have a quota . . . The same thing is true, for example, with regard to Negroes and Jews. I think that in all fairness to the national well-being and to our own ideals of democracy, all of these discriminations should be specifically barred whenever the federal government grants funds." *Ibid.*, 2249–50.

28. *Ibid.*, 2279.

29. Gunther, 331; Strickland, *Politics*, 27, quoting Bush.

30. Pepper hearings, 2253–55.

Surgeon General Dr. Thomas Parran also argued for keeping research programs within PHS, which already had authority to give fellowships; he also favored enlarging clinical facilities at the NIH to include a hospital that would bring patients, clinicians, and scientists "in close contact and result in more rapid progress in our studies" in the areas of cancer, nutritional disorders, mental diseases, degenerative diseases, dental decay, and the process of aging, "all of which should be intensively studied in the post-war period." Pepper hearings, 2284.

31. For this exchange, *ibid.*, 2256–59.

32. *Ibid.*, 2260.

Rhoads' civilian laboratory, according to his testimony, with a budget of $166,000 annually, at the time was conducting basic research on the chemical make-up of cancerous-versus-normal human cells.

33. *Ibid.*, 2264–65.

34. *Ibid.*, 2275.

35. *Ibid.*, 2276; Strickland, *Politics*, 19, quoting Pepper.

The hearings focused on the following themes: 1) the need for training more researchers; 2) allowing investigators freedom from government control; 3) the advantages of long-term funding; 4) the need for higher standards of pay for scientists; 5) coordination between the existing PHS and NAS-NRC; 6) support of basic as well as applied research; and 7) the need to survey research already under way and to plan future goals based on national interest and welfare.

36. Gunther, 319; Strickland, *Politics*, 20–21.

The Pepper hearings were followed by Bush's report, *Science: The Endless Frontier*, in July, 1945. Its recommendations were introduced as legislation by Democratic Senator Warren G. Magnuson of Washington, whose bill called for establishment of a National Research Foundation to coordinate all research activities in the nation. Another approach was introduced by Democratic Senator Harvey Kilgore of West Virginia. Although many scientists, even the American Medical Association (AMA), supported the National Research Foundation concept in Magnuson's bill, President Truman vetoed it in 1947 on grounds that it had inadequate controls over government spending. The bill was modified, setting up the National Science Foundation (NSF), and finally approved in 1950.

37. Strickland, *Politics*, 40–41; biographical draft, undated, FM Personal Papers, hereafter cited as biographical draft.

Mary Lasker contributed $1,000 to a committee of scientists supporting the National Science Foundation bill. Strickland believed that Mahoney and Lasker "changed their minds depending on which option seemed at the time most promising." Strickland, 85.

38. "Content Outline of 2nd Session, Mahoney Tapes," no date, FM Personal Papers, hereafter cited as Content Outline.

39. Strickland, *Politics*, 44–46; biographical draft, undated, 5; "Transcription of a tape recording of a meeting 9 February, 1967, in Lasker Foundation offices, to hear Mr. Mike Gorman of the National Committee against Mental Illness," 2, Gorman Papers.

40. Strickland, *Politics*, 44, 46; biographical draft, 10–11.

The lobbyist at the time was Lynn Adams.

The National Mental Health Act (PL 487) was considered by NIH officials as a model for other categorical institutes, the first legislation authorizing grants to educational institutions and the first major commitment to training health manpower; it authorized $10 million in grants to states for mental-health facilities and research projects. Mandel, 26.

41. Strickland, *Politics*, 46, 78; Starr, 346.

The PHS since 1930 had had the small Division of Mental Hygiene that operated the two federal narcotics hospitals and psychiatric services for federal prisons. The National Institute of Mental Health (NIMH), which replaced the division in 1949, represented a new federal approach by emphasizing research and training; it also gave states aid for mental-health clinics and other services.

42. Cox to ML, 20 August, 1946, Cox Papers.

43. ML to Cox, 29 August, 1946, Cox Papers.

44. FM to ML, "Saturday P.M.," 1944, M. Lasker Papers.

Ellis G. Arnall (1907–92), whom Cox and his newspaper backed against incumbent Eugene Talmadge, was Governor of Georgia 1943–47.

45. FM to ML, 4 September, circa 1944, M. Lasker Papers.

The National Committee on Mental Hygiene, which was separate from Mahoney's and Lasker's National Committee on Mental Health, had existed for some 34 years by 1944. Mahoney's other reference may have been to the American Foundation for Mental Hygiene, which had its 16th annual meeting in 1944, according to an article, "First Layman, [Eugene] Meyer [publisher of the *Washington Post*] heads Mental Hygiene unit," in the *Washington Post*, 16 December, 1944.

46. Strickland, *Politics*, 78–79.

Congressman Keefe (died 1952), while Republicans chaired the 80th Congress, pushed through a $1 million increase for research on tuberculosis in 1946. Mandel, 31.

47. Strickland, *Politics,* 29-31, quoting "NIH spokesman," no date.

48. See also note 149, which cites Mahoney's meeting Truman at a publishers' meeting in New York.

Truman, in his 20 January, 1946, inaugural address (written while he was in Key West), suggested a four-point foreign policy that called for "a bold new program for making the benefits of our scientific advances and industrial program available for the improvement and growth of under-developed parts of the world." M. Truman, 401.

49. Biographical draft, 5.

50. Clarence G. Lasby, "The War on Disease," in Robert A. Divine, ed., *The Johnson Years*, Volume Two, *Vietnam, the Environment and Science* (Lawrence, Kansas: University Press of Kansas, 1987), 186, 212 n8, citing Senator Brien McMahon to President Truman, 9 August, 1945, Box 466, Truman Library.

McMahon (1903–1952) was elected to the Senate in 1944 and 1950; he chaired the Joint Committee on Atomic Energy 1945–47 when he authored the Atomic Energy Act that led to establishment of the Atomic Energy Commission in 1946.

51. M. Truman, 577; Strickland interview, Gorman Papers.

52. Drew, 77.

In 1947 a change in the bill's administrative features was made to address criticism that health-care providers would be regimented by a government "health tsar." Senators Pepper, Glen H. Taylor of Idaho, and J. Howard McGrath of Rhode Island joined as co-sponsors of the 1947 bill. That bill's introduction was timed to coincide with Truman's second health message to Congress, an early move in his 1948 election campaign. Monte M. Poen, *Harry S. Truman versus the Medical Lobby: The Genesis of Medicare* (Columbia, Missouri: University of Missouri Press, 1979), 43, 45, 60, 98–99.

53. "President Truman's Health Plan would increase productivity, reduce disease, save lives," statement signed by some 200 people, published in the *New York Times* the first week of December 1945; Poens, 70, citing: Mary W. Lasker to author, 14 August, 1967; Lasker to H. Truman, 11 December, 1945, Official file, Truman Papers; Michael Davis to Samuel Rosenman, 26 November, 1945, President's Personal file, Truman Papers; biographical draft, 7–8; Strickland, *Politics*, 42.

Based on their experience with servants who had inadequate coverage, the Laskers had decided that a national system — patterned on unemployment insurance paid by employers and employees — was the only way to make medical care available for all citizens. It was clear that people who did not get care in a timely way got sicker, died prematurely, and cost industries and businesses untold millions in lost work time. Strickland, *Politics*, 32–42; Gunther, 319–20.

The Committee for the Nation's Health evolved out of an ad hoc committee created in February 1944. The Laskers contributed half of its initial $50,000 budget, and Mary Lasker contributed money and time to the committee's activities in efforts to get favorable publicity for the bill. Most newspapers, though, editorially opposed expanding Social Security to cover health care. Poen, 42–44, 83.

54. Poen, 62–64, citing author interview with Truman and "Special Message Recommending a Comprehensive Health Program," 19 November, 1945.

Truman also had learned that the conservative House Ways and Means Committee was about to consider ramifications of expanding Social Security coverage — which the committee likely would oppose — and decided to hasten his health message as a countermeasure.

The final version was the sixth draft of the health message. Truman advocated a single agency to, among other things, promote fundamental research in medicine, public health, and allied fields, provide scholarships and grants for promising young scientists, coordinate and control scientific activities conducted by different government agencies, and make publicly available to commerical and academic institutions the fruits of federally funded research. Much of the controversial proposal had been developed previously for Roosevelt, who had promised health reformers a similar message to Congress. Roosevelt staff were essential in formulating Truman's health message.

55. Strickland, *Politics*, 22–23.

56. Mrs. Albert Lasker, oral history interview by Charles T. Morrissey for John F. Kennedy Library, 18 April, 1966, 23–24, hereafter cited as M. Lasker oral history.

57. Poen, 70–71.

The view that Truman did not act aggressively was supported by later analysis, notably Poen's: "Support from the White House soon stalled. President Truman, in spite of his initial and decisive endorsement of national health insurance, simply did not follow through with the kind of articulate leadership the movement needed in order to gain additional adherents," *Ibid.*, 68.

58. M. Lasker oral history, 18 April, 1966, 24.

59. M. Lasker to Cox, 26 September, 1945, Cox Papers.

60. Poen, 60–61; FM memorandum, February 1992.

The different bill was designed to go to the Senate Education and Labor and its House counterpart committee, on which several sponsors like Murray and Pepper sat.

61. Senator Warren G. Magnuson, "The Medical Profession and the Congress Can Work Together," speech in U. S. Senate, 11 May, 1948, Papers of Oscar R. Ewing, Truman Papers, citing editorial, *Washington Post*, 7 May, 1948.

The contest offered eight prizes totaling $3,000.

62. FM to ML, undated, circa March 1947, M. Lasker Papers.

Clark Clifford, in his autobiography, *Counsel to the President*, with Richard Holbrooke (New York: Random House, 1991), 191, described Leslie Biffle as "the no-nonsense Secretary of the Senate, a powerful Washington insider who liked to travel around the country incognito in his old beat-up car, taking informal soundings of the popular mood."

63. Poen, 99.

64. ML to FM, 13 May, 1947, M. Lasker Papers.

65. FM to ML, undated, circa 1947, M. Lasker Papers.

66. FM to Senator Hayden (in Senate 1927–69), 4 October, 1947, M. Lasker Papers.

67. ML to FM, 24 July, 1947, M. Lasker Papers.

68. ML to Dan Mahoney, 16 July, 1947, M. Lasker Papers.

69. Poen, 106–07, citing Senate hearings on S. 545 and S. 1320 (the Murray-Wagner-Dingell-Pepper *et al* bill), 45.

Albert Lasker testified in July 1947 before the Senate Committee on Labor and Public Welfare as president of the Albert and Mary Lasker Foundation.

70. ML to FM, 24 July, 1947, M. Lasker Papers.

71. Poen, 130–31, citing Truman address, Indianapolis, 15 October, 1948.

Truman's GOP opponent, Thomas E. Dewey, was notably silent on the insurance issue because his running mate, California Governor Earl Warren, had publicly espoused a state-sponsored health insurance system, outlined in a *Look* magazine article, June 1948.

72. *Ibid.*, 132, citing correspondence between Lasker and Clifford, June-October 1948, Files of Clark Clifford, Truman Papers.

73. FM to Oscar Ewing, 8 July, 1950, Papers of Oscar R. Ewing, Truman Papers.

74. FM to Matt Connelly, 30 September, 1949, General file, Truman Papers; FM to Murphy, 23 September, 1950, Papers of Charles S. Murphy, Truman Papers.

75. FM to Murphy; "Lobbying against Human Needs," Committee for the Nation's Health, Bulletin #14, 25 July, 1950, and confidential memorandum, "The American Medical Association's Slush Fund to Defeat Democratic Candidates," 20 July, 1950, Papers of Charles S. Murphy, Truman Papers.

Gorman had pieced together the AMA expenditure figures from information printed in the *Congressional Record*, 14 July, 1950, noting that, because the existing lobbying law had no penalties for concealing information, it did not include what the lobbies chose not to reveal.

76. "Lobbying against Human Needs," quoting memorandum from Committee for the Nation's Health, 5 January, 1950, 5, and from confidential AMA "Slush Fund" memorandum, 5; Mike Gorman to Connelly, 31 January, 1951, Official File, Truman papers.

77. Memorandum from Committee for the Nation's Health, 5 January, 1950, 5, and confidential AMA "Slush Fund" memorandum, 5; "The American Medical Association and the 1952 Elections," 1950, Official File, Truman Papers.

78. Poen, 176–78, citing author interview with Mary Lasker; FM, journal, 25 January, 1966, FM Personal Papers.

Medicaid, a separate program covering health services for those with low incomes, funded by both federal and state governments, was enacted at the same time.

79. FM memorandum, February 1992, FM Personal Papers.

80. Drew, 77.

81. "Memoranda," FM Personal Papers.

82. M. Lasker oral history, 18 April, 1966, 24.

The AMA opposed another initiative supported by Mahoney and Lasker: direct federal aid to medical schools and students in the form of scholarships. The concept was based on growing fears that the nation soon would be faced with a severe shortage of doctors. In successive years, however, the AMA expressed skepticism about such a shortage, worried that federal aid would compromise medical schools' freedom. AMA opposition helped kill separate bills in 1949 and 1951. Legislation to subsidize medical education would not be considered for another 14 years. Biographical memorandum, "Reference: FM003," no date, 1, FM Personal Papers.

83. "Memoranda," and FM to Donald S. Dawson, 11 January, 1951, Official File, Truman Papers.

84. "Memoranda."

Mike Gorman, in a letter to the editor of *Atlantic Monthly*, February 1968, 45, wrote, "The idea for the commission originated in the minds of several key White House staffers who felt that the establishment of a non-partisan commission would keep most of the invective about the pros and cons of national health insurance out of the 1952 campaign. Dr. Rusk was instrumental in recruiting the chairman . . . Dr. Paul Magnuson, a distinguished surgeon and card-carrying Illinois Republican."

Dr. Lester Breslow, who was recruited by Dr. Russel Lee and others on the Commission to be its study director, had developed a chronic-disease program for California, where he subsequently became Public Health Director. He believed that the Commission's establishment "reflected Truman's frustration at not being able to achieve national health insurance because of AMA opposition, and his desire, in the last year of his term, to do *something* about health." Breslow, interview with author, 24 April, 1999.

85. "Memoranda."

Dr. Russel Lee was the father of Dr. Philip Lee, later an assistant secretary of health in the Department of Health, Education and Welfare (HEW).

86. Strickland interview, Gorman Papers; Drew, 77.

87. Dr. Paul B. Magnuson, chairman, President's Commission on the Health Needs of the Nation, speech, [1952], "PCHNN-SP-4," 14–15, 17, Official File, Truman Papers, hereafter cited as Magnuson speech.

88. Biographical memorandum, "Reference: FM003," undated, 2, FM Personal Papers.

89. Magnuson speech, 6–7.

The members of the commission were: Paul Magnuson, M.D., chairman, professor emeritus and former chairman, Department of Bone and Joint Surgery, Northwestern University, Chicago; Chester I. Bernard, chairman, National Science Foundation, New York; Lester W. Burkett, D.D.S., M.D., dean, School of Dentistry, University of Pennsylvania; Dean A. Clark, director, Massachusetts General Hospital, Boston; Donald M. Clark, M.D., lecturer in general practice, Boston University of Medicine, Peterborough, New Hampshire; Evarts A. Graham, M.D., professor emeritus of surgery, Washington University, St. Louis; Albert J. Hayes, president, International Association of Machinists; Joseph C. Hinsey, Ph.D., dean, Cornell University Medical College; Russel V. Lee, M.D., director, Palo Alto Clinic, clinical professor of medicine, Stanford University School of Medicine; Elizabeth S. Magee, general secretary, National Consumers League; Clarence H. Poe, president and editor, *Progressive Farmer*, Raleigh, North Carolina; Lowell J. Reed, Ph.D., vice president, Johns Hopkins University and Hospital; Walter P. Reuther, president, United Automobile Workers, CIO; Marion W. Sheahan, R.N., director, National Committee for the Improvement of Nursing Services, New York; Ernest G. Sloman, D.D.S., dean, College of Physicians and Surgeons and School of Dentistry, San Francisco.

Study director Breslow confirmed Magnuson's independence and determination to keep the commission apolitical. When FBI agents called on Magnuson to raise questions about Breslow's background, which included association with some organizations then consided suspect by anti-Communists, he reportedly ordered them out of his office, maintaining his right to run the commission and hire its staff until ordered otherwise by the president. "That's the kind of an independent-minded cuss he was — conservative in his views but not to be pushed around." Breslow to author, 24 April, 1999.

90. *Ibid.*, 7–8.

91. "The President's Commission on Health Needs of the Nation (1952 report), Statement by Dr. Paul Magnuson, Commission Chairman, on role of Mike Gorman in writing report," copy, FM Personal Papers.

92. Gorman, *Every Other Bed*, 31–32.

93. FM to Mrs. Truman, "Thursday," [1952]; text of address by Dr. Paul B. Magnuson, delivered at Lasker Awards in Medical Journalism banquet of the National Association of Science Writers, Chicago, Tuesday evening, 10 June, 1952, Official File, Truman Papers.

94. Truman to FM, 4 June, 1952, President's Secretary's files, Truman Papers; Truman to Magnuson, 23 June, 1952, Official File, Truman Papers.

95. Drew, 77, citing Gorman speech, circa 1967.

96. Strickland, *Politics*, 137.

97. India Edwards to "The Chairman" [DNC], 4 February, 1952, Papers of India Edwards, Truman Papers.

Edwards' memorandum continued: "Mary started paying his salary to give Bill Boyle [DNC chairman] time to make up his mind what he was going to do about supporting the President's Health Program. He did nothing so Mary has continued to pay Mike. Mike helped Dave Stowe in setting up the new Health Commission . . . . It was suggested that he [Gorman] be executive secretary of the Commission but, very properly in my opinion, he said that would be bad for the Commission and the Administration. I understand Dave Stowe has written the President a memorandum on Mike and that the President plans to discuss this matter with you on Friday. Hence this memorandum."

98. Strickland interview, Gorman Papers.

99. *Ibid.*

100. *Ibid.*

101. FM to ML, "Sunday 28th," [1949], M. Lasker Papers.

102. Gorman, *Every Other Bed*, 10.

Gorman had worked with governors in several states to change mental-health policy and with the National Governors' Conference to improve care and establish rights for the mentally ill, beginning in 1949, resulting in the first Governors' Conference on Mental Health in 1954.

103. Strickland, *Politics*, 41; biographical draft, 8–9; Gunther, 319; "Memoranda."

From 1947–48 funding for the National Institute of Health jumped from $8 million to $24.6 million.

104. Senate bill 720, "To authorize and request the President to undertake to mobilize at some convenient place or places in the United States an adequate

number of the world's outstanding experts and coordinate and utilize their services in a supreme endeavor to discover new means of treating, curing, and preventing diseases of the heart and arteries," introduced by Senator Pepper, 26 February, 1947, attachment to ML letter to Cox, 10 April, 1947, Cox Papers.

The simple two-page bill actually called for $1 million to be administered by the Surgeon General "or through an independent group appointed by him," to build "needed clinical and laboratory research facilities" for heart research.

105. ML to Cox, 10 April, 1947, Cox Papers.

106. Editorial, undated, circa 1947, with handwritten note, "Ran in April 15 issue and clip sent to Mrs. Lasker," Cox Papers.

Heart disease, the editorial stated, killed "587,314 people annually in the United States and caused disability to 7,840,000 more."

107. Biographical draft, 11–12.

108. Strickland, *Politics*, 84.

Gunther's book had been reprinted in *Ladies Home Journal* and *Reader's Digest*.

109. Gunther, 16; FM to ML, undated, circa 1946, M. Lasker Papers.

Lasker testified in 1946 before a Senate subcommittee as a member of the exeutive committee of the American Cancer society.

110. Mandel, 52; "Memoranda, book, personal," undated, FM Personal Papers; FM, "About People," by Mary Marley, *Miami Daily News*, 9 May, 1948, in Papers of Oscar Ewing, Truman Papers.

111. FM to Oscar Ewing, 24 May and 26 May, 1948, Papers of Oscar R. Ewing, Truman Papers.

112. FM to Ewing, 5 October, 1948, Papers of Oscar R. Ewing, Truman Papers.

113. FM and ML, telegram to Matthew Connelly, 3 November, 1948, President's personal file, Truman Papers.

114. Notes by Reathal Odum, citing gift with card bearing Mrs. Daniel Mahoney's name; Clifford to Odum, 30 November, 1948; H. Truman to FM, 2 December, 1948, President's personal file, Truman Papers.

115. Clark M. Clifford, "Memorandum for Mr. Connelly," 7 December, 1948, President's personal file, Truman Papers.

116. ML to Truman, 17 December, 1948, President's personal file, Truman Papers.

117. FM, telegram to "The President" from Miami Beach, 7 January, 1949; William D. Hassett, Secretary to the President, to FM, 11 January, 1949, President's personal file, Truman Papers.

118. "Memoranda."

119. FM to ML, "Sunday 28th," [1949], M. Lasker Papers.

120. FM to ML, "Mary darling, Thursday," undated, [1949], M. Lasker Papers.

World War I air hero Edward "Eddie" Rickenbacker, a friend of the Mahoneys from Miami although a political conservative, at the time was president and general manager of Eastern Airlines (1938–53) and later chairman of its board (1954–63).

121. Rufus E. Miles, Jr., *The Department of Health, Education, and Welfare* (New York: Praeger, 1974), 173; Starr, 343.

122. "Memoranda."

123. "6-billion health bill introduced in Congress," *Washington Evening Star,* 25 April, 1949.

124. "Memoranda."

The Arthritis Institute also was to study diabetes and obesity, and the Neurological Institute such things as multiple sclerosis, Parkinson's disease, epilepsy, cataracts, and glaucoma as they affected blindness.

125. Strickland, *Politics*, 84–85; Starr, 343.

126. "Memoranda."

The construction funds were the first for non-NIH facilities.

Clarence Cannon (1923–64) chaired the House Appropriations Committee in the 77th to 79th (1942–44), 81st to 82nd (1948–50), and 84th to 88th Congresses (1954–62).

127. Truman to FM, 30 October, 1951, copy in FM Personal Papers.

128. "Memoranda."

Congress in 1950 also created the National Science Foundation as well as a Division of Biological and Medical Sciences.

129. *Ibid.*

130. Biographical draft.

Leonard Scheele (1907–92), director of the Cancer Institutes, succeeded Dr. Parran as Surgeon General (S. G.) in April 1948 (at age 41) and served in that post for 10 years (twice reappointed by President Eisenhower). He resigned in 1958 to become a senior vice president of Warner-Lambert Pharmaceutical Company.

131. Strickland, *Politics*, 135.

Mahoney applied but was not appointed to the Heart Institute Council during Eisenhower's administration (1954–58).

132. John Foord Sherman, Ph. D. interview with T. Ray, 5 February, 1998, Washington, D. C.; interview with author, 6 July, 1999.

The event described took place when Mahoney joined the National Institute of Arthritis and Metabolic Diseases Advisory Council in 1959.

Sherman started at NIH in 1953 as a specialist in pharmacology, worked for many years in grants administration, and served as Deputy Director of NIH 1968–74, when he resigned to become vice president of the American Association of Medical Colleges. In that role, he appointed Mahoney to the association's advisory citizens' council.

133. Strickland, *Politics,* 136.

134. "Memoranda"; Starr, 347.

135. "Memoranda," and biographical memorandum, "Reference: FM003," no date, 1, FM Personal Papers.

136. "Memoranda."

Although defeated for the Senate in 1950, Pepper would return to serve for many years in the House of Representatives, beginning in 1963 until his death in 1989.

Congress ultimately gave the National Institutes of Health a record $44 million in 1950, almost twice what had been appropriated the previous year.

137. Biographical memorandum, 17, citing "Appendix 3.1, Figures requested by Mrs. Lasker and Mrs. Mahoney for National Institutes of Health in 1954 budget in meeting with President Truman in June of 1952."

The Korean War (1950–53) set back funding for NIH when Truman directed a curtailment of programs that did "not directly contribute to defense," resulting in reductions in NIH appropriations for 1952. Senators Pepper and Magnuson pressed for NIH increases, specifically for heart, cancer, and mental-health research, construction, and training, but their amendments failed. Mandel, 54; "NIH obligations and amounts obligated for grants and direct operations," NIH 1998 Almanac.

138. Mary Lasker, memoir notes, undated, copy in FM Personal Papers.

139. Biographical memorandum, "Reference: FM003," undated, 11–12, FM Personal Papers.

140. Mary Lasker, memoir notes, FM Personal Papers.

141. Biographical memorandum, "Reference: FM003," 13.

142. Gunther, 332; Pepper, 257; Starr, 343.

The NIH appropriation for 1954 was $11 million higher than for 1953. "NIH obligations."

The NIH by 1950 consisted of the National Cancer Institute (established 1937), National Heart Institute (1948, Lung was not added until 1969), National Dental Institute (also established in 1948), National Institute of Arthritis and Metabolic Diseases (which absorbed Experimental Biology and Medicine, 1950), and the National Institute of Neurological Diseases and Blindness (1950). The National Institute of Allergy and Infectious Diseases was created in 1955, absorbing the National Microbiological Institute. A Clinical Center was built in 1953, for which President Truman laid the cornerstone in the last days of his presidency. Other institutes would follow. Natalie Davis Spingarn, *Heartbeat: The Politics of Health Research* (Washington and New York: Robert B. Luce, Inc., 1976), 24; "NIH Chronology of Events (by year), Historical Data," NIH 1998 Almanac.

143. Truman's daily schedules for 1951–52 show that Mahoney and Lasker met with him a number of times, "off the record." President's Secretary's files, Truman Papers.

144. ML and FM to Truman, Truman to FM and ML, 19 February, 1949; FM, telegram to Truman, 26 April, 1949, President's personal file, Truman Papers.

145. Oscar R. Ewing to FM, telegram, 1 February, 1950, Papers of Oscar R. Ewing, Truman Papers.

146. Edith Allen, Secretary to Justice Douglas, to Connelly, 21 June, 1950, citing "What Forrestal Knew," *Chicago Daily Tribune*, 13 June, 1950, Official file,

Truman Papers; FM to Secretary of State Dean Acheson, 28 March, 1950; Acheson to FM, 7 April, 1950, Papers of Dean Acheson, Truman Papers.

147. Truman to Daniel J. Mahoney, *Miami Daily News*, 10 November, 1949, President's Secretary's files, Truman Papers.

The letter apparently concerned Truman's anger at a news story about him and his "cronies," according to an account by FM to Strickland:

"I cut things out of the papers, and I clipped something one time, and [Clark Clifford] apparently showed it to Mr. Truman, and Mr. Truman turned it over and on the back of that article was another one that talked about Mr. Truman and his cronies. Mahoney got a handwritten letter from the President explaining the facts of life about how he chose people; the cronies were people whom he played poker with, and not the way he ran the government. It was wonderful. So then Mahoney got the editorial writers of the papers, and the Governor [Cox], and they all answered this letter. I'd love to see the copy of it." Strickland interview with FM, no date, 17, copy in FM Personal Papers.

148. Connelly to Miss Reathal Odum, 14 February, 1950, Connelly to FM, telegram, 15 February, 1950; President's personal file, Truman Papers.

149. Margaret Truman Daniel, interview with author, 27 January, 1999; Dixon, "Mrs. Mahoney," *Washington Post* and *Times Herald*, 25 March, 1956, which said:

"Editor's Note: Mrs. Mahoney is a close friend of Bess Truman and was perhaps the one woman in Washington to know of Margaret's engagement to newsman E. Clifton Daniel, Jr. before it was announced. In his column last Tuesday, George Dixon told about Margaret and her fiancé spending the weekend of Feb. 18–19 at Mrs. Mahoney's Georgetown home a couple of weeks before their engagement was announced.

150. Mahoney permitted her house to be used for a crucial scene involving a child falling down steps in the 1973 film *The Exorcist*. According to Strickland, "The reason that Clifton Daniel didn't recognize Florence's house was that the filmmakers had added a left wing, which extended the left side of the house all the way over to the steep stairs, so that the child in the film could lean or fall directly onto the stairs. Florence, who never allowed her house to be part of the historic tours of Georgetown, permitted the use of her house this time for only one reason: The producer offered her [possibly] $150,000–200,000 for the use of the house for about two months (Florence moved out) and she wanted to give it all to the George McGovern campaign. My wife was an 'extra' in the film." Strickland to Ray, 14 February, 2000.

151. Dr. Howard Rusk's daughter, Martha Rusk Sutphen, related another account of one of their last nights in the Truman White House. Michael Mahoney remembers that only he, his mother and the newspaper columnist Leonard Lyons were present on the Truman's very last night there, however; Sutphen's account was as follows: "We were having dinner at Florence's house," and she said, 'You know, this is the last night that the Trumans are going to be in the White House. Let's give them a call.' She did, and they said, 'Come on over.'

'Well, I have Howard Rusk here and his daughter,' Florence told them. 'Well, bring them over,'" the Trumans replied. At the White House, Truman suggested, "'Let's go upstairs and really enjoy ourselves.' Up we went and had bourbon and branch water, or whatever — the three Trumans, Florence, Michael, Daddy and I. We just sort of laughed and talked" and Dr. Rusk gave the president some friendly advice: "You are going to have to be very careful, and wean yourself off this plain slowly — like a 'sand hog' [who builds tunnels under water in pressurized tanks], you're going to have to come up slowly or you'll get the bends," to which everyone laughed. Martha Rusk Sutphen, interview with author.

152. Michael Mahoney, memo to author, 13 October, 1998.

Julius and Ethel Rosenberg, convicted in 1951 of passing classified military information to the Soviet Union, were executed 19 June, 1953, the first U. S. citizens to suffer the death penalty for espionage.

153. Gunther, 331; also quoted in *NIHAA Update*, Newsletter of the NIH Alumni Association, Spring 1996, Vol. 8, No. 1, 11.

154. Margaret Truman Daniel, interview.

— CHAPTER 5 —

1. Miles, 176.

2. Between 1946 and 1956, U. S. government expenditures on medical research surged. From a modest $2.5 million in 1945, the biomedical research budget had risen to $47 million by 1952; it reached $67 million in 1955; by 1958, there would be eight institutes operating with $172 million — a 70-fold increase in 13 years. Gunther, 332; Mandel, 54; "NIH Obligations."

3. Biographical memorandum, 15.

4. Gorman, *Every Other Bed*, 11.

5. Miles, 173–75.

6. Gorman, *Every Other Bed*, 32–33.

7. Starr, 342–43; Gary Cohen and Shannon Brownlee, "Mary and her 'Little Lambs' launch a war," *U. S. News & World Report*, 5 February, 1996, 76; "Moving Force in Medical Research," *Medical World News*, 20 November, 1964, 83–84, 89.

8. Charles V. Kidd, "The NIH Phenomenon," review of Strickland's *Politics*, *Science*, 19 January, 1973, 271.

9. Laurence Stern, "Eyebrows raised over NIH," *Washington Post*, 3 March, 1963, E3.

10. "Moving Force," 88; Content Outline.

11. Strickland to FM, 25 July, 1972, FM Papers, National Library of Medicine (henceforth "FM Papers"); Spingarn, 27; Lee Langley, Ph.D., interview with author, 19 June, 1999.

Langley was chief of training grants, National Heart Institute, 1964–70, and associate director for extramural programs, National Library of Medicine, associate director for extramural programs, National Library of Medicine, beginning in 1970. After disagreeing with Mahoney on an issue, the subject of which he did not recall, he said he "didn't see much of her." Prior to that, Mahoney on several occasions asked Langley to act as messenger, once delivering a note to the Johnson White House en route to the airport ("I went to the wrong entrance," he said) and once transporting dishes to someone on the southeast coast when traveling there ("She just handed me a stack of dishes, which I took home and wrapped so they wouldn't break," he recalled with amusement). He also introduced Mahoney to E. Grey Dimond, who developed an accelerated medical-school curriculum at the University of Missouri, Kansas City. "They needed each other," Langley remarked of Mahoney's help when Dimond was setting up the new medical school in 1967–68.

12. Gorman interview with Strickland, Gorman Papers; Sana Siwolop, Jerry Brazda, "The fairy godmother of medical research," *Business Week*, 14 July, 1986, 67.

Pioneering heart surgeon Dr. Michael DeBakey (1908–), Baylor College of Medicine, Houston, Texas, was a Lasker Awards jury chairman. He received a Lasker Award in 1963 "for his brilliant leadership and professional accomplishments, which were responsible in a large measure for inaugurating a new era in cardiovascular surgery."

Dr. Sidney Farber (1903–73), a pediatric pathologist, in 1970 established the Children's Cancer Research Foundation (renamed after his death the Sidney Farber Research Center, later Institute). He was a Lasker awardee in 1966 for "original use of aminopterin and methotextrate in controlling acute childhood leukemia, and for his constant leadership in the search for chemical agents against cancer."

13. James Murphy, staff counsel (1970s) to Senate Subcommittee on Aging for Chairman Thomas Eagleton, Senate Labor and Public Welfare Committee, interview with author, 12 October, 1998.

14. Sherman, interview with author.

15. Gorman interview with Strickland, Gorman Papers; Strickland, *Politics*, 226; "Moving Force . . . ," 85.

New York Republican Kenneth B. Keating (1900–75) served in the House of Representatives (1946–58) and one term in the U. S. Senate (1959–65), losing re-election to Robert F. Kennedy; Keating subsequently served as Ambassador to India (1969–72) and was Ambassador to Israel at the time of his death in 1975. He was known as a moderate Republican who supported both conservative and liberal policies such as civil rights.

16. Content Outline.

17. Lasby, 187; Drew, 77; "Contributions, campaign 1970," list of donations by FM totalling $1,205, FM Papers; FM to author, interview, 1998.

The largest amount in 1970, $150, went to Congressman Andrew Jacobs, FM noting "Introduced bill for Inst. for Gerontology."

18. Lasby, 186–87; Drew, 78; Strickland, *Politics*, 137, citing e.g., *Facts on the Major Killing and Crippling Diseases in the U. S. Today*, National Health Education Committee, 1966; "Statistics: Death and Taxes," *Newsweek*, 21 August, [1959?], copy in FM Personal Papers.

19. ML to Rep. John Fogarty, telegram, 14 March, 1951, John E. Fogarty Papers, Phillips Memorial Library Archives, Providence College, Rhode Island, hereafter cited as Fogarty Papers.

20. David Bell, interview with Talton Ray, 19 January, 1999, Washington, D.C.

Bell, who died in 2000, was named by President Kennedy as his Bureau of Budget director, 1961–62. He then became director of the U.S. Agency for International Development, 1962–66.

21. Cohen and Brownlee, 77.

22. Gunther, 313–14.

Harriman owned a horizontal version of *White Roses*. Lasker bought a vertical one. The incident occurred in 1950.

23. "Moving Force . . . ," 83–84, 89.

24. Howard A. Rusk, M. D., "Time lag in research, international efforts pressed to speed data from laboratory to the patient," *New York Times*, 14 September, 1958.

Rusk believed that the AMA and "research purists" in 1953 had thwarted Rusk's proposal to try to curtail an epidemic of tuberculosis in Korea with newly discovered isoniazid tablets on grounds the drug had not been sufficiently tested. The drug had been discovered in a research project sponsored by Mary Lasker and David Heyman and subsequently was judged an effective prophylaxis and antidote to tuberculosis. "I am saddened to think of how many Korean lives could have been saved by an isonazid saturation campaign," Rusk wrote in his autobiography. Rusk himself received three Lasker Awards in international rehabilitation, medical journalism, and public health. Strickland, *Politics*, 201–02, based on interview with Rusk; Howard A. Rusk, M. D., *A World to Care For, The Autobiography of Howard A. Rusk, M.D.* (New York: Random House, 1977), 162–63.

25. Strickland, *Politics*, 228–29, 313, n 32; Spingarn, 27.

NIH Director Rolla E. Dyer and Deputy Director C. J. Van Slyke received Lasker Awards.

26. Lawrence K. Altman, M.D., "Why many trailblazing scientists must wait many years for awards," *New York Times*, 26 September, 1995; Cohen and Brownlee, 77.

27. Gorman interview with Strickland.

28. FM to Talton Ray, 14 August,1998.

29. Strickland, *Politics*, 125; FM to author, 1998.

30. FM to Connelly, 29 November, 1949, General File, Truman Papers.

31. Cohen and Brownlee, 76.

32. ML memoir notes, undated, copy, FM Personal Papers.

33. Drew, 77; Content Outline.

Bridges chaired the Appropriations Committee in the 82nd and 84th Congresses, 1951–53, 1955–57.

34. FM notes, "Memos - Book," "George Smathers' father and arthritis," no date, FM Personal Papers; Marquis Childs, "Millions for arms, pennies for health," 19 June, 1959, copy in FM Personal Papers.

35. Content Outline; Virginia Van der Veer Hamilton, *Lister Hill, Statesman from the South* (Chapel Hill: University of North Carolina Press, 1987), 205.

Senator Margaret Chase Smith (1897–1995) was the first woman to serve in both houses of Congress: the House of Representatives, 1940–49, succeeding her husband at his death, and the Senate, 1949–73. She began in the mid-1950s to urge NIH to develop five-year plans for major research activities. Smith was noted for speaking out against fellow Republican Joseph McCarthy's anti-Communist campaign in 1950. In a 1991 newspaper interview at age 94, Smith said of the issues in which she had been active, "Medical research is one that I've put a great deal of time in." Stanley Meisler, "Margaret Chase Smith, the nation's first woman Senator reflects back over a Capitol life," *Los Angeles Times*, 1991.

36. Donaldson, *Honolulu Star-Bulletin*, 8 March, 1955.

37. FM to ML, [December 1954], M. Lasker Papers.

38. FM to ML, [Spring 1954], M. Lasker Papers.

39. "Memoranda."

40. Drew, 78; "Mr. Public Health," *Newsweek*, 18 September, 1961, 62.

41. Strickland, *Politics*, 92, 303, n29, citing oral interview with Hill, 1967.

42. *Ibid.*, 92–93; Hamilton, 291.

Hill became chairman of the Labor-HEW Appropriations Subcommittee in January 1955 and was chairman of the full Labor and Public Welfare authorizing committee, 1955–67.

43. Strickland interview with FM, no date, 11, copy in FM Personal Papers; FM interview with Talton Ray, 29 July, 1998.

44. Strickland, *Politics*, 93.

45. *Ibid.*, 310, n8.

46. Drew, 78–79; Strickland, *Politics*, 229.

There were charges of conflicts of interest on the part of "citizen witnesses" who also were NIH grantees. Laurence Stern, writing in the *Washington Post* in 1963, noted, "These experts, comprising a 'Who's Who' of medical research, are in many cases advisers and consultants to NIH councils . . . they also turn up as major grantees . . . . [T]heir relationship to the Institutes makes it almost impossible for lawmakers to get disinterested advice on technically complex medical issues." Stern, "Eyebrows raised . . . "

47. Strickland, *Politics*, 305, n43, citing interviews with Fogarty and Hill.

48. Kidd, "NIH Phenomenon," 271.

49. Fogarty to FM and ML, 20 June, 1952, Fogarty Papers.

Other guests included Anna Rosenberg; Surgeon General Scheele; Dr. Van Slyke, head of NIH research grants; and four members of Congress.

50. Fogarty to ML, 20 June, 1952, Fogarty Papers.

51. FM to ML, postscript, 31 July, [1952], M. Lasker Papers.

52. Strickland, *Politics*, 124–25.

53. *Ibid.*, 225–26.

54. FM to Senator Hill, "Dear Lister," from Italy, 9 September, 1954, Lister Hill Papers, W. Stanley Hoole Special Collections Library, University of Alabama, hereafter cited as Hill Papers.

55. Hill to Oveta Culp Hobby, 14 September, 1954; Hill to FM, 14 September, 1954, Hill Papers.

56. Rockefeller to Hill, 1 October, 1954, Hobby Papers, Box 28, "M-(non-gov.)," Dwight D. Eisenhower Library, Abilene, Kansas, and Hill Papers.

57. Hill to Marion B. Folsom, 17 February, 1956; Hill to FM, 29 February, 1956, Hill Papers.

58. Hill to FM, 8 January, 1960, Hill Papers; list of members, National Advisory Arthritis and Metabolic Diseases Council, March 1961 meeting, identifying Mahoney's term as 10/1/59–9/30/63, and list of members, National Advisory Child Health and Human Development Council, 1 July, 1963, identifying Mahoney's term as expiring 30 June, 1967, FM Papers.

59. Miles, 173; Drew, 78.

60. Hamilton, 206.

61. Strickland, *Politics*, 139–40.

62. *Ibid.*, 138–40.

63. Drew, 79.

64. Strickland, *Politics*, 137–38.

Huggins received a Lasker Award in 1963 for "his role as catalyst in modern endocrine studies of tumor control in animals and men."

65. Dr. Kermit Krantz, interview with author, 19 April, 1999.

Krantz, professor of anatomy, obstetrics, and gynecology at the University of Kansas Medical Center, was noted for co-developing the Marshall-Marchetti-Krantz operation for stress urinary incontinence in women (1949). Of his appearance before Senator Hill's committee, Krantz said that Mahoney "sandbagged him with me. That's what she wanted to do. She wanted me to talk about population explosion and problems with family planning" related to Krantz's studies of the health impacts of sexual activity in young women. He and Mahoney, while serving on the NICHD Advisory Council in the early 1960s, shared a desire to increase basic research on reproductive biology.

66. FM interview with author, 1998; Hamilton, 206; FM note, "Mrs. Olson, Sen. Gruening's off., requested to send Krantz testimony to the following . . . ," 1964, FM Personal Papers.

67. George Dixon, "Mrs. Mahoney," *Washington Post and Times Herald*, 25 March, 1956.

Bricker (Senator from Ohio, 1947–59) was Republican presidential candidate

Thomas E. Dewey's vice presidential running mate in the unsuccessful 1944
contest against Franklin D. Roosevelt.

68. Strickland, *Politics*, 137–38.

69. *Ibid.*, 147.

The witness in 1958 was Dr. Isadore Ravdin.

70. FM to ML, 31 July, [1951?], M. Lasker Papers.

Even Republican Albert Lasker did not favor Eisenhower, who was known to
be unsympathetic toward federal aid for such things as medical education.
Gunther, 297.

71. Notes for biography, excerpts, undated, FM Personal Papers.

Atlanta businessman Frank H. Neeley in 1952 was chairman of Rich's, Inc.

Joseph Dodge, Eisenhower's first budget director, was quoted as saying that
his role was that of "dismantling the Christmas tree" that Truman had left with
his budget recommendations. Strickland, *Politics*, 158.

Floyd Odlum was a wealthy financier who suffered from arthritis and lobbied
for establishment of the National Institute for Arthritis and Metabolic Diseases.
Gunther, Appendix, 347.

72. Biographical memorandum, "Reference: FM003," 14; and early biographical draft, no date, 1, FM Personal Papers.

Oveta Culp Hobby (1905–95), Secretary of HEW 1953–55, was only the
second woman cabinet member after Frances Perkins, Secretary of Labor in the
Franklin Roosevelt administration. Hobby resigned in 1955 to succeed her ailing
husband as president of the *Houston Post*. Bart Barnes, "Oveta Culp Hobby dies
at 90; organized WACs, led HEW," *Washington Post*, 17 August, 1995.

73. Miles, 25–26.

74. Biographical memorandum, "Reference: FM003," 14–15; and FM
interview with author, 1998: "I had her come to dinner two times."

75. Early biographical draft, no date, 1, FM Personal Papers.

76. FM memorandum, "Inside the Cabinet," no date, FM Personal Papers.

Taft (1889–1953) was 64 at the time of his death.

77. Copy of memo signed "Hobby," 11 July, 1953, FM Personal Papers;
Strickland, *Politics*, 97–98, 101.

Hobby was pressing conferees to support lower House figures rather than the
Senate's, which authorized $32.6 million more for HEW's 1954 budget. "More
than $10 million of this difference is in the area of medical research," the note
stated.

78. Early biographical draft, no date, 2.

79. Murray Kempton, "Death and the Lady," *New York Post*, 5 August, 1953,
copy in FM Personal Papers.

80. *Ibid.*

81. Drew Pearson, "Mrs. Hobby urged research cut," *Washington Post*, 4
August, 1953.

82. FM to ML, 31 July, [1952], M. Lasker Papers.

Republican Senator Arthur H. Vandenberg died in 1951, McMahon in 1952 at age 49.

83. FM to Walter Locke, *Dayton Daily News*, 7 August, 1952, Cox Papers.

84. Transcript, "Meet the Press," Sunday, 24 October, 1954, guest, Mrs. Oveta Culp Hobby; interviewers Ernest Lindley, Mrs. Mae Craig, Roscoe Drummond, Lawrence Spivak, Ned Brooks, moderator, copy, FM Personal Papers.

85. The vaccine was developed with funds from the National Foundation for Infantile Paralysis.

86. Doris Fleeson, "Mrs. Hobby meets her critics," "States' rights vs. polio vaccine," [May 1955], "A triumph for Senator Hill, [1957]; Miles, 32–33; Drew Pearson, "'Bad words' enter Salk rhubarb," *Washington Post and Times Herald*, 18 June, 1955.

The National Foundation for Infantile Paralysis, which dramatically announced the vaccine breakthrough to coincide with the 10th anniversary of President Franklin Roosevelt's death (April 12) and supplied free inoculations to grade-school-age children, also came in for criticism for making the announcement before supplies and an administrative program of inoculation had been set in place. "Looking ahead on polio," editorial, *Washington Post*, 11 June, 1955; Murray Kempton, "La Belle Dame," *New York Post*, [July, 1955].

87. Drew Pearson, "The Washington Merry-Go-Round, Oveta tossed Dr. Scheele a curve," [1955], "Mrs. Hobby pressured on vaccine," 6 May, 1955, "'Bad words' enter Salk rhubarb," 18 June, 1955, *Washington Post and Times Herald*; Herblock cartoon, *Washington Post*, [1955], portraying Hobby riding in an open car during a March of Dimes parade carrying a sign reading, "No one could have foreseen the public demand for the Salk vaccine"; a banner on the car read, "Dept. of Not-Too-Much Health, Education and Welfare." The 204 polio cases were among 400,000 children inoculated with what turned out to be "live" vaccine shots. Mandel, *A Half Century*, 66.

88. Doris Fleeson, "States' rights vs. polio vaccine," [May, 1955], copy in FM Personal Papers.

89. Fleeson, "Folsom eyes Mrs. Hobby's job," 2 June, 1955, copy in FM Personal Papers.

90. Pearson, "Study of HEW urged on Congress," *Washington Post and Times Herald*, 3 June, 1955.

The Eisenhower administration in 1954, as part of its first formal science policy giving the National Science Foundation (NSF) oversight for all federal research and establishing a priority for basic over applied research, appointed a second Hoover Commission to investigate whether basic research could be centralized under the NSF. It also was asked by Senator John F. Kennedy, a member of the Labor and Public Welfare Committee, while recovering from back surgery in April 1955, to report on the backlog of approved but unfunded grants at NIH. Kennedy's father, Joseph Kennedy, was a member of the Hoover

Commission. Its findings — that up to 723 meritorious grants worth $7 million were expected to go unfunded in 1956 — justified the Appropriations Committee's increasing NIH's basic-research budget for that fiscal year, setting the stage for a 100-percent increase in fiscal year 1957. Mandel, 62–63, 67–68.

91. Letter to Mrs. Albert D. Lasker, copy to Mrs. Mahoney, 4 March, 1954, unsigned, presumably from Gorman, FM Papers.

92. Miles, 33, 36; Hamilton, 205; Strickland, interview with author, 24 September, 1998.

The Bayne-Jones report officially was titled "*The Advancement of Medical Research and Education through the Department of Health, Education and Welfare*, Final Report of the Secretary's Consultants on Medical Research and Education, Department of HEW, 1958." See Strickland, *Politics*, 159.

Folsom (HEW Secretary 1955–58) also favored federal aid to education, which Eisenhower had opposed; under urging from Folsom he agreed to the National Defense Education Act.

93. "The Resignation of Mrs. Hobby," editorial, Springfield, Ohio, *Sun*, 14 July, 1955, copy with FM's notations, FM Personal Papers.

The *Sun* was the morning paper, the Springfield *Daily News*, the afternoon Cox paper.

94. Strickland, *Politics*, 124, citing *Washington Post*, 23 November, 1965.

Cannon and Taber alternated as chairmen and ranking member of the House Appropriations Committee when Republicans briefly held a majority in the 83rd Congress, 1952–54: Cannon was chairman 1950–52 and 1954–62; Taber was chairman, 1952–54.

95. *Ibid.*, 124, 153.

96. *Ibid.*, 225, 313, n21–23.

97. "Excerpt from Drew Pearson broadcast, July 10, 1955," typed note, FM Personal Papers.

98. Mrs. Lyndon B. Johnson to FM, 14 July, 1955, FM Papers.

99. LBJ to FM, 12 November, 1958, 28 February, 1959, FM Papers.

100. Lasby, 187, 212, n11, citing Johnson to Mrs. Gordon Smith, 28 May, 1959, Senate subject files, box 676, 1959, Johnson Library.

101. Senator A. Willis Robertson to FM, 21 October, 1955, FM Personal Papers.

Robertson also was asking Mahoney if she could help find a house for him and his wife to rent in Washington when Congress convened January 1956.

102. Lasby, 188.

After Eisenhower suffered his heart attack in 1955, his administration proposed a comprehensive health program that the Senate Appropriations Committee called "wholly inadequate." It would have doubled the total NIH budget, which included manpower training. Mandel, 68.

103. Lasby, 212, n11, citing M. Lasker to Senator Johnson, 16 June, 1959, LBJ A file, box 6, Johnson Library.

104. *Ibid.*, 188, 212, n12; Drew, 78, quoting Johnson speech.

105. Drew, 78.

President Johnson also was given a Lasker Award in 1965 for "outstanding contributions to the health of the people of the United States."

106. Pearson, "Penny-pinching on health issues," 9 July, 1955; "Dewey does neat lobbying job . . . Battle over health," 3 August, 1955, *Washington Post and Times Herald.*

107. Gorman to ML, London, 4 August, 1955, Gorman Papers.

108. Pearson, "Dewey does neat lobbying job," 3 August, 1955, *Washington Post and Times Herald.*

109. Strickland, *Politics,* 152.

110. *Ibid.*, 137; *World of Winners,* Second Edition (1992), 448, listing Lasker Awards; Anna M. Rosenberg to John E. Fogarty, 19 October, 1959, Fogarty Papers.

111. Drew, 77.

112. George Dixon, *Leaning on a Column . . .* (Philadelphia & New York: J. P. Lippincott Company, 1961), 153–54.

113. Marlene Cimons, "4 Washington Women: A Study in Styles," *Los Angeles Times,* 17 February, 1974.

Cimons wrote of her profiles that they were "about four women whose talents, interests and individual life–styles are a part of Washington that is removed from the marble monuments and government office buildings." The three other women profiled were Sheila Isham, artist wife of a foreign-service officer; Elsa Rosenthal, a photographer; and Ann Hoopes, a concert pianist and health-food advocate.

114. FM to ML, [Spring 1954], M. Lasker Papers.

Sen. Prescott S. Bush (in Senate 1952–63) was the father of former President George H.W. Bush. Jackson served in the Senate 1953–83, Mike Mansfield, Democrat of Montana, 1953–77 and as Senate majority leader 1961–76 (longer than any majority leader to date), subsequently as U. S. Ambassador to Japan 1977–88.

115. Mandel, 64–66; J. Edgar Hoover to FM, "Dear Florence," 27 April, 1950, citing clippings from *Miami Daily News* and "the remarks which were published on April 7, 1950," FM Papers.

116. Mandel, 55.

NIH's Committee on Radiation Studies (a peer-review study section) tried to set up a monkey colony in Florida for a 20-year study of radiation effects in 1950–53. It was among other NIH efforts to obtain defense-related research money during the Korean War when funding for government programs that did "not directly contribute to defense" was cut back, at Truman's directive, in 1951.

117. FM interview with author, 1998; Strickland interview with FM, no date, 17.

The well-publicized incident referred to was in 1945 when three enlisted men were bumped off a military plane bound for California to make room for a dog that FDR's son Elliot was shipping to his new wife, actress Faye Emerson. Roosevelt Museum and Library, Hyde Park, N.Y.

118. FM to ML, "Saturday P.M.," [1950], M. Lasker Papers.

119. FM to Donald S. Dawson, 4 August, 1950, General File, Truman Papers.

120. Strickland interview with FM, no date, 17.

121. Gorman, *Every Other Bed*, 10, 32.

122. "Scheele calls for curbs on mental hospital stays," *Washington Evening Star*, 4 May, 1955.

123. Strickland, *Politics*, 153.

124. Connie Menninger, archivist, the Menninger Foundation, to Talton Ray, 21 October, 1998; Lawrence J. Friedman, *Menninger, The Family and the Clinic* (Lawrence, Kansas: University of Kansas Press, 1990), 258–60.

125. FM, interview with author; "Transcription of a tape recording of a meeting 9 February, 1967, in the Lasker Foundation offices, to hear Mr. Mike Gorman of the National Committee Against Mental Illness," 37–38, [M. Lasker Papers].

126. "Transcription . . . "; FM to ML, [Spring 1954], M. Lasker Papers.

127. Strickland, *Politics*, 138.

128. Chesler, 389–90.

The first U. S. Public Health Service–authorized family-planning programs were initiated by state health agencies, in cooperation with voluntary birth-control organizations, in 1942 for "child spacing for women in war industries, under medical supervision."

129. Esther Katz, Biographical Sketch, the Margaret Sanger Papers Project, Department of History, New York University, New York, N.Y., 1997.

Sanger served as the IPPF's first president until 1959. During the 1950s she also spearheaded privately funded research on a variety of contraceptives, including development of the first anovulant, or birth-control pill.

130. Chesler, 416–17.

Sanger's Lasker Award in 1950 was for "her heroic and singular role in founding the birth-control movement."

131. Shidzue Kato, *A Fight for Women's Happiness, Pioneering the Family Planning Movement in Japan*, Japanese Organization for International Cooperation in Family Planning (JOICFP), Document Series 11, 1984, 52, 101.

Sanger made several more visits to Japan into the 1960s (a total of seven in her lifetime). Her surname coincidentally transliterated in Japanese as "Sangai-san," meaning "destructive of production," which may account for why she was well known in Japan as an advocate of contraception; diaphragm kits reportedly were sold under that name. "Sanger, MacArthur and Birth Control in Japan," the Margaret Sanger Papers Project Newsletter, #7, Summer, 1994, citing Chesler, *Woman of Valor.*

Inspired by Sanger's efforts in the United States, Baroness Shidzue Ishimoto Kato (born 1897) in 1922 started a movement to introduce birth control to

Japanese women. Following the war, during which she was jailed for defying government policies, Kato became, in 1946, one of the first Japanese women to be elected to parliament. She was the first vice president of the Family Planning Federation of Japan in 1954, when she organized the IPPF's Fifth International Conference in Tokyo, which Mahoney and Sanger attended in 1955. Kato served on international Planned Parenthood organizations into the 1980s.

132. Tsunego Baba, *The Yomiuri Press*, to Sanger, 21 July, 1949, copy in FM Papers.

Repression of birth control had been fostered by right-wing Japanese leaders beginning in the 1930s and was still suppressed by 1949. The occupation forces, determined to discourage Communism in Japan, were reluctant to encourage any so-called radical reforms, including birth control. As a result, Japanese women resorted to abortion, which was one of the reasons Kato and others invited Sanger back to Japan in 1949, to promote reliable, safe contraception. "Sanger, MacArthur and Birth Control . . . "

133. William R. Mathews to Mahoney, 13 January, 1950, FM Papers.

134. *Ibid.*; "Statement by Margaret Sanger, released February 13, 1950," Planned Parenthood Federation of America, Inc., copy in FM Papers.

135. FM to Margaret Sanger, 14 February, 1950, Margaret Sanger Papers, Collected Document Series, Smith College, Northampton, Massachusetts, hereafter cited as Sanger Papers.

136. Margaret Sanger Slee to FM, 21 February, 1950, FM Papers.

137. Philip L. Graham to FM, 10 April, 1950, copy in Sanger Papers.

138. Tracy S. Voorhees to Mahoney, 7 March, 1950, Sanger Papers.

MacArthur told Scribner that no Japanese government agency had invited Sanger, and that he considered the private invitation from the newspaper editor "a publicity move to bring her to Japan for a lecture tour." He added that "none will fail to recognize the distinguished ability of Mrs. Sanger to counsel, support and defend the cause she has so long espoused." "Sanger, MacArthur and Birth Control . . .," citing MacArthur to Charles E. Scribner, 24 February, 1950, the British Library.

139. Margaret Sanger to FM, 15 April, 1950, FM Papers, Sanger Papers.

140. Sanger to FM, 11 May, 1950, Sanger Papers.

141. Sanger to FM, 15 March, 1954, FM Papers.

142. Sanger to ML, 27 May, 1955, copy in FM Papers; T. O. Griessemer, president, International Planned Parenthood Federation, to FM, 26 May, 1955, FM Papers; FM to Sanger, 9 June, 1955, Sanger Papers; Sanger to Mahoney, 5 July, 1955, FM Papers.

143. FM interview with author, 1998, and FM memo, "My first interest in birth control was as a volunteer worker [at a hospital] in New York . . . ," undated, FM Personal Papers.

144. Margaret Sanger documentary, 1998; "Wedding observers," photo and caption, *Japan News*, 5 November, 1955.

145. Chesler, 421, 436; Kato, 104–05.

146. Dixon, "Mrs. Mahoney."

Ambassdaor Allison served in Japan 1953–57.

147. Sanger to FM, 27 January, 1956, FM Papers.

148. *Ibid.*, and Sanger to FM, 23 February, 1956; FM to Sanger, 7 February, 1956, Sanger Papers.

149. Sanger to FM, 23 February, 1956, FM Papers.

150. Sanger to FM, 29 August, 1957, Sanger Papers.

151. Sanger to FM, 4 December, and FM to Sanger, 14 December, 1956, Sanger Papers.

152. Margaret Sanger documentary, 1998; Chesler, 414, 439.

153. Sanger to FM, 1 March, 1958, FM to Sanger, 4 March, 14 July, 1958, and 19 May, 1959, Sanger Papers.

154. FM to Sanger, 13 October, 1960, Sanger Papers.

155. FM statement dated December 1960, FM Personal Papers, with the heading, "This is the information I wrote . . . at the request of the Apostolic Delegate, Cardinal Vagnozzi, for him to send to the Pope. After the Pope had this information, he invited me to see him in a private audience at his summer residence in Italy. At that meeting he told me the problem would be the first thing on the agenda at the next Ecumenical Council. Unfortunately he died before the meeting."

Mahoney's audience with the Pope apparently was in 1961, as related in the succeeding 31 October letter to Sanger. See n156.

156. FM to Sanger, 31 October, 1961, Sanger Papers.

John XXIII (1881–1963), elected Pope in 1958, was noted for advocating social reforms for workers, the poor, orphans, and the outcast.

157. *Ibid.*

158. FM to Sanger, 7 March, 1962, Sanger Papers.

159. Max Freedman, "Margaret Sanger's Achievement," 22 March, 1965, copy in FM Personal Papers.

160. FM to Truman, 11 June, 1957, Post-presidential files, Truman Library.

161. Truman to FM, 1 July, 1957, Post-presidential files, Truman Library.

162. FM to Truman, 11 March, 1958, Post-presidential files, Truman Library.

163. Truman to FM, 20 March, 1958, Post-presidential files, Truman Library.

164. Truman to FM, 7 November, 1958, Post-presidential files, Truman Library.

165. Gunther, 332.

The NIH budget had grown from about $3 million in 1945 to $460 million by 1961. "NIH obligations."

166. Lasby, 187, 212, n11, citing William L. Laurence, "Four great medical triumphs just ahead," *Collier's*, 8 June, 1956, 25–27.

167. Mandel, 68, 70.

168. Senator Lister Hill, Senate speech, "United States research resources mo-

bilized," *Congressional Record*, 13 and 16 August, 1958; Hamilton, *Lister Hill*, 207.

Hill's proposal coincided with President Eisenhower's "framework of a plan for peace" in the Middle East, presented to the United Nations in August 1958.

169. Howard A. Rusk, "New war on disease," *New York Times*, 17 August, 1958, and "Time Lag . . . ."

170. Marquis Childs, "Millions for arms, pennies for health," 19 June, 1959, copy in FM Personal Papers.

171. Doris Fleeson, "A triumph for Senator Hill, popular lawmaker wins $32 million extra funds for medical research," [1959], copy in FM Personal Papers.

172. Strickland, *Politics*, 307, n44.

Congress had appropriated $547 million, $147 million more than the president had requested for NIH.

173. Starr, 347; Spingarn, 28–30.

The Heart Institute budget rose from $16 million in 1950, when the president requested $4.6 million, to $62 million in 1960 (when the president's request was for $45 million).

174. Drew, 79; "Moving Force . . . ," 88.

The Committee of Consultants on Medical Research (1960) was chaired by Boisfeuillet Jones, vice president for medical affairs, Emory University.

175. Strickland, *Politics*, 224, 227.

– CHAPTER 6 –

1. NIH's appropriations for fiscal year 1962 rose from $450 million in 1961 to nearly $630 million. "NIH obligations."

The Senate approved a record budget of $835 million for NIH for FY 1962 — $252 million and 43 percent more than the Kennedy budget request.

2. M. Lasker oral history.

Lasker helped find a new anti-malaria drug for Kennedy. During Kennedy's administration, the United Nations in 1962 articulated a policy of assistance for population control, and a National Academy of Sciences report on world population in 1963 recommended reversing Eisenhower's policy of not addressing the population problem.

3. JFK to FM, undated, FM Personal Papers.

Kennedy was hospitalized from 10 October until just before Christmas 1954 for spinal surgery, 21 October, from which he almost died; last rites were administered.

4. Gorman to FM, 15 September, 1960, FM Personal Papers.

5. M. Lasker oral history.

6. *Washington Post*, 20 January, 1961, with photographs of dinner party, Wednesday, 18 January, at FM's with guests including Trumans, Stewart Udalls (Secretary of Interior), Robert Frost, Kennedy advisor Arthur Schlesinger, Jr.

and wife, HEW Secretary Abraham and Mrs. Ribicoff, and Walter Lippman, who described the event as "rather friendly." Walter Lippman, oral history, JFK Library, 6–7.

Truman had successfully advocated a change in the line of succession to the Speaker of the House after the vice president instead of to a cabinet member (Secretary of State), which Truman disliked because it was not an elected post. That accounts for Kennedy's raising the subject with Truman.

7. Philip R. Lee, M. D., interview with author, 14 October, 1998, hereafter cited as P. Lee, interview with author. Lee served as assistant secretary for health and scientific affairs in HEW, 1965–69.

8. Theodore C. Sorensen, interview with author, 29 June, 1999.

Sorensen served as special counsel to President Kennedy, 1961–63.

9. P. Lee, interview with author.

10. E. Grey Dimond, M.D., interview with author, 15 June, 1999; Dimond, *Take Wing! Interesting Things that Happened on my Way to School* (Kansas City: University of Missouri-Kansas City School of Medicine and the Lowell Press, 1991), 206–08.

Dimond, a cardiologist by training, met Mahoney while a scholar-in-residence at the National Library of Medicine in 1967, when he conceived the idea of sending students directly from high school to medical school rather than through pre-medical undergraduate work, thus accelerating training of family practitioners. He subsequently served as special consultant on medical education to Dr. Philip Lee (1968–69) when he was assistant secretary of health for HEW. The accelerated curriculum was instituted at the University of Missouri, Kansas City, in 1971.

11. Spingarn, 27.

12. Dimond, *Take Wing!*, 207.

13. FM, "Memo about remembering Jackie," 6 April, 1994, FM Personal Papers.

14. *Ibid.*; Cimons, "4 Washington Women."

15. FM, interview with author; Barry Paris, *Garbo, A Biography* (New York: Alfred A. Knopf, 1995), 468–49.

Paris, in the Garbo biography, presumed that the first woman guest cited by Garbo was Irene Galitzine, with whom Garbo had cruised the Greek islands on Aristotle Onassis' yacht. It apparently was Mahoney, however.

16. "Food for Peace Council named by Kennedy," *Washington Star*, 7 May, 1961; George McGovern to FM, 9 May, 1961, Executive file, and McGovern to FM, 9 August, 1961, General file, John F. Kennedy Library, hereafter cited as Kennedy Papers; itinerary of official travel, Florence Mahoney, 1962, copy in M. Lasker Papers.

17. McGovern to FM, 3 May, 1962, FM Papers; invitation list for McGovern reception by Mrs. Florence Mahoney, 11 July, 1962, and acceptances from invitees, FM Personal Papers.

18. Gorman to M. Lasker, 7 August, 1961, FM Papers; "Rep. Fogarty assails cut in NIH fund," *Washington Post*, 4 November, 1961, A2.

Congress' $738 million appropriation for NIH in FY 1962 was $155 million above Kennedy's request. Ribicoff defended his action saying, "Since the budget proposals and estimates were made, it has been necessary to make unanticipated economics to meet extensive defense needs . . . against threats to world peace in Berlin, Southeast Asia and elsewhere, to avoid inflation and to be in a position to meet the administration's pledge to balance the budget in fiscal year 1963 . . . " NIH had not been treated differently from other across-the-board cutbacks, he said, and no current research would be cut. Charles G. Brooks, "Cutback in NIH brings attack on Ribicoff," *Washington Star*, July [?], 1961; "Mr. Public Health," *Newsweek*, 18 September, 1961, 62; Ribicoff to Fogarty, 4 November, 1961, copy in FM Personal Papers.

19. "Wanton Economy," editorial, *Washington Post*, 22 November, 1961.

Ribicoff proposed cutting NIH's budget for FY 1962 by $60 million from $738 million that Congress had approved.

Ribicoff picked a feisty, dedicated health-policy expert to be assistant secretary for legislation — Wilbur Cohen, then a professor at the University of Michigan with 20 years service in the Social Security Administration. Ribicoff resigned after a year and a half to run for the Senate, where he served from 1963–1981.

Kennedy's second HEW Secretary was former Cleveland mayor Anthony J. Celebrezze, who served for three years (1963–65), into President Johnson's administration. He was succeeded in 1965 by John W. Gardner, a respected educator, psychologist, author, and president of the Carnegie Corporation. Gardner was succeeded by Wilbur Cohen (1968). Miles, 41, 46–47.

20. Radio TV Reports, Inc., to National Health Education Committee, re: Huntley-Brinkley Report, 3 November, 1961, NBC-TV Network, FM Papers; Eleanor Roosevelt, "Victory at the polls," *New York Post*, 12 November, 1961.

21. FM to "Dear Bess," 26 March, 1963, Post-presidential files, Truman Papers.

22. Strickland, *Politics*, 166–69.

The president's budget request was cut from $930 million to $912 million.

23. *Ibid.*, 184.

24. Spingarn, 31.

25. Strickland, *Politics*, 169–77, 309 n40.

The president's budget request for NIH for fiscal year 1964 was reduced by $15 million.

26. "Jack" Kennedy to FM, 5 September, 1944, FM Personal Papers.

27. Walter Rybeck, "Kennedy inner circle to carry on," [*Dayton*?] *Daily News*, 1 December, 1963.

28. Strickland, *Politics*,178, citing *Biomedical Science and Its Administration* (Woolridge Report), White House, February, 1965, xv.

29. *Ibid.*, 180; Spingarn, 31, citing Woolridge report, 7.

30. Strickland, *Politics*, 180, citing *Congressional Record*, Senate, 5 August, 1965, p. 18868.

31. FM note, "All I could find in Dublin at that time," on "Declaration" of six antique silver marrow scoops purchased from John Morton, Limited, Dublin, dated 19 December, 1956. See also FM to Mrs. Johnson, 20 July, 1966, Social files; LBJ to FM, 14 December, 1966, Executive file; FM to Mrs. Johnson, 23 July, 1967, Social file; LBJ to FM, 21 September, 1967, Executive file; FM to Mrs. Johnson, 1 February, [1965]; FM to Ashton [?], no date, [1967]; Mrs. Johnson to FM, 26 April, 1967; FM to President and Mrs. Johnson, 17 November, 1966, Social files; LBJ to FM, 30 August, 1960, Public Activities/Greetings file, and 14 August, 1967, Executive file, Johnson Papers.

Acknowledging another letter from FM, Johnson wrote, "Your kind and generous letter made the day become brighter. I know of the consistency and the caliber of the work you do to help make lives healthier and more hopeful, and I am grateful to you for the thoughtfulness you always display." LBJ to FM, 14 January, 1966, Executive file, Johnson Papers. Mahoney also sent both Johnson daughters wedding gifts and was invited to their weddings. FM to Mrs. Johnson, 11 August, 1966, Social files, Johnson Papers.

32. FM to LBJ, 14 November, 1967, Executive file; FM to Mrs. Johnson, 13 November, 1967, Social file; Mrs. Johnson to FM, 17 November, 1967, Hand-writing and Social files, Johnson Papers, and 20 November, 1967, FM Papers.

33. FM to Juanita D. Roberts, personal secretary to the president, 12 March, 1964, General file; memorandum, Jack Valenti to LBJ, 16 March, 1965, Executive file, Johnson Papers.

34. LBJ to FM, 13 April, 1965, Executive file, Johnson Papers.

35. George E. Reedy to FM, 10 February, 1965, George Reedy file, Johnson Papers; FM to Mrs. Johnson, 23 February, 1965, Mrs. Johnson to FM, 7 April, 1965, Social files, Johnson Papers.

36. P. Lee, interview with author.

37. Joseph T. English, interview with author, 4 November, 1999.

English served in the Peace Corps, 1961–66, as Deputy Director and Director of Health Affairs, Office of Economic Opportunity, 1966–68, and as first Administrator of the Health Services and Mental Health Administration, 1968–70. English also credited Mahoney with introducing him to his wife, Ann Sanger, daughter of Dr. Paul Sanger, a prominent North Carolina vascular surgeon whom Mahoney knew.

38. FM to M. Lasker, 19 August, 1965, M. Lasker Papers; Gardner, interview with author.

Dr. William H. Stewart was chosen surgeon general. Aldrich was the first director of the National Institute of Child Health and Human Development. Gardner had 14 top positions to fill at HEW, with which John Macy, whom Gardner also admired, helped in finding candidates.

39. Strickland, *Politics*, 188–89, citing James A. Shannon, M. D., "The

Advancement of Medical Research: A Twenty-Year View of the NIH Role," Alan Gregg Memorial lecture, San Francisco, 22 October, 1966.

40. Spingarn, 32.

41. Strickland, *Politics*, 209.

42. *Ibid.*, 204–05; M. Lasker to Shannon, 17 July, 1964, and to Fogarty, 24 July, 1964, Fogarty Papers.

A congressional directive in 1955 had ordered emphasis on cancer chemotherapy despite scientists' objections. By the mid-1960s, little had resulted from the $250-million investment, although NCI Director Dr. Kenneth Endicott in 1963 called it "the largest single drug development program in the world." "The availability of money exceeded the availability of sound ideas," the Consultants on Medical Research had concluded, presaging a future fight over cancer research. See also Stern, "Eyebrows raised . . . "; Drew, 80; Daniel S. Greenberg, "Whatever happened to the war on cancer?" *Discover*, March 1986, 58.

43. Strickland, *Politics*, 196.

44. *Ibid.*, 202.

The Sabin polio vaccine was introduced five years after the Salk version.

The Heart Institute Advisory Council, on which DeBakey sat, had recommended as its highest priority a $100-million program to develop the artificial heart. Shannon, however, instituted a small, focused program aimed at finding what worked best for what problems. Drew, 80.

45. *Ibid.*, 205.

46. M. Lasker oral history, 5 April, 1967.

47. Spingarn, 31–32; Strickland, *Politics*, 207; Drew, 81; Lasby, 204–05.

NIH at the time was spending 60 percent of its funds for applied research.

48. Drew, 81; Lasby, 206; M. Lasker oral history, 5 April, 1967.

Clinical research includes testing the effects of therapeutic treatments on humans or animals. Lasker at that time was advocating the establishment of NIH "task forces" in specific disease areas to expedite applying research to treatments. Johnson did direct Secretary Gardner to appoint a Lung Cancer Task Force.

49. Strickland, *Politics*, 208–09.

50. Spingarn, 32–33; P. Lee, interview with author, 14 October, 1968; Lee, interview with David G. McComb, 18 January, 1969, Tape 1, 36, Johnson Library. Lee at the time was assistant secretary for health and scientific affairs, Department of HEW (1965–69).

Johnson's memorable visit to NIH was 21 July, 1967, his second trip to the campus. His first was in August 1965 to sign the Health Research Facilities Act. Neither Eisenhower nor Kennedy had visited the facility. Lasby, 185.

51. Lasby, 207–08.

52. P. Lee, interview with author, 14 October, 1968, and with McComb, 37–38.

53. Drew, 81; P. Lee, interview with author.

54. FM to LBJ, undated, [July ?, 1967] and LBJ to FM, 24 July, 1967, Executive TR 124, Johnson Papers.

55. FM to ML, 2 August and 19 August, 1965, M. Lasker Papers.

John W. Gardner (born 1912), president of the Carnegie Corporation and Foundation for the Advancement of Teaching at the time of his appointment as HEW secretary (he was sworn in 18 August, 1965, and served to March 1968), had served on President Kennedy's Task Force on Educational and Cultural Affairs, chaired Johnson's Task Force and White House Conference on Education (1965), and was a respected consultant to many government agencies. After resigning as HEW secretary, he chaired the National Urban Coalition and in 1970 founded Common Cause.

56. FM to LBJ, 9 November, 1967, Executive file, Johnson Papers and FM Papers.

57. John W. Gardner, interview with author, 2 September, 1998.

Mary Lasker, Gardner found, was more power-oriented than Mahoney, and Lasker's pressures to obtain appointments of people she wanted for government posts rankled him. "I consider appointments probably the most important organizational decision you make and gave a lot of attention to the top appointments, and I wasn't about to take pressure from anybody," he said in a 1998 interview. Gardner and Mahoney were mutually admiring of one another. "Any place would be lucky to have John Gardner as a public servant," she said of him.

58. Drew, 79; Lasby, 188–89.

59. Strickland, *Politics*, 196–98.

Shannon reduced the $31 million budgeted for the centers by half. He favored a mutli-categorical approach as less cumbersome for research institutions.

60. Drew, 79; Strickland, *Politics*, 204; Lasby, 189–90, n15, 23, 202; Myer Feldman, deputy special counsel to the president, to FM, 30 March, 1964, Executive file, Johnson Papers.

Lasker pressed Johnson hard to establish the commission, meeting and speaking with him numerous times, having Mrs. Johnson to lunch and the couple for dinner at her New York town house, and spending a night at the White House, all in the first two months of Johnson's presidency, according to Lasby. Johnson later said that he was convinced to set up the commission by the "grim facts" provided him by Lasker's National Health Education Committee that a million people would die of the diseases each year and by "the insistence of that lovely lady, Mrs. Mary Lasker." Johnson also believed that modern science had saved his life when he had had his heart attack nine years earlier.

61. Lasby, 190–94, quoting Dr. Philip Handler (later president, National Academy of Sciences) and DeBakey.

The Regional Medical Centers legislation (Heart, Cancer and Stroke Amendments of 1965) was only one among numerous programs enacted in the mid-1960s to expand health care accessibility, especially to the poor, including not only Medicare and Medicaid (1965) but also neighborhood health centers, Mental Retardation Facilities and Community Mental Health Construction Act of 1963, Health Education Development Act of 1963 (the first to subsidize training of health manpower), Maternal and Child Health Amendments of 1963, Civil Rights Act of 1964, and anti-poverty measures embodied in the Economic Opportunity Act of 1964. The result was a noticeable increase in the use of health services by the poor after 1965. Starr, 373; Miles, 45–46.

62. Drew, 80.

63. Lasby, 194–97; FM, journal or letter, undated, circa 1965 (summer), FM Personal Papers.

The RMP legislation initially included money only for planning and education, not for construction or development of the centers.

64. FM to Douglass Cater, 22 April, 1965, General health file, Johnson Papers; FM, journal or letter, undated, circa 1965 (summer), and FM memorandum, "Names Suggested to Douglas[s] Cater for Conference on Population," undated, FM Personal Papers.

The White House Conference on Health, November 3–4, 1965, during which Johnson was recuperating from gall-bladder surgery, pointedly involved practitioners from all state medical societies. "This was obviously a deliberate effort on our part to involve doctors in private practice in the affairs of the government, to have them as participants . . . so that they didn't feel that the government was doing something behind their back," as Dr. Philip Lee recorded in an oral history in 1969. Lee, interview with McComb, 4, 20, 23.

65. FM to ML, 19 August, 1965, M. Lasker Papers; Boisfeuillet Jones to FM, 12 December, 1964, FM Papers.

James Mackay represented a newly formed 4th District in Atlanta. "If you want a project, this is a good one," Jones had written Mahoney, enlisting her help in getting the committee assignment for Mackay, "a good friend of mine" whose district included Emory University.

66. FM, journal, undated, circa 1965 (summer), FM Personal Papers.

67. Lasby, 194–97; Lee, interview with McComb, 22.

According to Lee, "That was just another interesting illustration to what lengths the president would go personally to do something about getting a bill passed. It was just one of a number of bills. But he personally gave it this kind of attention."

68. LBJ to FM, 3 September, 1965, Executive file, Johnson Papers.

Cohen, in an oral history in 1969, said that he negotiated some 13 amendments with the AMA, mostly inconsequential changes, including changing words like "center," which the AMA objected to for fear it meant buildings where government doctors would be employed, to "program." "[C]ertain words used had formed an effect in their mind . . . that this was an attempt on the part of the federal government to organize the medical-care system in the United States under the medical schools, and by changing the words and . . . a few sentences and adding a few things, the AMA dropped its opposition to the bill, and it was successful in being passed. Everybody was amazed that the concessions were so minimal and, to some extent, verbalistic." Cohen oral history, tape 4, 10 May, 1969, 22–23.

69. Lady Bird Johnson, *A White House Diary* (New York: Holt, Rinehart and Winston, 1970), 326; Memorandum of invitation to Mrs. Florence Mahoney, National Committee against Mental Illness, for signing ceremony of HR 3140, Heart Disease, Cancer and Stroke Amendments of 1965, 6 October, 1965, Executive file, Johnson Papers.

70. Mrs. Johnson to FM, 19 October, 1965; LBJ to FM, 18 November, 1965, Executive file, Johnson Papers.

71. P. Lee, interview with author.

72. *Ibid.*

73. David Bell, interview with Talton Ray, 19 January, 1999. Both Bell and Lee credited Dr. Leona Baumgartner (the first woman to graduate from the University of Nebraska School of Medicine, who, according to Bell, had to sit outside classrooms to listen to lectures) with instigating AID's population-control policy. Adopted in December 1964, it provided for family-planning assistance to developing nations.

74. P. Lee, interview with author.

75. P. Lee, interview with McComb, 17–18.

76. The Johnson administration used task forces to develop legislation in many program areas. Dr. Urie Bronfenbrenner, a social psychologist at Cornell University, was on a task force set up by OEO Director Sargent Shriver in 1964 to discuss child-development initiatives that led to the creation of Head Start. Kay Mills, *Something Better for My Children, The History and People of Head Start* (New York: Dutton, 1998), 47; Lee, interview with McComb, 26–27.

77. FM Memo, "Dinner 3600 Prospect St., February 3, 1964, Dr. Bronfenbrenner showed slides . . . Russian educational system," listing 26 dinner guests, who included Mr. and Mrs. Drew Pearson, Members of Congress and their wives, and Mr. and Mrs. Boisfeuillet Jones, FM Papers.

78. Bess Abell, Mrs. Johnson's social secretary, to Mrs. Robert McNamara, 2 March, 1964; FM to Mrs. Johnson, 7 June, 1966, Mrs. Johnson to FM, 16 June, 1966, "Thank you for sending me the testimony of Dr. Bronfenbrenner, I found it quite interesting — particularly his remarks about the impact of Project Head Start," Social files, Johnson Papers; Mills, 49–50; Lyndon Baines Johnson, *The Vantage Point: Perspective of the Presidency, 1963–1969* (New York: Holt, Rinehart & Winston, 1971), 202–21; Lady Bird Johnson, 235.

79. FM, journal, 25 January, 1966, FM Personal Papers.

80. FM to LBJ, 11 September, 1967, Executive file, Johnson Papers.

81. Champ Lyons, M.D., to FM, excerpt, undated [circa 1962], ("Your suggestion for indoctrination of all girls during high school in nursing programs is a brilliant suggestion. I agree with you that the educational pattern must be revised . . . "), Kennedy Papers; FM to LBJ, 11 September, 1967, same; Memorandum for Honorable Douglass Cater from Office of the Secretary, HEW, 9 February, 1968, FM file, Johnson Papers; Joseph A. Califano, Jr., to FM, 7 March, 1968, Executive file, Johnson Papers.

82. Califano to FM, 25 March, 1968, Executive file, Johnson Papers.

83. Lasby, 198.

84. Strickland, *Politics*, 214–16, 312, n10; Morton Mintz, "Heart research and the 'lobby,'" *Washington Post*, 29 June, 1968.

The drug was Atromid-S (clofibrate), shown to be effective against ischaemic heart disease. At issue, critics of the targeted funding charged, was the use of federal funds to test a single, patented product; the drug already was being tested by the National Heart Institute in a $30-million, 10-year study of four coronary drugs.

85. Strickland, *Politics*, 216–17, 222; ML to Fogarty, 27 January, 1961, Fogarty Papers.

Between 1948 and 1968, Congress only four times failed to provide more for NIH than the president's request — in fiscal years 1951, 1952, 1964, and 1968. The FY 1968 NIH budget was cut by almost $20 million, the largest reduction in its history.

86. Nicholas Cavarocchi, former staff assistant, House Committee on Appropriations, Subcommittee on Labor-HEW Appropriations, interview with author, 20 July, 1999.

Democrat Flood (1904–94) served in the House 1945–47, 1949–53, 1955–80. Cavarocchi worked on Flood's subcommittee 1974–79.

87. Hamilton, 280–81, 290.

Texas Democrat Ralph Yarborough succeeded Hill as chairman of the Labor and Public Welfare Committee. Yarborough moved up because of the defeat of the more senior Oregon Senator Wayne Morse, an anti-war sympathizer, in 1968.

88. FM to Hill, 3 December, 1964; memorandum, "Mrs. Mahoney called to give Senator Hill the following suggested names as the director of the Child Health and Human Development Institute . . . ," 3 March, 1965; FM to Hill, 24 March, 1965, Hill Papers.

89. John F. Sherman, interview with author, 6 July, 1999; Miles, 176–77; Strickland, *Politics*, 222.

Shannon (1904–94) served as NIH director 1955–68. He was succeeded by Dr. Robert Q. Marston.

90. Drew, 75–76, 80–82.

91. Drew's theme was that the government was misplacing priorities to put so much emphasis on the elderly, those over 60 who comprised only one-eighth of the U. S. population but consumed half of the federal health budget, when nearly 50 percent of the population was younger than 25 years old and received considerably fewer federal health funds. She argued for more attention to preventable problems like those that affected children, and to maldistribution and lack of access to health care. She also disputed Lasker's claims that the large investment in research had increased U.S. longevity rates, noting that it had risen in other countries even more than in the United States.

92. Drew, 82.

93. ML oral history, 15 February, 1968, 155–57.

94. Drew, 77.

95. "Lasker Largesse," *Newsweek*, 20 November, 1967; Henry Turkel, M. D., to Editor, *Newsweek*, 13 December, 1967, copy in FM Personal Papers.

The Drew article was condensed and reprinted with the title, "How the Washington health lobby works" in *Medical Economics*, 11 November, 1968, 276–91.

96. Gorman letter to the editor, *Atlantic Monthly*, February 1968, 44–46.

97. Julian M. Morris, Washington, D. C., and Steven Lunzer, M. D., Durham, North Carolina, letters to editor, *Atlantic Monthly*, February 1968, 46.

98. Strickland, *Politics*, 151; Drew, 78.

Dr. Robert Q. Marston was NIH Director 1968–73.

Another critic, Joseph D. Cooper, Ph.D., in *Medical Tribune* magazine in 1968, called the "medical research lobby . . . one of the most powerful lobbying groups in modern times," but added that "the inexorable workings of time and tide have combined to diminish the lobby's political power . . . . All of this is now coming to an end, and it should, for we are moving into new times. Laskerism flourished because the right people were in place at the right time." Lasker and Mahoney were identified as principal activists in the lobby group. "The medical research lobby influence for NIH declines," *Medical Tribune*, 1968.

99. Strickland, *Politics*, 218–20, citing Fountain Committee report, October 1967.

The Fountain Committee charged NIH with concentrating grants on a few institutions, "weak central management," and with paying for many projects of less "than good quality."

100. Memorandum, "Mr. Cater has seen," 29 March, 1968, Executive file, Johnson Papers.

101. Lady Bird Johnson, 646.

Johnson's announcement came just two weeks after he appointed Wilbur Cohen as HEW Secretary to succeed John Gardner.

102. FM, notes, "Friday, 3 p.m., 4/15/68," and "Dinner Apr. 11 W. H.," undated, [1968], FM Personal Papers; Memorandum, list of guests for dinner with President and Mrs. Johnson, 11 April, 1968, Johnson Papers.

Secretary Gardner quit unexpectedly, "reportedly dismayed by budget cuts imposed by President Johnson," according to a report in the *Los Angeles Times*. Robert McNamara's resignation as Defense Secretary at the same time, like Gardner's, was effective March 1, 1968. "Gardner quits," *Los Angeles Times*, 28 January, 1968.

103. FM, notes, 16 May, 1968, FM Personal Papers; Memoranda, swearing-in for Cohen, 16 May, 1968; meeting in Oval Office with members of National Health Education Committee, 15 July, 1968; invitation to ceremony at the White House commemorating 20th anniversary of the National Heart Institute, 14 November, 1968; memorandum, Mrs. Florence Mahoney, Oval Office, 10 December, 1968, "12:06–12:15 p," Executive file, Johnson Papers.

104. LBJ to FM, 24 April, 1969, Public information/press file, Johnson Papers.

105. Mrs. Johnson to FM from Stonewall, Texas, 18 April, 1972, FM Papers.

106. Luci Johnson Nugent to FM, 12 March, 1973, FM Papers.

107. Lasby, 183, 209–11; Memo, "Mrs. Florence Mahoney, member, Board of Directors, Lasker Foundation, Receipt of the Albert Lasker Award," 7 April, 1966, Johnson Papers.

Clarence G. Lasby, in his essay in *The Johnson Years*, "The War on Disease," noted that Johnson actively backed federal medical-research programs for the five years of his presidency, not only with the presidential commission but White House conferences, a number of task forces, five special health messages, more than 50 statements, and signing ceremonies. His "leadership elevated the war against disease to a far-more-permanent position in American life, both for the people and for the government. He admittedly used extravagant rhetoric and promised far more than he could deliver; but this was not necessarily unfortunate," Lasby wrote.

Johnson with pride wrote in his autobiography, *The Vantage Point*, that during his administration, 40 national health measures were presented to and passed by the Congress — more than in all the preceding 175 years of the republic's history. Federal expenditures for health programs increased from $4 billion to $14 billion. He paid tribute to Mary Lasker as "a driving force in making the nation aware of the job to be done, in encouraging the Congress to appropriate funds, and in mobilizing public opinion." Johnson, *The Vantage Point*, 220.

Although the Johnsons' and Mahoney's papers contain numerous correspondences between them from the mid-1950s to the year of Johnson's death (1973), his autobiography does not mention her by name; Mrs. Johnson mentioned Mahoney once in her memoir, *A White House Diary*.

108. Nixon named Robert Finch, lieutenant governor of California and a close advisor, to be HEW secretary. Finch was succeeded in mid-1970 by then-Undersecretary of State Elliot L. Richardson. In the reshuffle, the research cause lost an important Republican ally in Congress when Melvin Laird left to become Nixon's secretary of defense. Miles, 57–59.

109. Strickland, *Politics*, 230; Spingarn, 33–34.

110. Strickland, *Politics*, 223, 231–32.

111. Strickland, *Politics*, 238–39.

112. Gardner, interview with author.

113. Strickland, *Politics*, 241–52.

114. Cohen oral history, tape 3, 2 March, 1969, 30, and tapes 1–2, 8 December, 1968, 10.

President Johnson gave Mary Lasker a Medal of Freedom. Lasby, 200–01.

Mathilde Krim, a scientist who had been a research associate at Sloan-Kettering, was the wife of Arthur Krim, a lawyer, friend and neighbor to the Johnson's in Texas and a fundraiser for the Democratic Party.

Cohen characterized the "women I worked with" as "populists" who, "while they were progressives, while they were strong believers in social legislation, were also strongly of the belief in the inevitableness of gradualism." They understood, "that the American people are much more pragmatic than they are ideological, and, if something works, they are willing to accept a sharp change in . . . principles." Nor were people like Mahoney and Lasker "the kind of people who are frustrated and dissatisfied by that process" of bringing about gradual change. Cohen likened it to slicing salami very thin, piling on "slice by slice so that eventually you have a very good sandwich."

115. *Ibid.*, tapes 1–2, 3–4.

116. *Ibid.*, tape 4, 10 May, 1969, 1–2.

– CHAPTER 7 –

1. Strickland, *Politics*," 230, 232.

2. Spingarn, 37; Cohen and Brownlee, 76.

For accounts of the NIH budget FY 1969–71, see also: Strickland, *Politics*, 230–32; Daniel Greenberg, "Whatever happened to the war on cancer?," *Discover*, March 1986, 58.

Lasker, in an oral history, blamed a religious bias for the less supportive position of the Nixon administration, noting that "six members of his staff are Christian Scientists, and consequently opposed to research and medicine." M. Lasker oral history.

3. Strickland, *Politics*, 231, 256.

4. Strickland, interview with author; Dr. Charles and Sue Edwards, interview with author, 8 July, 1999.

Doctor Charles Edwards served as FDA administrator, 1969–73, and assistant secretary for health, 1973–75 (through most of the administration of President Gerald Ford after he succeeded Nixon).

5. James T. Patterson, *The Dread Disease: Cancer and Modern American Culture* (Cambridge: Harvard University Press, 1987), 248; Cohen and Brownlee, 76.

6. Strickland, *Politics*, 260–63; Spingarn, 40-41; Cohen and Brownlee, *ibid.*

Bobst had arranged for Nixon to practice law in New York after his 1962 defeat for governor in California. Schmidt was a member of the board of the Sloan-Kettering Foundation for cancer research. Other members of the committee were: William McCormick Blair, a Mahoney and Lasker friend; Laurance Rockefeller; and clinical pharmacologist Solomon Garb, author of *Cure for Cancer: A National Goal* (1968), which predicted the conquest of cancer.

7. Sherman, interview with author; Edwards, interview with author.

8. Spingarn, 40.

9. Strickland, *Politics*, 264; Patterson, 243, 248–49; Starr, 381, 384.

The National Cancer Institute by 1969 was spending about $200 million.

10. Strickland, *Politics*, 263; Patterson, 252, quoting Sol Spiegelman, director, Columbia University's Institute of Cancer Research.

Among serendipitous discoveries benefitting cancer research were several drugs found to combat it, including methotrexate and prenisone to treat leukemias and lymphomas, the result of non-cancer basic research; information on cancer viruses had come from unrelated work on lysogenic phage. Senator Gaylord Nelson, testimony before House Subcommittee on Public Health and Environment on S. 1828, 92nd Cong., 1st sess., 16 September, 1971, reprinted in *Congressional Record*, 6 October, 1971; Lucy Eisenberg, "The Politics of Cancer," *Harper's Magazine*, November 1971, 105.

11. Gaylord Nelson served as Governor of Wisconsin (1959–63) and U.S. Senator, 1963–81.

12. Strickland, *Politics*, 266–67.

Richardson, assistant secretary under Marion Folsom, 1957–58, succeeded Robert H. Finch (1969-70) as HEW Secretary, serving from June 24, 1970 to November, 1972, when he became Nixon's Secretary of Defense; he was succeeded at HEW by Casper W. Weinberger who had been director of the Office of Management and Budget.

13. Nelson testimony to House subcommittee.

In response to Nelson's questioning, Richardson testified on 10 June, 1971: "The Administration regards it as vitally important that the cancer conquest effort go forward within the framework of the National Institutes of Health," despite, as Nelson said, "the fact that a 'compromise' had been worked out at staff levels with tacit high-level approval prior to his testimony." The "compromise" was a "face-saving" change in language "without changing the substance" of the original bill, Nelson charged, noting that the president had flip-flopped on the independent agency issue, which it initially opposed. In a letter to Chairman Kennedy 2 April, 1971, Richardson also stated that the administration intended to keep the cancer program as part of NIH. Strickland, *Politics*, 273.

14. Greenberg, "Whatever happened . . . ," 60; Ann Landers, *Washington Post*, 20 April, 1971, B5; Strickland, *Politics*, 271.

Landers' column appeared in 750 newspapers with a circulation estimated at 54 million.

15. Author's experience as legislative aide (1971–79) to Senator Nelson and professional staff member, Senate Labor and Public Welfare Committee.

16. Strickland, *Politics*, 270; Spingarn, 42–43; Senator Gaylord Nelson, "The Conquest of Cancer Act," statement accompanying amendment 109 to Senate bill 34, *Congressional Record*, 21 May, 1971; Nelson testimony before House subcommittee, 16 September, 1971, citing letter to *New York Times*, 29 July, 1971.

17. Author experience; Strickland, *Politics*, 276–77; Spingarn, 43; "Expanded attack on cancer," editorial, *The Milwaukee Journal*, 10 December, 1971; William Hines, "Nelson vindicated on cancer bill," *Chicago Sun-Times*, 24 December, 1971.

18. Nelson testimony to House subcommittee.

19. Strickland, *Politics*, 281, 283.

One article, "The politics of cancer," by Lucy Eisenberg, *Harper's Magazine*, November 1971, 100 and 105, called the "so-called Conquest of Cancer Act . . . the product of a high-powered PR campaign and a rather deceptive one at that. Its proponents, who are mostly laymen, claim that breakthroughs in cancer are imminent . . . . But scientists themselves dispute this assumption . . . . If NIH dies because of Mary Lasker's compulson to do something special about cancer, both science and medicine may suffer. Congress was bewitched by words, whipped into a rhetorical frenzy with talk of 'universal anguish and suffering.'"

The final act, approved 15 November and signed by Nixon 23 December, 1971, gave the Cancer Institute special budget privileges that bypassed HEW in-house review and went directly to the president's Office of Management and Budget; it also set up a presidentially appointed National Cancer Advisory Board and a three-person cancer panel appointed by and reporting directly to the president (Benno Schmidt was named its first chairman). The budget bypass provision of the 1971 act was largely ignored by NIH. Greenberg, "Whatever happened . . . ," 64.

Gorman claimed in a letter to Mary Lasker in 1986, "I cooked up the three-member Presidential Panel to get around Rogers. With the help of Phil Jaehle [lobbyist for] Smith Kline [pharmaceutical company], we sold it to [Representative] Ancher Nelsen [of Minnesota, the ranking minority member of the Rogers Committee]. Nelsen and I then went to Jim Cavanaugh [HEW deputy assistant secretary for health], who was then handling health matters for the Nixon administration. Cavanaugh bought the deal, the Democratic bill became a Republican bill, and Nixon signed it. I saw Cavanaugh [who later worked there] the last time I visited Smith Kline and he still laughs about the whole deal . . . . If people only knew how some of these things are done in Washington. Maybe I will have to do my memoirs." Mike Gorman to ML, 8 April, 1986, Gorman Papers.

Strickland posited an additional factor in Lasker's not prevailing with the cancer bill: She traditionally had not courted or worked closely with *authorizing* committees such as Rogers' subcommittee, concentrating her efforts over the years on *appropriations* committees. Strickland, *Politics*, 281.

Despite the controversy (one expert said "the war on cancer is a medical Vietnam"), federally funded cancer research moved forward in the 1970s. Among advances was a viral connection found in 1978; in addition, 17 comprehensive cancer centers were set up throughout the country for better diagnosis and treatment. Patterson, 251–52.

20. Spingarn, 45, quoting Irvine H. Page, Editor, *Modern Medicine*, "Another Crusade," *Science*, 2 June, 1972.

21. Kidd, "NIH Phenomenon," 272.

Marston, who succeeded Shannon in 1968, was replaced by Dr. Robert Stone, who served from 1973–75. Sherman and the other deputy director, Dr. Robert

Berliner, resigned soon after Marston's replacement, reflecting a period of demoralization among NIH staff in the 1970s. Stone was succeeded by Dr. Donald S. Fredrickson (1975–81), and he by Dr. James B. Wyngaarden (1982–89).

NIH's budget, though, continued to rise — reaching nearly $2 billion in 1972 (48 percent greater than in 1969). Spingarn, 45.

22. Spingarn, 47, citing, among other examples between 1972–76 (through the administrations of Nixon and his successor Gerald Ford), the appointment of singer-actor Frank Sinatra, a friend of Vice President Spiro Agnew, to the National Heart and Lung Advisory Council, whose meetings he never attended.

23. Strickland, interview with author.

24. Mahoney also said of the difference in perception over the cancer bill, "Mary knew an awful lot, but she hadn't had the elementary part of medicine that I had had. That doesn't mean anything except that you have a different understanding of things sometimes."

25. Gorman, interview with Strickland.

26. Cimons, "4 Washington Women."

27. Edwards, interview with author.

28. Dimond, 207; Robert N. Butler, M.D., interview with author, 30 September, 1998.

29. A Center for Research on Child Health had been established in 1961, in part due to the Kennedy family's personal interest in research on mental retardation, which afflicted a sister (Katherine). The center was upgraded to the National Institute of Child Health and Human Development in 1963 by executive order of President Kennedy, incorporating research on mental retardation, child health, population control, and aging. Miles, *HEW*, 172.

30. Ghita Levine, "Reversing the irreversible," *Baltimore Sun*, 11 May, 1975.

31. Senator Thomas Eagleton, statement on Research on Aging Act of 1972, *Congressional Record*, 12 October, 1972, 35407.

The Center, located at Baltimore, was operating at 50 percent of its intended capacity by 1972. About 11 percent of the NICHD budget (some $15 million) was earmarked for gerentological research (out of NIH's $2 billion budget); 58 percent went to child health, and 31 percent to population research. It was "reflective of the relatively low priority accorded this kind of research within the present organizational structure of the NIH," Eagleton stated.

32. Eagleton, *ibid.*; Butler, interview with author.

33. FM to ML, undated, circa 1960s; FM diary notes, January 1965, "Dr. Schnaper & Dr. Myers here for lunch & 4 hours discussion on how to get 2 mil. $ for aging program in Veterans," FM Personal Papers; FM to ML, 2 August and 19 August, 1965, M. Lasker Papers.

34. P. Lee, interview with author.

35. FM to John Macy, White House, 26 August, 1965, FM Papers.

Mahoney was recommending Russel Lee (1895–82) for a Medal of Freedom at the time. He was a principal behind the then-innovative concept of a moderately priced retirement home in a hotel-like environment with a full range of medical care — Channing House in Palo Alto, founded about 1962, one of the first of its kind in the nation. It was set up as a privately funded, nonprofit entity and continued to operate as of 1999 with about 350 residents. Lee also wrote a book on aging.

36. FM to Macy, 26 August, 1965; Paul F. Glenn to FM, 4 February, 1965, FM Papers.

37. FM to Glenn, 1 April, 1965; Glenn to FM, 31 December, 1965, FM Papers.

38. Levine, "Reversing the irreversible."

39. Gorman, Strickland interview.

40. Eagleton was first elected to the Senate in 1968.

Responding to a series in the Cox-owned Palm Beach *Post-Times* on nursing homes that Mahoney sent Eagleton, he wrote her in May 1972: "I wonder what the tangible results are of a series such as this. Does this kind of publicity actually spark some action in a community? In any case, there cannot be real progress until the sad facts are more widely known and there is a better appreciation of what the neglect of the aged implies about the value of our society." Eagleton to FM, 4 May, 1972, FM Papers.

41. Thomas F. Eagleton, letter to Talton Ray, 26 August, 1998.

42. Lister Hill to FM, 27 November, 1972, FM Papers.

43. *Longevity*, June 1991, reprinted in *Charter 100 News*, September-October 1991, 2.

44. James Murphy, interview with author, 12 October, 1998.

45. Floor debate, Research on Aging Act, *Congressional Record*, 18 July, 1972, 24125.

46. Eagleton, *Congressional Record*, 12 October, 1972, 35407-8.

47. FM to ML, 2 March, 1973, FM Personal Papers.

48. ML to FM, 9 February, 1973, FM Personal Papers.

49. Helen K. Neal to FM, 5 May, 1974, FM Personal Papers.

50. Levine, "Reversing the irreversible."

The institute was authorized by Public Law 93-296 and officially established 7 October, 1974. Mahoney served on the advisory council from 1974 to 1978. After the bill's enactment, Eagleton was named to the appropriations committee and successfully argued for substantial funding of the Aging Institute in its first years.

51. Lola Romanucci Ross, Director of Contemporary Issues, Cultural Traditions and Interdisciplinary Studies, Professor of Community Medicine, University of California, San Diego, to FM, 25 June, 1974, FM Personal Papers.

52. FM, interview with author, 1998; FM, "Content Outline," undated, FM Personal Papers.

53. FM to David Pryor, 29 July, 1974, FM Papers.

Democrat Pryor served in the U.S. House of Representatives, 1966–73; as Governor of Arkansas, 1975–79; and as U.S. Senator, 1979–97. He chaired a Special Committee on Aging in the 101st and 103rd Congresses.

54. FM to Lister Hill, 29 July, 1974, FM Papers.

55. Butler and FM, interviews with author.

56. Butler's previous experience at NIH had been as a resident and principal investigator on a human-aging study at the National Institute of Mental Health (1955–66); he subsequently was a research psychiatrist and gerontologist, Washington School of Psychiatry (1962–76). He served as NIA "director designate" 1975–76 and Director 1976–82.

57. Butler, interview with author.

58. Cavarocchi, interview with author.

59. FM to ML, 6 June, 1976, FM Personal Papers.

60. FM to ML, 13 November, 1981, FM Personal Papers.

61. Murphy, interview with author.

62. Butler, interview with author.

63. "Focus on the old," unidentified published article, circa 1990s, FM Personal Papers.

64. "Focus on the old"; NIH, Alzheimer's disease budgets, 1996–99. NIH 1998 Almanac, "The Organization, National Institute on Aging, Important Events in NIA History."

More than two million people were estimated to suffer from Alzheimer's disease in the 1990s.

65. Edwards, interview with author.

66. "The first five years of the National Advisory Council on Aging," National Institute on Aging and Josiah Macy, Jr., Foundation, cosponsors, NIA accouncement, 29 May, 1980; Claude Pepper to FM, 25 April, 1984, FM Personal Papers.

Mahoney was active in a number of private organizations in addition to the Glenn Foundation: the Institute for Advanced Studies in Aging & Geriatric Medicine, of which she was a founding member with Mary Lasker and Jonas E. Salk; the American Federation for Aging Research, in which grants to support talented young scientists' research were named in her honor; and the American Aging Association, of which she was a board member.

67. NIA announcement, Florence Mahoney Lecture on Aging.

68. NIH, National Institute on Aging budget obligations, 1976–99; president's budget request for 2000 ($614.7 million); Doctor Richard J. Hodes, director, National Institute on Aging, testimony on NIA FY 2000 President's Budget Request, to House of Representatives, Appropriations Committee, 1999, NIA.

In the 1990s the aged consumed one-third of the nation's health costs, largely from Medicare and Medicaid, the largest funder of nursing home beds.

69. *Longevity.*

The article portrayed Mahoney as "one of those rare individuals who changed the course of government policy by organizing, sometimes singlehandedly, one of the most effective lobbying efforts Congress has ever seen."

70. "Focus on the old."

Geriatrics training, a subspecialty of internal medicine and gerontology (the study of aging), combined medicine, psychiatry, social work, and pharmacology. Similar programs were established at Harvard, Johns Hopkins, and the University of California at Los Angeles. One outgrowth of the Aging Institute was the establishment of training fellowships; the Veterans Administration, partially in response to Mahoney's pressure, financed the first of such fellowships in the early 1970s. A shortage of geriatricians continued by 2000, however, their number not keeping pace with the needs of the nation's aging population (expected to rise from almost 35 million, nearly one of every eight people 65 or older, to 70 million by 2030). There also were shortages of other health-care workers like nurses, social workers, and aides to serve the elderly. Beth Frerking, Newhouse News Service, "Severe shortage of doctors for the elderly," *San Francisco Examiner*, 20 February, 2000.

71. *Ibid.*

72. *Longevity*; Hubert Pryor, "Theory into practice, gerontologist Robert Butler shows how research into aging can work," *Modern Maturity*, [month?] 1994, 12, copy in FM Personal Papers; Dr. Isadore Rosenfeld, "The best medicine of the century," *Parade Magazine*, 12 December, 1999, 16, and Rosenfeld, "Why we're healthier today, your chances for survival, longevity and well-being are better than ever," *Parade*, 19 March, 2000, 4.

From 1900 to 2000 the average U.S. life expectancy increased by 30 years (from 48 to nearly 80 for both men and women), and the number of centenarians was expected to exceed 800,000 by the middle of the 21st century.

73. Dimond, 208–09.

74. Jack Nelson, "Arthur Fleming, 60 years of fighting for social programs — within the Republican Party," *Los Angeles Times*, 18 June, 1995, quoting Fleming, former U.S. Civil Service commissioner and long-time public servant active in aging issues and organizations.

75. FM notes, "F.M. Personally, re: conversation with Clark Clifford, 5/22/72," "Memos," 29 and 30 June, 1972, FM Personal Papers.

76. FM "Memorandum," 11 December, 1976, citing March 1, 1976; FM journal excerpt, "Friday, 12th," April, 1976, FM Personal Papers.

77. English, interview with author.

78. Sherman, interview with author.

79. FM to ML, 22 December, 1976, FM Personal Papers.

80. FM, "Expense Voucher," 1977, 1978; Thomas E. Bryant, President's Commission on Mental Health, to FM, 10 June, 1977, FM Personal Papers.

81. Rosalynn Carter to FM, 2 January, 1 May, 1981, FM Personal Papers.

82. FM to Lister Hill, 29 July, 1974, FM Papers.

The Lister Hill Center for Biomedical Communications was approved by Congress (P.L. 90-456) 3 August, 1968, and dedicated as part of the National Library of Medicine 22 May, 1980.

83. Gorman to FM, 20 January, 1978, FM Personal Papers.

The Harrington bill was not enacted.

84. Marjorie Sun, "A new arthritis institute nears approval," *Science*, 13 August, 1982, 610; Gorman, interview with Strickland.

Lasker at the time was on the NIH director's advisory board.

85. Sun, *ibid.*; Siwolop and Brazda, "Fairy godmother."

The National Institute of Arthritis, Metabolic and Digestive Diseases, first established by the 1950 Omnibus Medical Research Act, was renamed the National Institute of Arthritis, Diabetes, and Digestive and Kidney Diseases (NIADDK) 23 June, 1981; it was converted to "bureau" status 22 April, 1982. A separate National Institute of Arthritis and Musculoskeletal and Skin Diseases was approved by Congress 20 November, 1985, and in May 1986 split off from the NIADDK, which became the National Institute of Diabetes and Digestive and Kidney Diseases, thus giving diabetes its own institute.

86. Greenberg, "Whatever happened . . . ," 64.

87. ML to FM, 31 July, 1986, FM Personal Papers.

88. FM to Gore, 28 September, 1992, FM Personal Papers.

89. FM, notes for letter, "I always think of Avent;" FM to David Pryor, circa 1993, FM Personal Papers.

– CHAPTER 8 –

1. FM to ML, undated, circa 1960s, FM Personal Papers.

2. Michael Mahoney to author; FM to ML, 6 June, 1976, FM Personal Papers.

3. Andrew Jacobs, Jr., to FM, 23 June, 1969, and 2 January, 1973, FM Papers.

4. William R. Roy to FM, 25 June, 1971, FM Papers.

Democrat Roy served in the House 1971–75; he was nominated to run for the Senate in 1990 but declined and returned to practice medicine in Topeka.

5. Eagleton to FM, 30 March and 3 June, 1992; Bentsen to FM, 11 December, 1992; Atkins to FM, 29 August, 1991; Moynihan to FM, 30 December, 1994, FM Personal Papers.

6. John D. Dingell to FM, 13 August, 1992, and FM to Dingell, 28 September, 1992, FM Personal Papers; Fallows, 66.

7. "National Institutes of Health Alumni Association (NIHAA) 1996 Public Service Award presented to Florence Stephenson Mahoney," announcement of award presented 15 June, 1996; *NIHAA Update*, "Florence Mahoney chosen 1996 Public Service Awardee," Spring 1996, 1–2, 9, 11; John F. Sherman to FM, 16 December, 1995, FM Personal Papers.

8. Jeffrey L. Fox, "Mary Lasker enshrined eponymously at NIH," *Science*, 1 June, 1984, 969; Barbara J. Culliton, "Congress, NIH dedicate Center to Mary Lasker," *Science*, 12 October, 1984, 151.

Congress in 1983 appropriated funds to purchase a former Catholic convent adjacent to the NIH campus and in May 1984 (Public Law 98-297) designated it the Mary Woodward Lasker Center for Health Research and Education. The

Center was to house medical students interested in spending a year at NIH in research training under a program jointly sponsored by NIH and the Howard Hughes Medical Institute.

9. Siwolop and Brazda, "Fairy godmother."

10. "Thomas F. X. Gorman, Administrator, 75," obituary, *New York Times*, 14 April, 1989; "Thomas Gorman, mental health leader, dies," *Washington Post*, 13 April, 1989.

Among other accomplishments for which he was lauded, Gorman had been with the first U.S. mental-health delegation to visit the Soviet Union in 1967, resulting in a book, *Psychiatry in the Soviet Union* (1969). He had served on the NIH Science Board and the Menninger Foundation board. Besides the Lasker Award, he received a number of others, including the William C. Menninger Award.

11. Claudia Levy, "Philanthropist Mary Lasker dies at 93, *Washington Post*, 23 February, 1994; Eric Pace, Mary W. Lakser, philanthropist for medical research, dies at 93," *New York Times*, 23 Feburary, 1994; Cohen and Brownlee, 77.

In addition to the Presidential Medal of Freedom (1969), the highest U.S. civilian award, Lasker received a Congressional Gold Medal (1989) and other honors; a new variety of pink tulip was named for her in 1985 and a health sciences professorship at the Harvard School of Public Health in 1989.

12. Sarah Booth Conroy, "Celebrating a century of health, research advocate Florence Mahoney, living to the fullest," *Washington Post*, 26 April, 1999.

13. These data are derived from the website of the National Center for Health Statistics, Centers for Disease Control and Prevention (http://www.cdc.gov/ nchs/products/pub/has/00tables). The mortality rates for the three diseases are those for "All ages, age adjusted."

14. Jane Ciabattari, "New weapons in battle against flu," *Parade Magazine*, 8 November, 1998, 13; Rosenfeld, "The best medicine . . . " and "Why we're healthier today"; Keay Davidson, "Dramatic leap in life span from small advances," *San Francisco Examiner*, 19 September, 1999, B-5; Jane Kay, "Miraculous medicine: UCSF at the forefront," *San Francisco Examiner*, 5 October, 1999, C-1.

15. "Killer bugs," editorial, *San Francisco Examiner*, 20 June, 1999.

16. "World population nears 6 billion," *San Francisco Examiner*, 12 July, 1999; James O. Clifford, "Tracking idealists in the class of '69," *San Francisco Examiner*, 30 May, 1999; Charles J. Lyons, president, U. S. Committee for UNICEF, "Plagues persist despite century of miracles," *San Francisco Chronicle*, 15 August, 1999.

Stephanie Mills, valedictoran at Mills College, Oakland, California, in 1969 (the same year that future President Bill Clinton's wife, Hilary Rodham, had been an outspoken speaker at Wellesley College), interviewed in 1999, said that she had upheld her vow not to have children.

17. Fallows, 67, 74.

Politically conservative and Catholic "pro-life" groups objected to using public funds for research involving aborted fetuses and embryos, in response to which Congress prohibited NIH from funding experiments that created or destroyed human embryos.

18. "News Hour," Public Broadcasting System, 25 September, 1998.

19. Sherman and Cavarocchi, interviews with author.

20. Geraldine Baum, "Clinton vows to increase efforts to fight cancer," *San Francisco Examiner*, 27 September, 1998.

The Clinton administration proposed a 65-percent increase for NIH cancer research over five years, beginning in 1999, greater involvement by patients and their advocates in setting research priorities, and congressional approval for Medicare to cover clinical trials. More than 1.2 million new cancer cases were diagnosed annually, and 564,800 Americans were expected to die of it at the rate of 1,500 each day, according to American Cancer Society statistics in 1998.

21. J. Michael Bishop, Marc Kirschner, Harold Varmus, "Science and the new administration," *Science*, Vol. 259, 22 January, 1993, 444.

The authors, all on the faculty at the University of California/San Francisco School of Medicine, were presenting views of a Joint Steering Committee for Public Policy representing the American Societies for Cell Biology, Biochemistry and Molecular Biology, the Biophysical Society, and the Genetics Society of America.

22. *Ibid.*; Fallows, 72.

23. Bishop, Kirschner, and Varmus, *ibid.*

24. Fallows, 66.

25. *Ibid.*, 72–73.

26. P. Lee and Edwards, interviews with author.

William H. Natcher, Democrat of Kentucky, served in the House 1953–94.

27. Butler, interview with author.

28. Sherman, interview with author.

29. Cavarocchi, interview with author.

30. Dimond, 208.

31. English, interview with author.

32. Boisfeuillet Jones, interview with author, 15 June, 1999.

33. Eagleton, letter to T. Ray, 26 August, 1998.

34. Butler, interview with author.

35. Charles and Sue Edwards, interview with author.

36. FM, note, fragment, undated, circa late 1960s, FM Personal Papers.

37. Dimond, 207.

38. FM to Larry Levinson, 13 October, 1967; Levinson to John Robson, 16 October, 1967, "Please give me a call after you have looked at the attached material," Executive file, LBJ Papers.

39. Dimond, 207.

40. FM, letter to "Mr. President, I hope you have missed my clippings," undated, FM Personal Papers.

41. Fallows, 66–68, 72.

NIH also included the National Center for Research Resources and the John E. Fogarty International Center for Advanced Study in the Health Sciences.

42. NIH 1998 Almanac, "Forward," "The National Institutes of Health."

Index